# PRIMAL
## ENDURANCE

MARK SISSON
AND BRAD KEARNS

Library of Congress Control Number: 2015945804

Library of Congress Cataloging-in-Publication Data is on file with the publisher

Sisson, Mark 1953-  ; and Kearns, Brad 1965-

Primal Endurance/Mark Sisson and Brad Kearns

ISBN: 978-1-939563-08-8

1. Endurance training 2. Physical fitness 3. Weight loss 4. Exercise physiology

**Design and Layout:** Caroline De Vita
**Illustrations & Cartoons:** Caroline De Vita
**Cover Design:** Janée Meadows
**Cover photography:** Leslie Klenke
**Editor:** Penelope Jackson
**Copy Editor:** Kate Kennedy
**Index:** Tim Tate

**Other photos used by permission and courtesy of:** Dr. Peter Attia, Robina Bennion, Nick Borelli, Katy Bowman, Suzanne Cardenas, RunDMC Curley, Jacques DeVore, Doug Ellis Photography, Johnny G, Richard Graham (professional quality triathlon photos of Pigg, Allen, Kearns, etc.), Joe Grant, Brad Kearns, Maria Kearns, Dr. Steven "E" Kobrine, Lauren Lobley, Dr. Phil Maffetone, Betty Melocotón, Colleen Conners-Pace, Dr. Cate Shanahan, Carrie Sisson, Mark Sisson, Mike Stahlberg, Jon Stahley, Dr. Kelly Starrett, Sweetwater Health LLC, Lindsay Taylor, US Government DMSP, and the featured athletes in Chapter 7.

**Shutterstock images-©:** EpicStockMedia, Foodpics, Jane Halmes, Vadim Ivanov, Sebastian Kaulitzki, Kayo, ruigsantos, TigerForce, Dennis Van de Water, vlad.georgescu, Davydenko Yuliia. **iStock images-©:** angelhell, Matthias Drobeck, kickers, Steve Krull, Lorado, Jason Lugo, mihtiander, Joe.Potato, sangfoto, stockstudioX, strauski, swetta, thelinke.

**Publisher:** Primal Blueprint Publishing, 1641 S. Rose Ave., Oxnard, CA 93033

For information on quantity discounts, please call 888-774-6259,
email: info@primalblueprintpublishing.com,
or visit PrimalBlueprintPublishing.com.

# TABLE OF CONTENTS

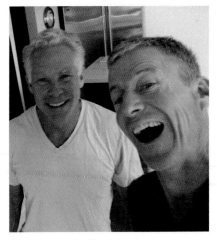

# PREFACE

*Welcome from Mark and Brad!*

**NOTE FROM MARK:** As you probably already know or will find out soon, I enjoyed some success in marathon and triathlon back in my day, but I struggled and suffered so much in the process that I was compelled to rethink many of the standard assumptions about endurance training and racing. You know, stuff like "more is better," "consistency is key," and other such complete nonsense. I've been talking, coaching, and writing about this stuff for many years, but in recent years I've been diverted to a bigger calling than the niche community of endurance athletes in my quest to counter conventional wisdom about diet, exercise, and lifestyle with the evolutionary health principles, and my particular spin on evolutionary or ancestral health practices that I call the Primal Blueprint.

This book feels like I've come full circle, able to return to my roots in the endurance scene while acquainting the community with my passion for primal living. Since there is so much disparity between the conventional approach to endurance training and the Primal Blueprint way of life, this endeavor is a challenge in many ways.

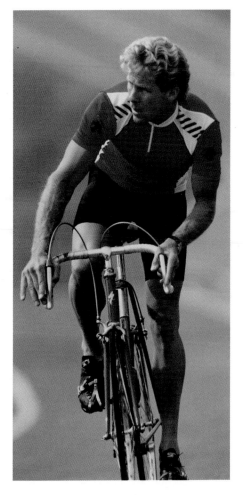

*Okay, I've "come full circle" in spirit, but not in body. I can't drop any more 100-milers before lunch like this guy did back in the day.*

v

Along those lines, we have made a sincere commitment to pull no punches and give you the real scoop at all times in this book. I know you've been exposed to a ton of training and racing philosophies through your eager consumption of books, magazines, internet resources, coaching advice, and peer banter. Sometimes this overstimulation makes it difficult to distill what's most important, or make sense of conflicting viewpoints. Throughout this project, Brad and I have been mindful of keeping our commitment to giving you the very best we've got on this subject. If you feel chapped at commentary about why endurance athletes are too fat or the like, please remember that we're speaking to you from the perspective of having been through a similar journey.

Even though my days on the starting line have long since passed, I have a deep appreciation and respect for the goals you are pursuing and working toward each day, and I want the very best for you. With my natural coaching instincts such a big part of who I am, I'm going to push and challenge and second guess you in the process of helping you be the best you can be. So get ready for a wild ride with *Primal Endurance*!

**NOTE FROM BRAD:** Well said, Mark! I too am overjoyed to have this opportunity to work with Mark and present this story to you on a topic that is near and dear to both of our hearts. As an athlete, my association with Coach Mark transformed my career, allowing me to reach the top level of triathlon while at the same time protecting my health much more than I could have following the conventional approach. When I stopped competing and Mark stopped coaching in the mid-1990s, we pursued separate career paths for many years, but reconvened when I was compelled to assist Mark with the phenomenal growth of the Primal Blueprint movement that he started with the launch of MarksDailyApple.com in 2006.

Mark and I always kept in touch over the years, and I'd paid a casual interest in his MarksDailyApple.com musings in the early days. But when he published his groundbreaking article, "A Case Against Cardio," in 2007, I was absolutely thrown for a loop. Here was my coach and mentor, a former elite marathoner and Ironman triathlete himself, calling out the entire endurance community as engaging in unhealthy, even dangerous, behavior in the form of chronic cardiovascular exercise!

At the time the article was published, I had been retired from the pro triathlon circuit for over a decade. I was a busy husband, father, youth sports coach, and working stiff trying to stay a little bit fit and healthy to preserve my legacy (existing mainly in my own mind) as a legendary *(The older I get, the faster I was,* as the saying goes) former pro triathlete. I'd meet the gang for an hour-long run once or twice a week, and hit the mountain bike trails for a two-to-three-hour session (including some gnarly climbs!) on the weekend.

I considered myself fit and healthy, and kept near my competitive weight and all that, but some disturbing signs of aging were taking hold. Those hour runs didn't cover nearly as much ground as I could in my racing days, and often left me feeling a little bit depleted afterward. I'd definitely feel fried after those hilly bike rides, sometimes for days, even though I stayed at what I thought was a comfortable pace. One day I tore my meniscus with no distinct attribution; I was walking my dog and noticed my knee swell up like a grapefruit and lock up.

I had to limp home a quarter-mile, collapse in exasperation on the couch, and summon my physical therapist friend over for a house call. "Dude, what the heck—you tore your meniscus!" Jeff exclaimed. I Googled and discovered that "males around age forty often experience a torn meniscus with no distinct attribution" (and I was only thirty-nine!). Another day, I threw my back out bending down to the kitchen counter to chow down some scrambled eggs before rushing out the door. The pain sent me to the deck immediately (my wife and kids thought I was goofing around as usual), and I could barely walk for a week. I never even comprehended what the term "throw your back out" meant until that fateful ingestion of eggs.

After reading "A Case Against Cardio," I immediately talked at length with Mark, absorbing his message deeply. Later we talked some more, and then more again. In a matter of days, I was convinced I should completely reject the major tenets of the endurance training/fitness/health paradigm I had operated in for decades. I accepted the harsh reality that while I still possessed some measure of cardiovascular fitness as a has-been pro, I was grossly deficient in total fitness (I considered a single set of twelve pullups to be a good strength workout), and furthermore my faithful efforts to get out on the road and peg my heart rate at 155 for a few hours might possibly be challenging my health in assorted ways.

Meanwhile, Mark and I were both experiencing the horror of seeing a shocking number of the world's elite endurance athletes, friends and former peers of ours on the racing scene, become stricken with serious heart problems that were not well explained by mainstream medicine. We'll talk more about the heart disease risks of chronic endurance exercise in Chapter 1.

I took that fork in the road and started getting more primal: sprinting, ramping up my strength training, and slowing down the pace, duration, and frequency of my endurance workouts. I've been exercising primal-style for nearly ten years now, and feel better physically at the age of fifty than I did when I was twenty-five. I was at the top of my game as a triathlete back then, but my fitness capabilities were extremely narrow, and I was constantly battling fatigue, injuries, illnesses, and burnout trying to keep pace with the pack on the circuit.

My wish for you is to enjoy peak performance the right way, in a manner that protects your health, and to also enjoy something that I didn't think at all about during my days as a pro: longevity—*longevity*, for some measure of peak performance and competitive passion for the rest of your life.

*Raising the bar: At age fifty in 2015, I cleared the USA Masters Track & Field Age 50 All-American high jump standard of 5'3" (1.6 meters). This was just as satisfying as winning a race on the pro circuit a lifetime ago (albeit with fewer spectators observing).*

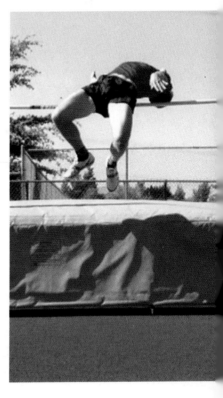

**WHO IS THIS BOOK FOR?** The primal approach to endurance training is based on simple, health-promoting, life-balancing principles that are applicable to a variety of endurance goals. Whether you are doing a Spartan race, a community 10K run, or entering your first ever all-women's mini-triathlon relay team with a couple of training buddies, you must approximate the challenge of your performance goals in training in a manner that protects your health. You must balance stress and rest and be intuitive about your workout decisions and scheduling. And you must honor the fundamental principles of aerobic base building, nutritious eating, complementary lifestyle practices, and correct implementation of high intensity exercises in order to reach your potential and avoid the health hazards of an overly stressful approach. Obviously, the particulars of your goals, workout schedule and overall time commitment to training will vary wildly, but you will apply the same success principles as an Olympic athlete toward even the most modest endurance goals. On the flip side, if you use the all-too-common flawed, overly regimented approach, you will be on the same highway to burnout as a globetrotting pro who's gone over the edge.

**ABOUT THE BOOK:** The chapters are obviously meant to be read in sequence, but they also stand alone if you can't help yourself and need to jump straight into topics like diet, sprinting, or strength training. If you're a cut-to-the-chase, short-attention-span kinda person, we have thoughtfully prepared the following "115 Things You Need To Know" section offering an excellent sneak preview—the "Glyph Notes" (corny primal joke, get it?) of the content that follows. We thought about presenting the diet information right out of the gate, since it's so critical to your health and your endurance progress to escape carbohydrate dependency, mitigate chronic inflammation, and reprogram your genes to prefer fat as fuel. However, you are going to have a really difficult time escaping carbohydrate dependency until you slow down and eliminate chronic patterns in your training, so that's what we tackle first.

We hope you have great fun reading this book, and great success implementing the Primal Endurance principles into your training and overall healthy life. Thank you for your interest!

Mark Sisson
Brad Kearns
Malibu, CA
December 2015

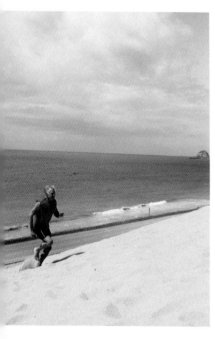

*Cover shot, take 24... Told ya it was steep!*

# 115 THINGS YOU NEED TO KNOW

*(and Will Learn in This Book)*
*as a Primal Endurance Athlete!*

## AEROBIC TRAINING

1.  Endurance athletes on the whole carry too much body fat—a consequence of carbohydrate dependency eating and overly stressful training patterns.

2.  The fundamental elements of the Primal Endurance approach are to slow down and emphasize aerobic workouts, balance stress and rest, and adopt an intuitive, flexible approach to training.

3.  The conventional approach to endurance training is deeply flawed, resulting in widespread burnout and excess body fat among even the most dedicated athletes.

4.  The flawed conventional approach can be characterized as "chronic cardio"—too many moderate-to-difficult-intensity workouts with insufficient rest and recovery.

5.  Chronic cardio can cause permanent damage to the heart by promoting chronic inflammation, and scarring/hardening of the arteries from repeated micro tears.

6.  A moderate exercise schedule (e.g., running ten-minute miles for a total of 1–2.5 hours per week) can dramatically increase longevity in comparison to more arduous and time-consuming training schedule, which—when it gets chronic—can accelerate aging.

7.  The critical distinction for endurance workout intensity is *aerobic vs. anaerobic*. Aerobic workouts emphasize fat burning, and are energizing and minimally stressful. Anaerobic workouts emphasize glucose burning and elicit a significant stress response.

8.  Emphasizing aerobic workouts delivers the best return on investment for endurance athletes, because endurance competitions—even as short as one hour—are fueled almost entirely by aerobic energy systems.

9.  Developing an efficient aerobic system is like building a powerful, clean-burning Tesla engine. Excess anaerobic training with an insufficient aerobic base is like fine-tuning a small, inefficient, dirty-burning car engine.

10. Aerobic development is best accomplished by training exclusively at aerobic heart rates for a sustained period of time. This enables a steady progression in fat-burning efficiency without interruption from stressful high-intensity workouts.

11. The cutoff point for aerobic training is the *maximum aerobic heart rate*, defined as the point where maximum aerobic benefits occur with a minimum amount of anaerobic stimulation. To calculate your maximum aerobic heart rate, use Dr. Phil Maffetone's formula of: *180 − age = maximum aerobic heart rate*.

12. Endurance athletes have extreme difficulty slowing down into what feels like a disturbingly slow aerobic heart rate zone. But massive improvements can occur over time by becoming more efficient (faster) at the same comfortable, conversational aerobic heart rate.

13. Aerobic improvement can be tracked by conducting Dr. Maffetone's Maximum Aerobic Function (MAF) test. You complete a fixed course (e.g., run eight laps) at a fixed heart rate (max aerobic: 180 − age) and obtain a finishing time.

14. Improvement in MAF test results means training is working—you are more efficient at burning fat at aerobic heart rates. Regression in MAF test results suggests you are overtraining and/or overstressed.

15. High-intensity workouts are not advised until a strong aerobic base is built, as evidenced by steady improvement in MAF test results.

16. Even a slight stimulation of anaerobic metabolism during a workout can accelerate sugar burning for up to seventy-two hours after the workout, compromising fat reduction efforts.

17. Besides exceeding aerobic maximum heart rate with chronic cardio, endurance athletes are often guilty of an overly regimented, overly consistent approach, which brings a high risk of overstress and burnout.

18. Aerobic and anaerobic workouts, as well as primal-aligned eating, all help improve mitochondrial function, protecting you from stress-induced oxidative damage and delaying the aging process.

19. Mitochondria burn fat and ketones more cleanly than they do glucose. Glucose burning generates more free radicals, causing oxidative damage and accelerated aging.

20. Nose breathing during exercise ensures the most efficient exchange of oxygen on each breath, and helps you maintain an aerobic pace.

21. The "black hole" designates an exercise intensity that is slightly too strenuous to be aerobic, but not difficult enough to qualify as a peak performance speed workout. Unfortunately, the black hole heart rate range is the default landing area for many exercisers, from novice to competitive athletes.

22. A wireless heart rate monitor is essential to conducting proper aerobic workouts, because intensity at aerobic maximum is so comfortable that it's easy to drift into the black hole.

**The seven habits of highly effective primal endurance athletes are:**
1. **Sleep**
2. **Stress/rest balance**
3. **Intuitive and personalized schedule**
4. **Aerobic emphasis**
5. **Structured intensity**
6. **Complementary movement and lifestyle practices**
7. **Periodization.**

*Don "Dewey" Weaver (1960-2006) running in Auburn, CA — national age group triathlon champion and one of the most intense competitors, and hilarious training partners, of all time.*

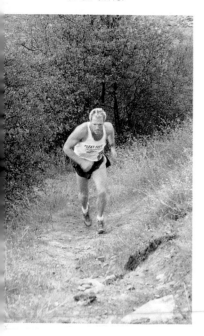

23. *Slowing down* to perform better in endurance competition has been proven effective by the world's leading athletes for over fifty years, but it's still difficult to convince many casual enthusiasts about its effectiveness.

24. The seven habits of highly effective primal endurance athletes are: sleep, stress/rest balance, intuitive and personalized schedule, aerobic emphasis, structured intensity, complementary movement and lifestyle practices, and periodization.

## PERIODIZATION

1. Periodization entails focusing on different types of training during specific blocks of time over a calendar year. The broad annual schedule is: aerobic base period, mini-periods of intensity/competition bookended by mini-periods of rest and aerobic, and finally a lengthy rest period to end the season.

2. Consistency in the context of endurance training is ill advised. You are better off being intuitive, varied, and flexible in your workout patterns. The process of fitness progress is dynamic and unpredictable, not linear.

3. A good strategy for intuitive training is to align workout difficulty with your subjective evaluations (1–10 score) of daily levels of energy, motivation, and health.

4. The aerobic base period to commence the season should last at least eight weeks, and possibly much longer if progress with aerobic function stalls or overstress symptoms are present (e.g., illness, injury, fatigue).

5. Intensity should be introduced only after a successful aerobic period, and last a maximum of four weeks (with greatly reduced total training volume during that time) before a mini-rest period is observed.

6. Mini-periods of high intensity during the competitive season should be followed by a period of nearly equal duration composed of rest and aerobic exercise.

7. The season-ending rest period should be diligent and comprehensive. No training, no thinking about training, and extra attention to rest, sleep, and neglected hobbies and social connections.

8. Tapering with a huge reduction in training volume and intensity promotes peak performance. It's very difficult to lose fitness if you maintain even a fraction of normal training.

9. True detraining from inactivity due to illness or injury causes rapid fitness losses, but you can regain fitness at approximately a one-to-one exchange of time off to time returning to training.

10. The specific nature of high-intensity workouts is of minimal importance. All anaerobic exercise (intervals, time trials, hill repeats, Tabata, etc.) has a similar effect on the body.

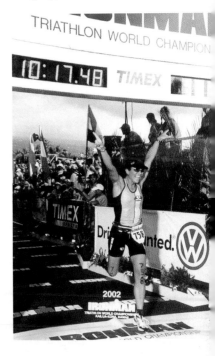

*Dr. Diana Hassel, Hawaii Ironman world age group champion and excellent horse doctor. If your horse needs surgery, call Diana.*

A GOOD STRATEGY FOR INTUITIVE TRAINING IS TO ALIGN WORKOUT DIFFICULTY WITH SUBJECTIVE EVALUATIONS OF DAILY LEVELS OF ENERGY, MOTIVATION, AND HEALTH.

## PRIMAL EATING

1. The Standard American Diet is based on excessive intake of grains and sugars, which stimulates excess insulin production, leading to lifelong insidious weight gain, chronic inflammation, and elevated disease risk factors.

2. A high carb, grain-based diet leaves endurance athletes nutrient deficient, inflamed, and more susceptible to oxidative damage from the stress of training, general life, and poor nutrition.

3. Grains, or "beige glop," are a cheap source of calories that are immediately converted to glucose upon ingestion and offer minimal nutritional value. There is no good reason for humans to consume grains, and many good reasons not to, especially for those sensitive to gluten and other anti-nutrients.

4. Everyone is sensitive to the health-compromising effects of grains at some level, especially the pro-inflammatory effects of gluten and the propensity for the lectin proteins in grains to cause leaky gut syndrome.

5. Carrying excess body fat despite careful attention to diet and a high volume of training hours is largely due to carbohydrate dependency—caused by a grain-based diet and chronic training patterns.

6. Endurance athletes can dial in optimal carb intake by first asking the question: "Do I carry excess body fat?" Any excess body fat calls for a reduction in dietary carbohydrate intake to accelerate fat burning.

7. Weight loss through portion control and devoted calorie burning is ineffective. Calories burned through exercise stimulate a corresponding increase in appetite. The secret to weight loss is *hormone optimization*, primarily through moderating excess insulin production.

8. Endurance athletes with optimal body composition looking to improve performance and recovery should choose high-nutrient-value carbs like abundant vegetables, sensible amounts of fruit, sweet potatoes, wild rice, quinoa, and dark chocolate.

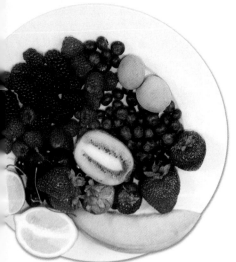

9. High-calorie-burning endurance athletes with optimal body composition can enjoy occasional treats, but the habit of unbridled intake of nutrient-deficient refined carbohydrates should be eliminated in the interest of health and performance.

10. Even lean people suffer from the negative health consequences of carbohydrate dependency, such as chronic inflammation, oxidative damage, and accelerated aging and disease risk factors.

11. Carbohydrate dependency leads to burnout because the body perceives fluctuating blood sugar as a stressful event, leading to an overstimulation of the fight-or-flight response and eventual burnout.

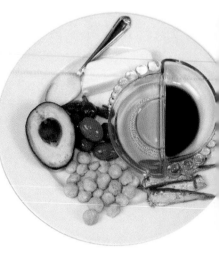

12. The carbohydrate dependency cycle looks like this: consume high carb meal > elevate blood sugar > stimulate insulin response > shut off fat metabolism and promote fat storage > experience fatigue and sugar cravings > consume more carbs > stimulate fight-or-flight response to regulate blood sugar > disregulate and exhaust assorted hormonal processes > end up in burnout and lifelong insidious weight gain.

13. Primal-style eating is fractal and intuitive. When escaping carbohydrate dependency and becoming fat-adapted, you don't have to rely on ingested carbs for energy. Eating patterns can be driven by hunger, pleasure, and maximum nutritional benefit.

14. Once fat-adapted, Intermittent Fasting (I.F.) can be used to accelerate fat loss, fine tune insulin sensitivity, and improve cellular repair for an anti-aging, immune-boosting effect.

15. A suggested entry strategy for Intermittent Fasting is to wait until you experience hunger before eating in the morning. This enhances appreciation for food and provides feedback on your progress with fat adaptation.

16. Your excess body fat is a function of your genetic predisposition to store fat *combined with* the amount of insulin you produce in your diet. Losing excess body fat involves moderating insulin production by ditching sugars and grains.

17. Primal-style eating minimizes the importance of genetic predispositions and enables you to achieve your personal ideal body composition.

18. Escaping sugar dependency and becoming fat-adapted gives you a cleaner burning engine, since glucose burning promotes inflammation and oxidative stress.

19. Ketones are an internally manufactured, energy-rich byproduct of fat metabolism in the liver when blood glucose and insulin levels are low due to carbohydrate restriction. Ketones are burned efficiently by the brain, heart, and skeletal muscles in the same manner as glucose.

20. Ketogenic endurance training represents an exciting new frontier for peak endurance performance. Ultra-low-carb athletes can perform amazing feats and literally become bonk-proof by remaining in a fat- and ketone-burning state.

21. Ketogenic endurance training is an advanced strategy that requires a strict devotion to very low dietary carbohydrate intake. However, it's acceptable to waver in and out of this fragile state and still enjoy the overall performance benefits of being fat-adapted instead of carb dependent.

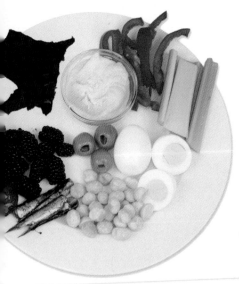

22. A bonk-proof ketogenic athlete is preserving ketones for use by the brain (relieving it of glucose dependency) and prioritizing fat for muscular fuel.

23. Ketones burn cleaner than carbohydrates, minimizing free radical damage and delivering a potent anti-inflammatory effect. Ketogenic endurance athletes recover faster from stressful training, improve cognitive function, and minimize the disease risk factors associated with a pro-inflammatory high carb diet.

24. The new "fat-burning beast paradigm" offers great promise to endurance athletes, but can have an even more profound effect on the global obesity epidemic. Reduce carb intake (in favor of fat) and you reduce excess body fat, period.

25. Dr. Jeff Volek's vaunted FASTER study, and the well-chronicled personal experiments of Dr. Peter Attia and Sami Inkinen, suggest that any endurance athlete can quickly become fat-adapted and deliver performances superior to carb-fueled efforts all the way up to anaerobic threshold intensity.

26. Being carb dependent sucks on several levels: your performance hinges on the tenuous ability to assimilate additional carbs during exercise; you produce more inflammation and oxidative damage from burning a dirty fuel source; you risk muscle catabolism (via gluconeogenesis), and you have difficulty reducing excess body fat.

27. Step 1 to going primal is to ditch sugars, grains, and industrial vegetable/seed oils for twenty-one days. Step 2 is to emphasize highly nutritious primal foods, such as meat, fish, fowl, eggs, vegetables, fruits, nuts, and seeds, and supplemental carbs like sweet potatoes—the natural plant and animal foods that fueled human evolution.

28. While transitioning to primal involves eating rich, satisfying meals, some can expect to struggle initially due to lifelong carbohydrate dependency and the drug-like addictive properties of sugar and wheat.

29. Eating primally and losing excess body fat does not involve any suffering, struggling, or sacrifice. The high satiety factor of primal foods will prevent the cravings and binges that derail calorie restriction dieters.

30. Primal eating can improve endurance performance by improving fat metabolism, moderating the overstimulation of fight-or-flight hormones, improving immune function, improving digestion, and reducing inflammation, oxidative damage, and muscle breakdown from training.

31. You can accelerate the process of fat adaptation in a depleted post-workout state, when your appetite hormones are most sensitive to rewiring. Instead of habitually pounding sugary treats, fast for a stretch and/or choose high fat, low-insulin-producing foods. You will rewire your brain to be less dependent on carbs at all times.

32. The Primal Blueprint Carbohydrate Curve predicts the results of body composition goals based on different levels of carb intake. One hundred grams per day or less promotes fat loss; 150 grams is primal maintenance level; over 150 promotes lifelong insidious weight gain; and over 300 promotes metabolic disease patterns.

STEP 1 IS TO DITCH SUGARS, GRAINS, AND INDUSTRIAL VEGETABLE/SEED OILS. STEP 2 IS TO EMPHASIZE HIGHLY NUTRITIOUS PRIMAL FOODS, SUCH AS MEAT, FISH, FOWL, EGGS, VEGETABLES, FRUITS, NUTS, AND SEEDS, AND SUPPLEMENTAL CARBS.

# STRENGTH AND SPRINT TRAINING

1. Strength training is essential to success in endurance sports. Putting your muscles under load by lifting heavy things, whether weights, machines, or just bodyweight resistance exercises, stimulates positive hormonal adaptations, and helps you preserve good technique and maximum power output as muscles fatigue during endurance workouts.

2. Strength training can help athletes identify functional weaknesses that lead to poor technique, overly stressful workouts, and delayed recovery.

3. Many endurance athletes err by conducting "blended" workouts that deliver both a cardiovascular training effect (unnecessary in light of the extreme cardiovascular training already) and fall short of developing the absolute power that endurance athletes are deficient in.

4. Endurance athletes with excellent cardiovascular endurance should focus on brief, high-intensity strength sessions that increase raw strength and explosiveness. Emphasis should be on maintaining excellent technique, and workouts end when fatigue inhibits reaching max power level.

5. Endurance athletes over age forty will particularly benefit from strength training, since strength declines more steeply than endurance with aging. High-intensity strength sessions will deliver a profound anti-aging effect by preserving muscle mass and optimizing adaptive hormones.

6. The Primal Essential Movements represent a safe, simple, effective, full-body workout sequence consisting of pushups, pullups, squats, and planks. A series of progression exercises allow athletes of all fitness levels to perform an appropriate number of reps and increase competency over time.

7. Maximum Sustained Power (MSP) training represents a cutting edge strategy to improve absolute power and explosiveness. These sessions involve popular functional movements like deadlifts, squats, and leg presses—lifting heavy weights for few reps, and taking frequent mini-rest periods to sustain maximum power output.

8. MSP sessions enable you to lift more total weight than the traditional "light weights, high reps, multiple stations till exhaustion" blended workouts. The MSP strategy is to go max or go home—you never reduce weights, and you stop when you can't lift the "five-rep max" baseline MSP heavy bar due to accumulated fatigue.

9. All-out sprinting is widely disregarded by mileage-obsessed endurance athletes who don't see the connection between short sprints and endurance performance. But becoming competent in sprinting will improve endurance performance in many ways: reduced perceived fatigue, enhanced fat metabolism, enhanced mitochondrial function and oxygen utilization, improved muscle buffering capacity, and strengthened muscles and connective tissue.

10. Sprinting, like strength training, delivers a potent anti-aging effect by flooding the bloodstream with adaptive hormones and actualizing the anti-aging maxim of "use it or lose it."

SPRINTING, LIKE STRENGTH TRAINING, DELIVERS A POTENT ANTI-AGING EFFECT BY FLOODING THE BLOODSTREAM WITH ADAPTIVE HORMONES AND ACTUALIZING THE ANTI-AGING MAXIM OF "USE IT OR LOSE IT."

11. Maximum intensity sprinting significantly increases your resilience to physical and psychological fatigue at lower intensity levels. Your muscles regenerate energy faster (through improved calcium-potassium pump function) and your central nervous system recalibrates so slower paces feel easier.

12. One of the most important benefits of sprinting is how it "cuts you up" like nothing else. Primal-adapted eaters who experience stalled weight loss progress can send an intense message to the brain to ramp up fat metabolism as an adaptive response to sprinting—an effect that continues for up to twenty-four hours after the workout. Ever seen a fat sprinter? Nope!

13. Endurance athletes must adopt a different mindset for sprint workouts—rejecting the "suffering" ethos of endurance sessions in favor of striving for *consistent quality* performances. Perform at max or go home—workouts end when time gets slower, form gets compromised, or effort increases to maintain the same times.

14. Consistent quality sprinting means a similar time and similar perceived exertion for each effort. If it becomes harder to deliver the same time, or if time slows at the same perceived exertion, the workout must end. As fitness progresses, strive to increase speed before considering increasing the number of reps.

15. Sprinting in a pre-fatigued state is not only harmful for muscles, but also the central nervous system. Athletes should only sprint when 100 percent rested and energized to deliver a peak performance. Extensive warmup and technique drills should be performed before delivering maximum efforts.

16. A proper warmup entails dynamic movements that elevate your temperature, lubricate your joints (no cracking or creaking), and get your central nervous system focused on good technique with form drills. A deliberate cooldown will minimize the stress impact of the session and facilitate faster recovery. No abrupt endings!

17. Running is the best sprinting choice due to the benefits of weight-bearing intense activity. If you have joint or injury concerns, or specific competitive goals, you can sprint with low or no impact exercises. Ideal duration of sprints is between ten and thirty seconds, and four to six reps are plenty. Since running is harder, shorter and fewer work efforts are advised.

18. The rest interval between sprints should be sufficient to ensure respiration returns to near normal, muscles feel reinvigorated, and that mental energy is refreshed. This will probably be achieved in thirty to sixty seconds of rest consisting of slow movement.

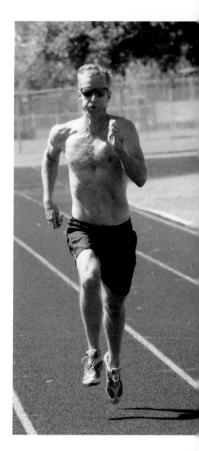

*"Running in the 50s, in my 50s." 400-meter time trial in 59.8 seconds (2015). Can you say "piano on back?" Brad can, during the final 100-meter straight...*

## COMPLEMENTARY MOVEMENT AND LIFESTYLE PRACTICES

Getting adequate sleep is not as simple as logging eight hours per night. Sleep requirements vary by the seasons, training workload, overall life stress levels, and genetic factors.

1. Optimal sleep starts with mellow, dark, calming evenings that minimize artificial light and digital stimulation after dark. This allows for the circadian influenced dim light melatonin onset (DLMO) to happen on cue, making you feel sleepy soon after it gets dark.

2. Awakening naturally, near sunrise, feeling refreshed and energized, is indicative of adequate sleep. Feeling less than perky in the morning suggests you must minimize artificial light and digital stimulation in the evenings.

3. An ideal sleeping environment is quiet, clutter-free, cool (68°F or less), and completely dark. Even tiny light emissions (LED devices, etc.) can disturb the highly sensitive release of melatonin into the bloodstream.

4. Napping is especially effective for catching up on evening sleep deficiencies, refreshing brain neurons after sustained periods of peak cognitive function, and generating a pulse of adaptive hormones into the bloodstream.

5. The "active couch potato syndrome" describes an actual medical phenomenon of devoted fitness enthusiasts nevertheless suffering from elevated disease risk factors due to predominantly sedentary lifestyle patterns

6. Walking will improve many aspects of your general health and also contribute to aerobic fitness by stimulating the complete range of aerobic muscle fibers and energy-producing enzymes.

7. Extended periods of sitting/stillness can compromise musculoskeletal function, cellular health, cardiovascular function, and fat metabolism—negating many of the benefits of endurance training.

OPTIMAL SLEEP STARTS WITH MELLOW, DARK, CALMING EVENINGS THAT MINIMIZE ARTIFICIAL LIGHT AND DIGITAL STIMULATION AFTER DARK.

8. Taking frequent movement breaks throughout the day improves insulin sensitivity/fat metabolism, improves muscular balance, flexibility and bone density, and enhances cognitive function through improved circulation.

9. The "athlete's mindset" of being lazy in everyday life on account of compiling an impressive workout log must be reframed to emphasize the importance of increased everyday movement to speed recovery and optimize metabolic function.

10. Cardiovascular fitness is the ability to challenge the heart and certain muscles to perform extreme athletic efforts. Cardiovascular health is the ability to efficiently deliver oxygen to 100 percent of the cells in your body (Katy Bowman, MS).

11. Creating a standup desk environment is great, but the primary goal should be to create more variation in workplace positions— switching back and forth from standing to sitting, sitting on the ground, and going mobile whenever possible.

12. Brain science confirms that humans are incapable of focusing for longer than twenty minutes without a break. Taking a five-minute break for every twenty minutes of peak cognitive focus, and longer breaks every few hours, will improve metabolic health and cognitive performance.

13. Complementary movement and mobility exercises like yoga and Pilates improve athletic performance by allowing you to preserve correct technique and optimal power output even as you fatigue during workouts.

14. Neglecting complementary movement and mobility practices can compromise athletic performance by allowing inefficiencies and imbalances to occur from narrowly focused training patterns, leading to accelerated fatigue, diminished power output, and increased injury risk.

15. Deliberate movement practices also help improve your ability to focus during challenging endurance efforts, and provide a calming balance to the high-stress nature of endurance workouts.

16. Play is a fundamental element of human health, and a key factor in the success of human evolution. Play is a critical stress release from the pressures, schedules, and responsibilities of daily life, and promotes the development of a "cognitively fluid mind."

17. Play can take many forms, but ideally involves unstructured, outdoor physical activity to balance the structured, confined, and sedentary forces in modern life.

18. Primal thrills can deliver a healthy burst of adrenalin to counter the mundane and predictable nature of modern life. Choose challenges that are well managed and just outside of your comfort zone.

## RECOVERY

1. Cold therapy can help speed recovery by delivering a refreshing psychological sensation and recalibrating the central nervous system and muscle metabolic activity back to calm, cool resting levels.

2. Full body immersion into water at 50°F to 60°F (10°C to 15°C), for five to ten minutes, is believed to be the optimal strategy for post-exercise cold therapy.

3. The old injury treatment protocol of RICE (Rest, Ice, Compression, Elevation) is being replaced in the eyes of many experts with ECM (Elevate, Compress, Move). Icing of injuries can retard the natural healing process.

4. The new RTX cooling glove can rapidly cool core temperature by acting upon the extremely temperature sensitive vein network in your hands. Quickly lowering core temperature with this portable device can extend workouts beyond the natural limitations of overheating.

5. Compression wraps or garments act like pumps to squeeze blood vessels open with force, allowing more blood and oxygen into the area and improving removal of waste and excess fluid. Studies suggest reduced muscle soreness and improved performance using compression garments.

6. Post-exercise hydration is essential to ensuring that assorted recovery mechanisms work without interference from the immediate urgency of needing to rehydrate.

7. Movement is also an important element of recovery. Athletes should refrain from prolonged stillness periods after workouts, and throughout the day. Over time, efforts to move more will result in improvements in the familiar morning stiffness that many athletes experience.

8. For post-workout refueling, forget the synthetic bars, gels, beverages, and sweets. Instead, focus on getting wholesome, nutritious food—like a salad!

9. Self-myofascial release is an effective recovery technique. Using rollers or balls, you can apply deep pressure to trigger points that represent the origination of stiffness and mobility problems, which possibly refer pain elsewhere.

10. Self-myofascial release delivers the added benefit of stimulating the parasympathetic nervous system, allowing you to truly unwind after workouts.

11. Releasing your attachment to the outcome can alleviate the psychological stress of missing workouts or performing below expectations. Instead, relax, be patient, and focus on the enjoyment of the process of getting fit. Take what your body gives you each day and nothing more.

12. Heart Rate Variability (HRV) is an excellent method of monitoring your state of stress and recovery—it provides a direct window into the functional state of your autonomic nervous system. HRV is a great complement to monitoring resting heart rate for tracking recovery and making optimal training decisions.

13. HRV measures the fluctuation in your beat-to-beat intervals. Surprisingly, more variation in beat-to-beat intervals indicates a fit, healthy, recovered cardiovascular system, and is represented by a higher HRV score on a 1–100 scale. A more metronomic heartbeat is a sign of overstress or an unfit cardiovascular system.

# PRIMAL
## ENDURANCE
### IS FOR YOU!

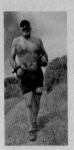
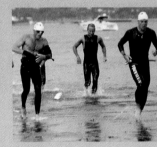
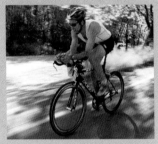
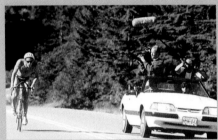
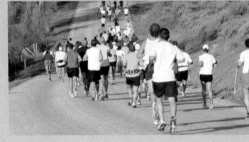
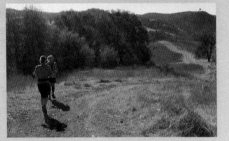
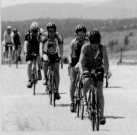
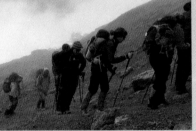
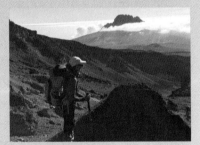
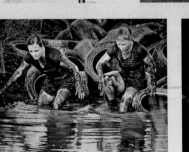
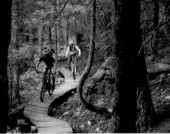
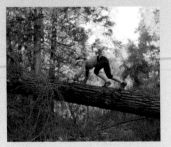

# INTRODUCTION

*Conventional endurance training*
*is making you fat, tired, and unhealthy.*
*It's time to go primal!*

Congratulations on your interest in health, fitness, and the pursuit of ambitious endurance goals! Okay, now that the pleasantries are out of the way, we want to get right down to the elephant in the room: *fat*. As in, too much of it. On your body. On your hard-training, disciplined, devoted, healthy-eating-conscious body. Training ten, fifteen, or even more hours per week while still carrying a spare tire or junk in the trunk is a major disconnect, don't ya think?

TRAINING TEN, FIFTEEN, OR EVEN MORE
HOURS PER WEEK WHILE STILL CARRYING
A SPARE TIRE OR JUNK IN THE TRUNK IS
A MAJOR DISCONNECT, DON'T YA THINK?

Not only are the extra pounds bumming you out and compromising your performance, they are an indicator of something even more disturbing—a very serious problem that pervades the endurance scene as a whole. The problem is that the conventional approach to endurance training and racing is not healthy, and it's not effective. Yep, there's another elephant in the room, and the poor thing is overstressed and in poor health. For some reason, endurance athletes tend to engage in overly stressful chronic train-

1

ing patterns. Their workouts routinely exceed comfortable intensity and reach the medium-to-difficult intensity category. They are slightly too difficult to optimize aerobic development, too long in duration, and conducted too frequently, with insufficient rest and recovery before the next dose of chronic stress.

The Primal Blueprint calls this type of training pattern "chronic cardio." Many passionate endurance enthusiasts object to this negative characterization, because we have been socialized to believe that "consistency" is the key to success in endurance sports. We're here to convince you that this mentality is dead wrong, it's destructive to your health and fitness, and it's the reason you aren't as lean, fit, healthy, or fast as you dream of being.

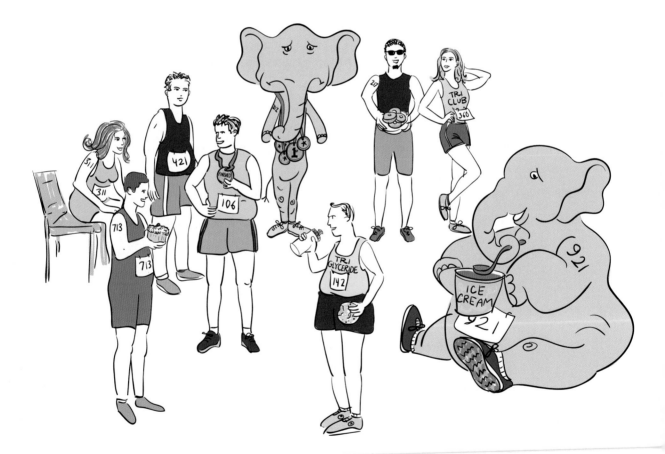

Elephants in the Room

Your devoted efforts to follow the principles espoused by your coach, your training group, or the magazines and books on your shelves are partially responsible (along with your poor decision-making and possibly obsessive/compulsive behavior tendencies) for making you not only fat, but tired, injured, and unhealthy, and quite possibly elevating your risk for those inactivity-driven diseases that you believe you are successfully running away from.

Our apologies if the message here is starting off a bit harsh. First of all, we're not making this stuff up. Dr. Timothy Noakes, long considered the world's pre-eminent endurance exercise physiologist and whom you'll read about frequently in this book, cites a study showing that a full 30 percent of the participants in the Cape Town Marathon were classified as overweight or obese. That's the same overweight/obese percentage as the world's population as whole, as reported in the 2013 Global Burden of Disease Study. So the roadside spectators at a marathon are physically indistinguishable from the participants? Sounds more like a golf tournament than a marathon!

Secondly, we want you to know that we're speaking to you from experience and deep empathy. The authors have both compromised health in the name of fitness, and now we know better. We're urging you to do as we say, learn from the mistakes we and millions of other well-intentioned, highly disciplined endurance athletes have made, and immediately and decisively correct the flawed course that you have been sailing on with the rest of the pack.

## PRIMAL ENDURANCE IS ABOUT REPROGRAMMING YOUR GENES AWAY FROM CARBOHYDRATE DEPENDENCY AND BECOMING A FAT-BURNING BEAST!

As you follow the traditional path of high-carbohydrate eating and chronic endurance training, you are getting yourself stuck in a round-the-clock pattern of sugar dependency and fat storage (or at least lack of fat reduction). Primal Endurance is about recalibrating your approach to endurance training and competition to escape the disastrous sugar-burning trap and reprogram your genes so that you can become a "fat-burning beast." This is the framing principle of the primal/paleo/ancestral health diet that has become popular among ordinary and athletic folks alike in recent years.

When you "go primal" as an endurance athlete, you can expect, in shorter order, to:

- Easily reduce excess body fat and keep it off permanently, even during periods of reduced training

- Perform better by reprogramming your genes to burn fat and spare glycogen during sustained endurance efforts

- Avoid overtraining, burnout, illness, and injury by improving your balance of stress and rest, both in training and everyday life

- Spend fewer total hours training and get more return on investment with periodized and purposeful workout patterns

- Have more fun, be more spontaneous, and break free from the obsessive-compulsive mindset that is common among highly motivated, goal-oriented endurance athletes

- Follow a varied, integrated lifestyle approach to training, in which assorted elements of your daily routine, like ordinary movement and play, hone your competitive fitness

- Have more energy and better focus during daily life, instead of suffering from "active couch potato syndrome," where cumulative fatigue from incessant heavy training makes you lazy and sluggish in between workouts

## DO YOU REALLY WANT TO STRUGGLE?

Sir Roger Bannister, the first human to break four minutes for the mile run, uttered these profound words back in 1954: "Struggle gives meaning and richness to life." It's a deep thought that requires some drilling down. It seems what Bannister meant was that pursuing ambitious goals that require discipline, sacrifice, and overcoming setbacks and roadblocks have tremendous intrinsic value. Struggle promotes personal growth and deep fulfillment, while a life of ease can make you soft, atrophied, and disenchanted. Endurance athletes know this, and embody it with their high-achieving lifestyles.

However, we can only appreciate the magnificent intention of Bannister's message by defining the term *struggle* clearly. Bannister wasn't talking about manufactured struggle through self-sabotage, nor immersion into an unbalanced, overstressed lifestyle that makes mere existence a struggle. No, Bannister was talking about struggling to stretch the outer boundaries of human peak performance. In a 2015 *New York Times* article called "The Moral Bucket List," journalist David Brooks touched on the topic, noting that people "on the road to inner light" have lives that "often follow a pattern of defeat, recognition, redemption. They have moments of pain and suffering. But they turn those moments into occasions of radical self-understanding."

## "STRUGGLE GIVES MEANING AND RICHNESS TO LIFE." —SIR ROGER BANNISTER, FIRST SUB-FOUR-MINUTE MILER

Running enthusiasts know that in Bannister's day, the sub-four-minute mile was considered by many medical experts to be humanly impossible. There was talk in respected scientific circles that the human heart might explode if pushed beyond sensible limits in pursuit of this mythical performance barrier. These notions were harbored as the mile world record (after a steady reduction for decades) stagnated at a shade over four minutes for *nine years* until Bannister's record run in 1954. Immediately after Bannister posted his 3m:59:4, the floodgates opened and numerous runners across the globe broke the four-minute barrier in short order.

Because Bannister had an evolved, process-oriented mindset, he wasn't hindered by what was obviously an artificial mental performance barrier. Like other great achievers and innovators, he was consumed by the honor and the beauty of the struggle, rather than fretting whether he would miss out on a lucrative shoe contract if he *failed* to break four minutes. Bannister was one of the last truly amateur world champions, as he balanced his record-setting running with full-time studies as a medical student at Oxford. Soon after his performance, he retired from competition to focus on his medical career. Unlike so many modern athletes who cash paychecks long after their passion and peak abilities have faded, Bannister realized that he had a higher calling in medicine.

Reflecting on Bannister's athletic journey, it's clear that for your struggles to give meaning and richness to your life, they must be well-formulated, you must have a true passion for them, and they must be endeavors that nurture your overall physical and mental health.

Let's make a clear distinction here between this and the catch-all term *fun*. Indeed, it's important to have fun in life, but it's not the end-all. It's hard to argue that racing a marathon or triathlon—especially at a competitive level where you are pushing your absolute physical limits—is ever fun. Certainly other ideas come to mind besides hoofing it for 26.2 miles if you are looking to have some real fun. Obviously, your athletic journeys as a whole offer many elements of fun, and struggle, and assorted other components that stimulate a range of emotions and contribute to your personal growth and generate an overall positive experience—even if lots of pain is involved!

SETTING TANGIBLE GOALS IS FINE, AS LONG AS EVERYTHING IS COUCHED IN A SENSIBLE BIG-PICTURE, PROCESS-ORIENTED, HEALTH-SUPPORTING PERSPECTIVE.

It's important to reflect on the true meaning of Bannister's message because it seems many endurance athletes are simply looking for an outlet to suffer, perhaps to balance the many other elements of their lives that are safe, secure, predictable, and, ahem, boring. The fact that your life might be easy and relatively affluent is not a strong rationale for completing a thirteen-miler with flu symptoms, or thrashing up and down the pool lane, refusing to get a technique lesson.

Similarly, pursuing ambitious endurance goals mainly for the sake of the finisher medal or some other arbitrary performance milestone can easily lead to disappointment—it's struggle in the name of struggle instead of personal growth. Sure, sports shrinks want you to get specific and measurable with your goals to better predict success. That's fine, as long as everything is couched in a sensible big-picture, process-oriented perspective. Your ultimate goal really should be to achieve your performance standards in a manner that supports your health instead of compromises it, and builds your character rather than just providing an outlet for excess energy and aggression. Similarly, any bloke trying to climb Mount Everest might want to clarify the goal a bit. The ultimate goal of conquering Everest should be not just reaching the 29,028-foot summit, but also *making it back down safely!*

If you're with us so far, let's get into the nuts and bolts of how to become a Primal Endurance athlete—a fat-burning beast. One thing this might require at the outset is a leap of faith. This book is going to shatter many of the core beliefs and strategies that endurance athletes have trafficked in for decades. Some of them are just plain wrong, outdated, or based on the flawed assumption that what works for elite professionals will work for the average athlete with a busy life and an assortment of other stressors. In other cases, we'll apply breaking exercise science to implement exciting new strategies like ketogenic eating patterns to extend endurance, Maximum Sustained Power workouts to build pure strength with less risk of exhaustion or unnecessary bulking up, or using Heart Rate Variability technology to better monitor overtraining and recovery.

## THE PRIMAL ENDURANCE APPROACH

Here are the main elements of the Primal Endurance approach that will be detailed in the coming chapters. These pretty much all slap conventional wisdom in the face, so we'll provide not only step-by-step instructions for implementation, but a detailed rationale for why you are going to boldly venture out beyond the confined and dated thinking of conventional endurance training.

**1. Slow Down!** (We almost said, "Slow the F&@*! Down," but we don't know you well enough yet to tease you that hard.) We've discovered over the years that this admonition is not eagerly embraced by the typical highly motivated, Type-A endurance athlete, even though success in endurance sports is all about increasing your aerobic capacity—teaching your body to burn fat and process oxygen more efficiently. Improving your aerobic capacity is achieved at low intensity, where fat is the predominant fuel choice, ample oxygen is available, and minimal stimulation of your alternative anaerobic (sugar-burning) energy system occurs.

When you get really good at burning fat, through sensible training and dietary patterns, you are able to go faster and faster while still staying aerobic—technically, burning predominantly fat in the presence of ample oxygen. When it's time to go really fast and enter anaerobic intensity at a race or occasional breakthrough workout, your aerobic base gives you a higher platform from which to launch your peak performance effort. Consider that elite marathon runners can jog along comfortably, carry on a conversation, and barely break a sweat while running at a pace of better than six minutes per mile. This is the same pace that many accomplished amateur runners and triathletes strive to achieve during high-intensity interval workouts!

What's going on here? How can one human with two lungs and two legs be chatty-chatty at a six-minute pace for twenty miles, while another person is fighting for his life to stay with the pack for just a couple of laps around the track at that pace? Superior aerobic capacity is the answer. It really is that simple. The fast guy burns fat better than the struggling amateur, who is quickly burning up glucose and running low on oxygen at a six-minute pace, and can thus only run two laps before needing to stop and rest.

# SCIENTIFICALLY SPEAKING, AEROBIC CAPACITY IS THE END-ALL IN ENDURANCE PERFORMANCE. A FAST ATHLETE BURNS FAT BETTER THAN A SLOW ATHLETE, PERIOD.

Scientifically speaking, aerobic capacity is the end-all in endurance performance. Unfortunately, most endurance athletes train too frequently at a heart rate that is slightly too elevated—outside of the aerobic maximum and into what exercise scientists call the "black hole." It's not as hard as a proper anaerobic threshold workout or competitive event, but it's just hard enough to stimulate anaerobic metabolism, over-activate the fight-or-flight response, and consequently teach your body to prefer burning glucose over fat. This up-regulation of sugar-burning genes happens not only during the workout, but for up to seventy-two hours after the workout.

If aerobic workouts are helping you patiently and steadily build an incredibly powerful, clean-burning Tesla engine over time, then going a little too hard, too frequently is fine-tuning a smaller, less powerful, less efficient SmartCar engine…or maybe we should say a DumbCar. Sure, doing workouts that are slightly too hard, too frequently, with insufficient rest between sessions, will deliver a certain measure of results in comparison to living as a couch potato, and in fact it's not a big concern for novices to train with undisciplined heart rates. Anything you do beyond an unfit starting point will generate results. The approach presented here is directed toward experienced athletes who are interested in peak performance, and avoiding injuries, burnout, and serious health risks that come from chronic training patterns and undisciplined heart rate zones.

**2. Balance Out, Chill Out.** Striking an optimal balance between stress and rest is the quintessential challenge of endurance sports. We all know that marathons and triathlons are not completed on visualization and ab-roller sessions alone; you need to put in the miles to prepare your body for what you will face on race day. However, the collective efforts of endurance athletes to successfully balance stress and rest has been a dismal failure. The newsflash here is that we err on the side of overstress perhaps 99 percent of the time. Forget the clinically undertrained clowns who enter a marathon to impress the front desk girls at the gym and end up panhandling for cab fare at mile eight: We're talking about sophisticated, experienced athletes striving for peak performance and drifting into chronic patterns again and again in pursuit of a P.R. or age group placing.

Primal Endurance promotes a more severe fluctuation of stress and rest patterns—higher highs and lower lows.

With the Primal Endurance approach, you will challenge yourself with occasional breakthrough workouts that approximate the challenge of race day and stimulate a fitness breakthrough, and you will rest and recover much more diligently than before. In essence, your training program will evolve from an emphasis on "consistency" (ill-advised in this context, because it means a consistent application of stress) to having a much more severe fluctuation of stress and rest patterns. You'll have higher highs and lower lows, because this is how your body actually becomes stronger and fitter with less risk of burnout.

**3. Eat Primally**. Your dietary habits are the main reason you are carrying excess body fat; namely, the overconsumption of processed carbohydrates driving excess insulin production and locking you into a fat-storage pattern. The Standard American Diet (SAD) compromises endurance performance in many ways. First, grain-based meals and snacks train your system to prefer sugar for fuel, a huge disadvantage in comparison to an aerobically efficient fat-burning beast. Second, high-carbohydrate eating patterns promote system-wide inflammation in the body. Your favorite bar, gel, drink, and post-workout pizza fests promote fat storage, prolong your recovery, suppress your immune system, and elevate disease risk factors—yep, even if you are super fit.

CONSUMING TOO MANY CARBOHYDRATES LOCKS YOU INTO A PATTERN OF FAT STORAGE, CHRONIC INFLAMMATION, INCREASED OXIDATIVE DAMAGE, NUTRIENT DEFICIENCY, AND DELAYED RECOVERY.

Third, the high-carb endurance athlete diet is nutrient deficient in comparison to a primal-style eating pattern. The 4,500 calories you slam down each day from cereal, bread, pasta, cookies, crackers, cakes, macchiatos, Tostitos, bars, gels, and free soda refills may reload your liver and muscle glycogen for more chronic exercise the next day, but beyond that they offer no added value and create plenty of problems. The lack of vitamins, minerals, antioxidants, and essential fatty acids in the go-to meals of even the most health-conscious endurance athlete is especially troublesome because of the stress that hard training inflicts on the body. Nutrient-deficient high-carb diets make you more susceptible to the oxidative damage caused by training and other forms of life stress. The seemingly healthy, enjoyable practice of eating tons of carbs and burning up tons of carbs during chronic exercise essentially accelerates the aging process in the body.

When you go primal, you will transition out of a high-carbohydrate, grain-based diet in favor of emphasizing nutrient-dense meat, fish, fowl, eggs, vegetables, fruits, nuts, and seeds—the foods that fueled human evolution and promote optimal gene expression. Granted, as a hard-training athlete, you'll need an appropriate amount of carbs to fully reload glycogen after challenging workouts. But instead of processed junk like sugary beverages, bars and gels, and heaps of bread, oatmeal, muffins, pasta, and rice, you will restock glycogen by empha-

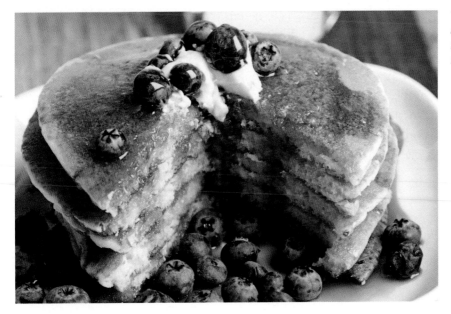

sizing highly nutritious, easy-to-digest carbs like sweet potatoes, fresh fruit, wild rice, quinoa, and dark chocolate.

Eating primally will also deliver the fringe benefit of making you more efficient at burning fat and sparing glycogen during workouts and even peak performance racing efforts. That's right, your everyday dietary choices can make you faster! We'll explain just how in the diet chapter.

**4. Add Strength and Speed.** While maximizing your aerobic output is the key to peak endurance performance, fantastic fitness breakthroughs can be made when you introduce some carefully structured brief, high-intensity workouts into your routine after you have built a strong aerobic base. Strength training will enable you to generate more power and resist fatigue and technique breakdown at all intensity levels—yep, even long, slow efforts. Sprint training will turbo-charge your cardiovascular function, accelerate fat reduction, improve lean muscle development or maintenance, and reduce perceived exertion at all intensity levels.

Adding strength and speed work (including not just intervals and tempo workouts, but also all-out sprints) into your regimen will make a huge difference in your ability to maintain proper technique for the duration of your endurance workouts and competitions. This is an often overlooked element of the complete training picture. When you get tired, your technique falls apart. You're still mustering the energy to progress toward the finish line, but every time you swim a stroke, crank the pedals or the oars, take a step running, or push off the skis, that energy output is less efficient and less productive than the energy you generated with correct technique when you were fresh. Basically, things get ugly out there on the race course! For example, when you get the shuffles late in the marathon, more of your energy collapses into the pavement instead of generating explosive forward propulsion with each footfall, which is what happens when you have excellent technique and a nice soft, quick, snappy footstrike.

# STRENGTH AND SPRINT WORKOUTS HELP YOU MAINTAIN BETTER TECHNIQUE AS YOU FATIGUE, AN OFTEN OVERLOOKED ELEMENT OF THE COMPLETE TRAINING PICTURE.

When you occasionally perform squats, deadlifts, and upper-body work in the gym, and conduct brief, all-out sprint efforts, you will preserve efficient technique longer amidst the inevitable fatiguing of your cardiovascular system, central nervous system, and oxidative muscle fibers (the slow-twitch fibers used for prolonged aerobic efforts). Furthermore, as you may know, you can train certain types of fast-twitch fibers to take over for slow-twitch fibers when the slow-twitch fibers conk out after a couple hours. These are called oxidative fast-twitch fibers.

While high-intensity strength and sprint workouts can generate fitness breakthroughs faster and more significantly than any other type of exercise (yep, even long, slow overdistance workouts), it's extremely important to understand that these benefits will only occur if you have established a solid aerobic base. Then, in literally just a few weeks, you can make astonishing breakthroughs. We're talking about going from the guy or gal who's barely hanging on at the back of the pack to going off the front and making your training partners suffer royally. Seriously!

If you struggle to develop a sufficient aerobic base and then jump into high-intensity training anyway—because it's that time of year, or because you hit week eleven in the training schedule article in the magazine—you will likely get fatigued, injured, or sick. Similarly, if you get greedy and do more than the optimal amount of high-intensity workouts, you will negate almost all of the potential benefits and end up feeling tired and going slower. If you escape the major risks of an aerobically deficient, intensity-excessive training pattern, the very best possible outcome will be a fine-tuning of that DumbCar engine instead of fine-tuning the Tesla that you patiently built during the previous training phase that emphasized aerobic development.

**5. Add Complementary Lifestyle Practices.** Endurance athletes with daunting goals tend to apply a narrow focus to their training, and understandably so. If you are enlisted to cover twenty-six miles on foot or seventy miles by water, bicycle, and foot, you are going to have a lengthy to-do list of workouts that directly apply. However, even an elite athlete training at ultra-high volume only spends a small percentage of her total time training over the course of a week. Instead of paying lip service to the peripherals ("Get plenty of sleep, my friends, it's important for recovery!"), Primal Endurance emphasizes a big-picture approach in which what you do off the roads plays a major role in your success.

This includes allowing yourself to have a little fun with spontaneous, unstructured "play." Play is a fundamental element of the Primal Blueprint (law number seven, as a matter of fact!), and has played a critical role in the evolution and survival of our ancestors. So when you take a surfing lesson instead of hitting the pool for more laps, enter a geocaching competition instead of logging another long run, or jump in for a Capture the Flag battle with a pack of rowdy middle school kids, you are honoring the primal approach—and getting an edge on the race course.

We'll treat sleep with the respect it deserves, and get into a focused plan of practical steps to ensure that you are optimally rested, refreshed, and recovered. And we'll examine the importance of increasing general everyday movement and variation, because our lives are so heavily influenced by sedentary forces like commuting, office work, and digital entertainment leisure time. This will prevent you from falling victim to the "active couch potato syndrome," an actual observed medical phenomenon whereby devoted fitness enthusiasts nevertheless suffer from inactivity-related disease risk factors by virtue of leading an inactive lifestyle outside their workout commitments.

# MAXIMUM RETURN ON MINIMUM INVESTMENT

In the *Primal Blueprint* book, I detail the sad story of destroying my health in the process of competing at the elite level in marathon and Ironman triathlon. But the story turns inspiring after I formally retired from pro competition and became a personal trainer. Suddenly, instead of killing myself every day to hit my mileage goals, I was spending hours walking, jogging, or pedaling side-by-side with my clients—very comfortable, very low-intensity aerobic exercise.

Since I had precious little time for my own workouts, I'd go all out for brief sessions (running sprints at the track, doing bicycle hill repeats, or redlining on my favorite gym machine, the VersaClimber) and jump right back into the groove with my next client. You might recognize this exercise pattern as the foundation of the Primal Blueprint fitness philosophy, as modeled by our primal ancestors. They blended frequent movement at a slow pace (foraging for food or scouting their terrain), regular lifting of heavy things (to build shelter and so forth), and occasional all-out life-or-death sprints (secure dinner, or become some other creature's meal). They became exceptionally fit and suffered none of the illness, breakdown, and burnout that come from following today's chronic training.

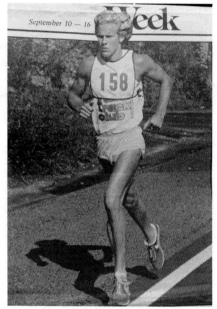

**2h:18 Marathon or Bust! (...or is it, "*and* bust?"):** *I was the fittest guy my friends knew, but inside my body was inflamed and falling apart. Knowing what I know now, I speculate I could have run just as fast, maybe faster, and stayed much healthier in the process.*

As I stumbled into this primal training pattern, some amazing things happened. First, I reclaimed my health in short order. The arthritis in my feet resolved, the tendonitis in my hips disappeared, and I didn't get sick every other month as I had during my racing days. Second, I started to feel stronger and stronger when I did push myself, like I'd somehow not even lost a step after departing from my extreme high-mileage training patterns.

I was coaching a group of professional triathletes in LA at the time, and for fun started jumping into some of their liveliest workouts on the running trails or bicycle climbs through the canyons. To my surprise—and theirs—this old coach (I was pushing forty by that time) was able to hang tough with world-ranked guys on their hardest days of the week. If they weren't fully receptive to my counter-cultural training philosophy at first, they started to pay more attention to my commentary after we'd finish these sessions together!

I carried this momentum from my strange new "training" program to the race course and excelled beyond my expectations. I went to the world duathlon championship series out in Palm Springs and easily disposed of guys my age on the grueling 10K-62K-10K route, quietly slotting into the final results in around the middle of the pro field. Now, it's hard to

THE NEXT-BEST THING TO WINNING IS TO BE THAT
GUY OR GAL WHO TRAINS THE LEAST, LIVES THE MOST
NORMAL LIFE, BUT STILL PERFORMS AT A HIGH LEVEL.

compare anything to the incredible sensation of winning an event, but I'd say the next best thing is to be that guy or gal who trains the least, lives the most normal life, can maintain a respectable job instead of just bumming around like a typical pro, but still perform at a high level. Ah, the backhanded compliments dripping with envy or excuses; the point-blank interrogations to the tune of, "Come on, you have to be training more than that!" and the satisfaction of feeling like you performed at your peak with a minimal amount of pain, suffering, and sacrifice, and protected your health in the process.

This is what I wish for you—to compete hard, have fun, continually improve, struggle, suffer, and sacrifice less than 90 percent of your peers do, but still finish in the top 10 percent of the field!

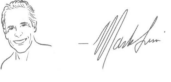

— Mark Sisson

## DON'T FORGET—YOU DA BOSS!

In the coming chapters, we will present a detailed plan to transform your approach to endurance exercise, primal style. First, we will examine the flaws of the conventional strategy, or "chronic cardio." Next, we will cover each component of the Primal Endurance program: slowing down to emphasize aerobic exercise; rejecting a chronic, overly stressful approach in favor of a periodized, intuitive approach; getting off the carb dependency cycle in favor of a primal eating style that helps control inflammation and reduce excess body fat; and finally adding high-intensity strength and sprint workouts to help you break through to the next level (apologies in advance to your current training partners).

Unlike many training modalities that are complex and regimented, Primal Endurance is simple, self-directed, open-ended, and intuitive. We're giving you the skills and tools you will need to succeed, but we're not mandating that you follow predetermined workout schedules to the letter. It's important for any coach, author, or know-it-all training partner to respect that you are the world's foremost expert on your own training program and urge you to create your own vision for how your training and competitive efforts take shape each season.

You must apply your intuitive sense of what feels right and what doesn't as you ponder every single workout that you conduct, and every bit of training advice you encounter. Call upon that little voice inside you that has a sense for the right thing to do before you start workouts ("I'm feeling tired and stressed today"), during the actual sessions ("I'm really dragging and my shoulder hurts; I'm gonna get out of the pool early," or "Wow, I feel incredible today; I'm gonna keep going all the way to the summit!"), and also after workouts ("My foot is hurting more now, I better take some time off," or "I'm really feeling strong and comfortable even after my longest ride of the winter. I think I'm ready to introduce some intensity sessions!").

# PRIMAL ENDURANCE REQUIRES THAT YOU HAVE AN OPEN MIND AND A WILLINGNESS TO ENGAGE IN SELF-EXPERIMENTATION; IT'S THE BEST WAY TO PROVE THAT THIS NEW APPROACH REALLY WORKS!

The one commitment we ask of you is that you retain an open mind and a willingness to engage in self-experimentation to prove effectiveness in the most memorable and impactful way possible. This may require reigning in some hyper-competitive, instant-gratification urges that influence the motivations and behaviors of many endurance athletes. Building an awesome aerobic engine requires patience and restraint. Few things are more frustrating than hearing the heart rate monitor beeper alarm go off during what you think is a comfortably paced workout. But the heart doesn't lie, and nor do the performances of the world's elite athletes who spend years and decades patiently developing their huge aerobic engines. Even the most hardcore hammerhead will be assuaged by the incredibly rapid improvement that occurs when you build a base properly and teach your body to become a fat-burning beast.

# THE FAT-BURNING BEAST

Mike Pigg, one of the greatest triathletes in history and the undisputed king of the bicycle segment during his career, was as driven and hyper-competitive as any athlete in the history of sports. Known for his prodigious work ethic and solo training habits in remote Arcata, CA, Pigg experienced a serious case of burnout and chronic digestive illness after several intense years at the top of the world Olympic distance rankings.

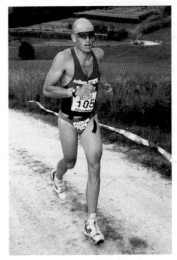

In search of a solution, Pigg decided to consult with Dr. Phil Maffetone, author of many health and fitness books, including *The Big Book of Endurance Training and Racing,* and a pioneer in advocating aerobic training and balancing health in pursuit of fitness. In *The Big Book of Endurance Training and Racing,* Pigg relates how exasperated he was at the outset of his aerobic training "experiment." At first, when he limited his heart rate to 155 beats per minute during all workouts, he felt like he was crawling. He'd have to walk up steep hills during a run or zig-zag on steep bicycle climbs to keep his heart rate in range. But as his aerobic efficiency improved over months and years of devoted attention to training within the aerobic limits, Pigg experienced an incredible revelation on a training ride one day.

*After destroying all comers, all over the globe, for many years, but slowly falling apart from the stress of superhuman training and heavy traveling, Mike Pigg rescued his health and prolonged his career by slowing down.*

Often, Pigg would ride a sixty-five-mile hilly course from his home in Arcata to a family cabin in the nearby national forest lands. One day early in his career, he and fellow pro Chris Hinshaw put the hammer down from start to finish, setting an impressive record time of 3h:15. Pigg's heart rate during the ride ranged from 165 to 182. This maximum effort—delivered by the number-one athlete in the world, mind you—culminated at the cabin with he and his training partner stuffing their faces with all available food, then collapsing in exhaustion to sleep for the rest of the day.

As Pigg started to emphasize aerobic development and limit his heart rate to 155, this same route would take over four hours of pedaling. After three-and-a-half years of patiently building his aerobic engine, moderating his overall stress, and improving his general health, Pigg became vastly more efficient at aerobic heart rates—swimming faster interval times, running a faster pace per mile at 155, and of course cycling more efficiently. One fine day he followed that same route to the cabin, never exceeding 155 beats per minute—even on the big climbs—and was astonished when he reached the cabin in 3h:09! Incredibly, Pigg was now entirely aerobic, comfortable, conversational, and arrived to the cabin a few minutes sooner then when he went balls-to-the-wall using his sugar-burning, high-stress engine from years past. After that perspective-altering aerobic performance, Pigg relates that he was neither hungry nor sleepy, and in fact was inspired to park his bike and head out for a ten-mile training run in the forest. This is what being a fat-burning beast is all about!

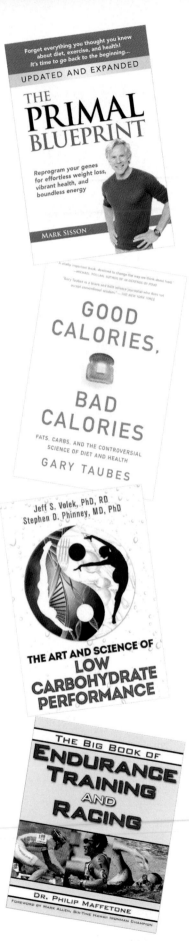

## STREAMLINING THE MESSAGE

Our goal with this book is to give you a streamlined education about the Primal Blueprint diet and lifestyle principles applied specifically to endurance training and competition, and to inspire you to take decisive action to improve your health and performance. Most importantly, we want to help you escape the destructive chronic cardio/sugar-dependency trap that you are possibly now trapped in to a mild or severe extent. We want to help you avoid the disastrous mistakes we made that compromised not only our athletic performances but also our general health, caused our endurance careers to end early, and accelerated the aging process in our bodies. And we want to present you with an exciting and simple alternative approach that will generate immediate positive feedback that you are doing something that really works, and that keeps you energized, motivated, and healthy as you pursue ambitious endurance goals within fast-paced, high-tech modern life.

We want this to be an easy, entertaining read instead of a chore or a bedtime sleeping aid. Consequently, we're not going to get bogged down with extensive scientific references or overly detailed discussions about the rationale for the rules and guidelines presented. If you object from time to time that we're asking you to take our word for something without detailed explanation, we beg your pardon in advance. And then, we encourage you to dig deeper into the science that frames the ancestral health movement and primal-aligned endurance training. The *Primal Blueprint* book provides further detail on primal living as a whole, while the Primal Blueprint Expert Certification Program will give you a comprehensive education on primal living akin to a semester-long upper division college course in the health sciences. We've also compiled a list of internet resources and suggested reading, which is available online at PrimalBlueprintPublishing.com on the *Primal Endurance* book page.

If you are a science-y type looking for exhaustive validation for the primal/paleo/ancestral health tenets such as "Saturated fat isn't bad for you" and so forth, you can check out Gary Taubes's 640-page tome (with over a hundred pages of scientific references), *Good Calories, Bad Calories*. When it comes to the scientific aspects of low-carb endurance performance, Dr. Steven Phinney and Dr. Jeff Volek have been generating incredible work for several decades. They present compelling evidence and detailed science validating the benefits of low-carb endurance training in their book *The Art and Science of Low Carbohydrate Performance*. If you require further convincing about the importance of emphasizing aerobic exercise heart rates, you will appreciate the detailed rationale and real-life success stories in Dr. Phil Maffetone's *Big Book of Endurance Training and Racing.*

It's also amazing to note that Dr. Timothy Noakes of the University of Cape Town, South Africa—author of many books, including the epic *Lore of Running* (a 944-page opus that is widely regarded as the most informative book ever written on the physiology of endurance performance), and founding member of the IOC's Olympic Science Academy—is a recent convert to Primal Blueprint–style eating and training.

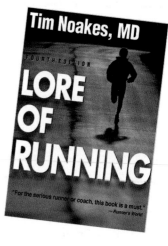

What's notable about Professor Noakes living and promoting a primal lifestyle is that much of mainstream endurance exercise physiology has for decades operated in the carbohydrate dependency paradigm—the science of how to ingest, store, and burn carbohydrates for energy during endurance exercise. Accordingly, in recent years Dr. Noakes has had to reject many of the important assumptions that frame his life's work and that of his colleagues. Here in the twilight of his exceptional academic and scientific career, he is absorbing a ton of heat from his brethren and even the mainstream media in South Africa and abroad for his aggressive refutation of conventional wisdom about diet and endurance performance in the carbohydrate paradigm—which he played a big role in shaping!

With so many health, fitness, and science professionals wedded to and heavily invested in the status quo, Dr. Noakes is a true hero for speaking and living his truth. In fact, Noakes was inspired to challenge his beliefs and investigate a new path when weight gain and health concerns revealed (via a self-diagnosis) a pre-diabetic condition. Despite a lifetime of long-distance running and over seventy marathons and ultramarathons under his belt, Noakes was headed down the same unfortunate path that claimed his father before his time. If arguably the most accomplished exercise scientist in the world can flat-out reject the carbohydrate-eating and -burning paradigm and embrace a new approach, we venture to say it's worth having an open mind yourself!

*Dr. Timothy Noakes went primal, lost twenty kilos (forty-four pounds) of excess body fat, got a handle on his type 2 diabetes, and in the process shook up the exercise physiology community deeply immersed in the carbohydrate paradigm.*

"WE HUMANS ARE THE ONLY MAMMALS THAT SUFFER FROM CHRONIC ILL HEALTH. ONE CRITIC SUGGESTS IT'S BECAUSE WE ARE THE ONLY ANIMALS CLEVER ENOUGH TO MANUFACTURE OUR OWN FOOD—AND STUPID ENOUGH TO EAT IT." —DR. TIMOTHY NOAKES

Perhaps when you experience your initial success with the Primal Endurance approach, you will become inspired to learn more about primal living and ancestral health and dive into the books, websites, and articles listed in the online resources guide (PrimalBlueprintPublishing.com/books/primal-endurance).

# CONVENTIONAL WISDOM VS. PRIMAL ENDURANCE

## COACHING/WORKOUT PROGRAMMING

**CW:** Find an expert coach, group training program, book, or magazine article. Follow a regimented schedule with linear progressions and built-in rest periods. Or go big time and hire an online coach to get a new customized workout grid every six weeks.

**PE:** Adhere to sensible, intuitively sound principles and allow the workout specifics to occur in an intuitive, spontaneous, and fractal manner. Coach rides shotgun, you get veto power on all workout decisions. Be flexible, with higher highs and lower lows!

## FOOTWEAR

**CW:** Sturdy, cushioned shoes minimize injury. Get a shiny new pair every three hundred miles—keep track of "shoe mileage" in your log. Beware the barefoot craze due to high risk of injury.

**PE:** Free your feet! Pursue gradual transition to a barefoot-dominant lifestyle through increased barefoot time around the house, foot strengthening and stretching exercises, and embracing minimalist footwear. Try short duration barefoot/minimalist workouts and increase carefully over time.

## CARBOHYDRATES

**CW:** High carb diet, grain-based diet are essential for high-volume endurance training. Carbs fuel working muscles and brain. Restock glycogen after workouts. Consume carb supplements during long workouts and races.

**PE:** Escape carb dependency by ditching grains and sugars and eliminating chronic training patterns. Emphasize fat burning to improve endurance performance and boost general health. Consume appropriate levels of high-nutrient-value carbs to optimize body composition and workout recovery.

## PRIMAL/PALEO REPUTATION

**CW:** Low carb primal/paleo is a crazy fad like Atkins—especially destructive for endurance athletes. Besides, fat and cholesterol will clog your arteries and cause heart disease. Low-fat, grain-based diets are "heart healthy," nourish working muscles and brain, and are essential for endurance athletes.

**PE:** Fat is the preferred human fuel, scientifically proven by two million years of evolution! High carb/high insulin, grain-based diets will cause oxidation and inflammation—the true catalysts for heart disease.

## INJURIES

**CW:** Treat with rest, ice, ibuprofen and perhaps visits to an orthopedist for Rx anti-inflammatories. After rest period, gradually return to training and hope for no recurrence.

**PE:** Identify functional weakness that caused injury and engage in targeted movement exercises to shore up imbalances/weaknesses. Treat injury with new "MCE" protocol: Move, Compress, Elevate. Don't ice! Icing dulls pain but inhibits the functioning of the lymphatic system to clear waste products and speed healing.

## LOSING EXCESS BODY FAT

**CW:** Pursued through portion control (especially limiting calorically dense fats) combined with high-calorie-burning workouts and increased training volume. It's all about the simple math of "calories in vs. calories out," right?

**PE:** Excess body fat is 80 percent dependent upon diet, specifically your level of carb intake/insulin production. Increased training volume (especially chronic patterns) simply increases appetite and reduces general daily activity levels. It's all about calories burned vs. calories *stored*. Fat loss comes from hormone optimization, not math equations.

## MILEAGE OR INTENSITY?

**CW:** Traditional, high mileage LSD approach conflicts with burgeoning intensity movement (e.g., CrossFit Endurance), which suggests gym and sprint sessions can deliver similar benefits to aerobic work. Many athletes blend both overdistance and intensity into weekly training routines.

**PE:** Both…and neither! It ain't as simple as either/or. Prioritize stress/rest balance, periodization (aerobic base before brief, high-intensity sessions), and intuitive training patterns. Reductions in mileage *and* intensity often deliver performance breakthroughs.

## PERFORMANCE NUTRITION/REFUELING

**CW:** Use sugary drinks and gels to sustain performance during long workouts and races. Take advantage of the thirty-minute post-exercise "window of opportunity" to restock muscle glycogen with carbohydrates and a bit of protein.

**PE:** Become fat-adapted through primal-style eating and stress-balanced, aerobic emphasis training. Fat adaptation negates the importance of supplemental carbs during exercise and obsessive post-exercise carb reloads. Favor wholesome, natural foods instead of synthetic "designer" energy products. Consider supplemental fats or "super starch" products for workout fuel.

## STRENGTH TRAINING

**CW:** Blended workouts (with both strength and endurance elements) featuring high reps, light weights, short rest periods, and lifting to "failure" on numerous isolated body part machines. Frequent sessions lasting 45–60 minutes that leave you feeling tired—a good sign you've worked hard enough for a beneficial workout.

**PE:** Go explosive or go home. Brief, intense, functional, full-body movements (squats, deadlifts, etc.), with heavy weights, few reps, and ample rest between sets (to preserve explosive performance). Twenty-minute sessions, conducted only during specific high-intensity/low-volume training periods.

## STRESS/REST BALANCE

**CW:** Strive for consistency. Adhere to time-tested maxims like one rest day each week, a winter "off-season" of cross training, and steady, linear progressions in mileage. Weekly schedule features workouts that stimulate disparate energy systems to cover all the bases.

**PE:** Prioritize rest. Align workout choices with daily energy and motivation levels. Strive for "inconsistency" to prevent overstress and burnout. Increased volume produces better performances…sleep volume, that is!

# SLOW DOWN!

*Escaping the Trap of Chronic Cardio*
*and Carbohydrate Dependency*
*and Becoming a Fat-Burning Beast*

# CHAPTER 1

## IN THIS CHAPTER

The Primal Endurance approach offers a refreshing alternative to the sugar-dependent, overly stressful "chronic" approach to endurance training. The typical workout pattern of doing workouts that are slightly too hard, too frequently, with insufficient rest between them, coupled with a pro-inflammatory high-carb diet and hectic lifestyle practices, leads to burnout, elevated disease risk, and accelerated aging.

The Primal Endurance approach focuses on comfortably paced aerobic workouts to build an endurance base over a period of weeks or months without the stress of moderate- to high-intensity workouts. Aerobic workouts and training periods entail exercising at or below your *maximum aerobic heart rate,* as determined by Dr. Phil Maffetone's simple calculation: 180 – age = maximum aerobic heart rate (with some adjustment factors). Be disciplined to avoid drifting above this very comfortable intensity level and entering the so-called "black hole," where aerobic development and recovery are compromised by workouts that are slightly too stressful. Aerobic development has been a hallmark of every elite performer in every endurance sport for more than fifty years.

The seven habits of highly effective Primal Endurance athletes are: getting adequate sleep, expertly balancing stress and rest (in workout patterns and in life), implementing an intuitive and personalized approach to training, emphasizing aerobic development, carefully structuring high-intensity workouts and training blocks, engaging in complementary movement and mobility practices, and following an annual periodization program.

• • • • • • • • • • • •

**CONVENTIONAL WISDOM ABOUT** endurance training has long emphasized more, more, more: a firm belief that more raw mileage and hourly volume equates with more competitive success. Over the past several decades, world record holders and Olympic gold medal winners fed this beast by attributing their success to the prodigious workloads they performed in training. With no better options pondered, the masses fell in line and doggedly tried to complete as much volume of work as possible in the name of peak performance. What resulted over decades of trial and error was a harsh realization that elite athletes are elite for a reason, and that the training schedule of a champion has little relevance to the optimal approach for an amateur competitor balancing endurance goals with real-life responsibilities and stressors.

The pure mileage fad faded as the road-weary endurance community came to the realization that it's not as simple as filling the logbook and then setting records on the race course. As endurance training and racing became a pop culture phenomenon, a much wider audience joined the old war horses on the marathon, triathlon, and ultra run starting lines. Slick magazines and books appeared everywhere, filled with all manner of "expert" training advice. As an evolution from the flawed linear assumption that mileage is king, the catch-all phrase "quality over quantity" rose to prominence. On the surface, this sounds great. How can you argue with an adjective like "quality" to describe your training program?

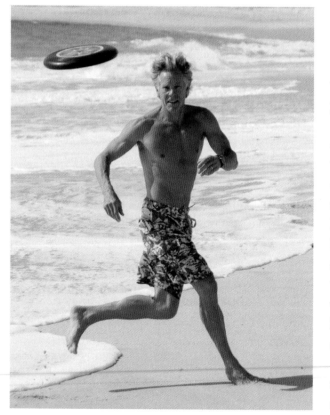

*Imagine: slowing down, having more fun (in workouts and in life), and going faster too!*

Unfortunately, the practical application of this maxim was essentially to speed up workout pace into the high-stress, sugar-burning intensity ranges and generate, yet again, burnout, illness, and injury. Indeed, there are many roads that lead to burnout, and the endurance movement seems to have found every single one over the years. What's more frustrating is that we seem to continue down the burnout highway even when confronted with huge caution signs all along the way.

Okay, perhaps it's not fair to say we blatantly ignore the warning signs of the chronic approach, because they are often nuanced and easy to misunderstand. It feels good to elevate your heart rate into a zone where you are breathing hard, sweating, and feeling a sense of accomplishment from making a respectable exercise effort. It feels good to enter those impressive figures into your online database or handwritten training journal. Also, we mustn't forget the chemical "endorphin" high that occurs after a sustained vigorous effort.

# TODAY, WE ABUSE THE DELICATE HORMONAL FIGHT-OR-FLIGHT RESPONSE WITH UNRELENTING STRESS.

When we experience a stressful event, whether it's a tempo run, a road rage incident, or an important sales presentation in the conference room, the fight-or-flight response is triggered in the body. Our bloodstream becomes flooded with feel-good hormones and neurotransmitters like cortisol, dopamine, serotonin, epinephrine, and norepinephrine, and the function of all of our senses is heightened.

This so-called "adrenalin rush" is part of our ancient hardwiring. When we faced the life or death environmental stressors of primal times, these feel-good chemicals interacted with opiate receptors in the brain, flooding the space between nerve cells and inhibiting neurons from firing. This masked sensations of pain and fatigue, inspiring our ancestors to continue to run away from the lion that was trying to eat them—literally—rather than give up. The same chemicals help today's marathon runners get their depleted bodies through those final miles to the finish line.

After the chase—the stressful event—is over, these chemicals linger in the bloodstream and we experience a blissful state that today's endurance athletes call the endorphin high, buzz, or rush. The term *endorphin* literally means "endogenous (internally manufactured) morphine." In this chemical state, messages of pain and exhaustion are not fully appreciated and you feel surprisingly chill, even (or especially) after pushing your body to a maximum effort. The high you obtain validates you doing this crazy extreme endurance stuff, while your ordinary neighbors just shake their heads and wonder why.

Today, the demand for life or death physical efforts are rare, but our brains and bodies don't know the difference between the ancient lion chase and the modern triathlon starting line. And we tend to engage in the latter more than the former, abusing this delicate hormonal process that was designed for life or death matters only. Those of us who take satisfaction in conducting tough workouts are literally addicted to the chemical high that comes as a consequence of these efforts.

We realize that "addicted" is not a complementary term, but it's important to recognize the chemical payoff you enjoy when you push your body through challenging individual sessions, training blocks, or even crazy six-month pushes to get your startup company to IPO day. Then you can sit back and utilize your higher reasoning skills to conclude that you might not want to abuse this fight-or-flight, endorphin-high programming, because your body will eventually become exhausted if you do it too frequently. Certainly you can relate times when you have become overtrained and fried your central nervous system to the extent that instead of a pleasant endorphin buzz after a vigorous session, you feel like taking a nap…and not waking up for fourteen hours!

So, we have some major influences conspiring to repeatedly plunge us into chronic patterns. First, we have the cultural influences, the prevailing philosophy that encourages "chronic" training, macho-ing out on mileage totals, never missing a workout, or always leading the group down the trail or up the mountain. We also have our own highly motivated, goal-oriented mindsets—really our ego demands—that mandate we do something productive and impressive toward our fitness goals and high standards every single day.

Finally, we have that chemical stuff going on, that compelling, hardwired desire to seek pleasure and dull pain through the release of adaptive fight-or-flight hormones. Well-meaning and enthusiastic as we may be to become fitness pillars in our community, the chronic patterns we engage in destroy health, compromise performance, and lock us into a sugar-burning, fat-storing metabolic state.

## CHRONIC CARDIO ELEVATES DISEASE RISKS

Chronic cardio is a *sustained pattern* of overly stressful endurance workouts: sessions that are a bit too long, a bit too hard, and conducted too frequently with insufficient rest in between. A chronic approach will lead to poor competitive performance, lingering fatigue, suppressed immune function, persistent stiffness and soreness, increased injury risk, failed weight loss efforts, and finally—when your fight-or-flight resources become exhausted from chronic stimulation—burnout.

Mileage versus intensity—the age-old debate has raged for decades. The truth is that a lot of mileage will get you really fit, and a lot of intensity will also get you really fit. But the big question is how endurance training will affect your long-term health, your longevity, and your stress hormone balance—that's what people forget when they get obsessed with the intricacies of how to stress your body in training.

CHRONIC CARDIO PATTERNS CAN INFLAME AND SCAR ARTERIES, AND DAMAGE THE VULNERABLE RIGHT VENTRICLE—LEADING TO ARRHYTHMIAS, ATRIAL FIBRILLATION, AND SUDDEN DEATH IN ATHLETES.

It's bad news for your race results, but the news is worse deep inside. When you live a life of chronic stress, you develop serious hormonal abnormalities that impede cognitive function, sexual performance, and immune function. Your cardiovascular system is especially vulnerable to chronically stressful, pro-inflammatory diet, exercise, and lifestyle patterns. Strange as it may seem, your misguided fitness efforts trigger the development of oxidation and inflammation in your arteries, setting the stage for heart disease.

Dr. Peter Attia is a physician, endurance swimmer and cyclist, blogger (eatingacademy.com), and president and co-founder (with Gary Taubes) of the non-profit Nutrition Science Initiative (NuSI). He is fond of performing extreme metabolic "human guinea pig" experiments on himself, and is one of the leading advocates for the health and performance benefits of doing fat-adapted endurance training. Attia explains how heavy training can potentially damage your heart, as long bouts of exhausting cardiovascular exercise actually create a stretch in the heart.

"When we engage in an extreme effort like an all-out time trial," says Attia, "we increase both heart rate and stroke volume [amount of blood pumped out per beat of the heart], by stretching the heart larger to pump more blood per beat. This amazing organ can quickly go from pumping three to five liters of blood around our body per minute at rest to thirty liters per minute during very intense exercise. Unfortunately, the right side of the heart, which pumps only against the low-resistance lungs, and is far less muscular than the left ventricle, is more vulnerable to damage from chronic amounts of high cardiac output training. So while short bouts of this intensity don't appear to cause lasting damage on the heart, prolonged activity does—at least in susceptible individuals. The so-called chronic cardio patterns can cause the right ventricle to become scarred from excessive use and insufficient recovery. This scarring can lead to cardiac arrhythmias, especially atrial fibrillation, and even sudden death in athletes who have no evidence of atherosclerosis."

Something called the "excessive endurance exercise hypothesis" is gaining traction in scientific circles. One of the leading voices is Dr. James O'Keefe, a sports cardiologist in Kansas City (look up his TED talk titled "Run For Your Life—at a comfortable pace, and not too far") and co-author of four bestselling books, including *The Forever Young Diet & Lifestyle*. O'Keefe mentions how seasoned marathon runners, sporting good bodyweight and blood profiles, nevertheless show increased scarring, thickening, and literal searing of the arterial walls from chronic inflammation. Their heart and entire cardiovascular system are aging at an accelerated rate. They have markedly elevated levels of calcified and non-calcified arterial plaque compared to a control group of sedentary folks. An adverse coronary artery calcium value, known as the Agatson score (after *South Beach Diet* author Dr. Arthur Agatson), is linked to higher future mortality rates. Some of the medical folks deeply involved in this disturbing issue are using the sobering nickname of "Pheidippides cardiovascular disease."

Keep in mind that the heart is damaged not by vigorous exercise, but from chronically excessive vigorous exercise. Dr. O'Keefe explains in his TED talk that after you do something extreme like a marathon, the micro tears occur in the arteries and your heart becomes inflamed and burned—just like any other muscle challenged through extreme use. This is why you may have heard that if a marathon finisher strolled into an emergency room and had some blood panels run, he or she would have levels of inflammation markers like troponin and C-reactive protein high enough to diagnose acute myocardial infarction—a heart attack. Thankfully, the heart and arteries are good at healing up and the damage heals in a couple days. However, if you engage in chronic exercise patterns, you get stiff, thickened, scarred, calcified arteries; your heart becomes prematurely aged as a direct consequence of your running.

Dr. O'Keefe's firm conclusion is that moderate exercise patterns are healthier than extreme ones. "The fitness patterns for conferring longevity and robust lifelong cardiovascular health are distinctly different from the patterns that develop peak performance and marathon or superhuman endurance. Extreme endurance training and racing can take a toll on your long-term cardiovascular health. For the daily workout, it may be best to have more fun and endure less suffering in order to attain ideal heart health," he explains in his talk.

While being able to break the hour barrier for 10K might get you laughed out of age-group contention, O'Keefe suggests that reaching such a modest fitness capability makes you "bulletproof" when it comes to disease risk. "We're not born to run. We're born to walk, and to move more in general," O'Keefe tells his TED audience. He goes on to make a specific recommendation that running two to five days per week for a total of ten to fifteen miles, at around a ten-minute-per-mile pace, is ideal for bulletproof cardiovascular health. The vaunted Copenhagen heart study concurs, saying two to three runs per week for a total of 1 to 2.5 hours gives you a 44 percent reduction in mortality compared to sedentary folks. O'Keefe and the Copenhagen study and many other experts assert that when you go beyond these modest standards, you start to compromise the many extraordinary health benefits of moderate exercise. The secret is out, and into mainstream media—such as the *Wall Street Journal*'s 2012 article "One Running Shoe In The Grave."

Most of you might be cringing by this point, and it's interesting to note that both Dr. O'Keefe and Dr. Attia report taking some heat from naysayers who challenge the assumptions that extreme exercise is unhealthy. But we must all take a step back and admit that this laundry list of cardiovascular lousiness absolutely should not be happening in a community of the fittest, most energetic, most accomplished modern humans. And it doesn't have to. Contrary to what you might believe after spending however many years in the game, struggling to attain your mileage goals and consistent workout patterns, you do not have to struggle or suffer or constantly straddle the red line between race-ready and broken down in order to succeed in endurance sports. You can pursue even the most extreme competitive goals in a manner that supports your health, or at least doesn't out-and-out destroy it every step of the way. Interestingly, Attia says he somewhat ignores his own moderation advice because he gets tremendous enjoyment from his endurance cycling pursuits, which extend far beyond moderate. Acknowledging the health risks associated with chronic exercise instead of being cavalier about them can be extremely helpful when you face the nuanced daily training decisions of when to back off and when to push on.

> *"We're not born to run. We're born to walk, and to move more in general. For the daily workout, it may be best [for longevity] to have more fun and endure less suffering."*
>
> —Dr. James O'Keefe

Metabolically, chronic cardio workouts are slightly too strenuous to emphasize fat as a fuel source, and instead emphasize glucose burning. While this makes the workout more difficult and generates more fatigue and sugar cravings right afterward, the truly damaging effects of chronic workout patterns occur around the clock. Workouts elevate metabolic function multiples higher than your resting metabolic function. This is measured by a figure called "Metabolic Equivalent of Task

(MET)." For example, an all-out sprint workout can go up to an amazing 30 MET—you are generating energy at thirty times your resting rate. Running a steady pace (e.g., 7m:30 per mile) is 13.5 MET, while even a casual bike ride (10–16 mph), easy swim, or vigorous hike will still elevate the function of the various body systems up to between 6–10 MET. So when you are pumping blood and processing oxygen and fuel to the tune of ten, twenty, or thirty times your resting rate, you send a powerful signal to your genes for how to regulate metabolic function for many hours after the workout.

# EVEN A SLIGHTLY ANAEROBIC WORKOUT PROMOTES SUGAR BURNING FOR UP TO SEVENTY-TWO HOURS AFTERWARD.

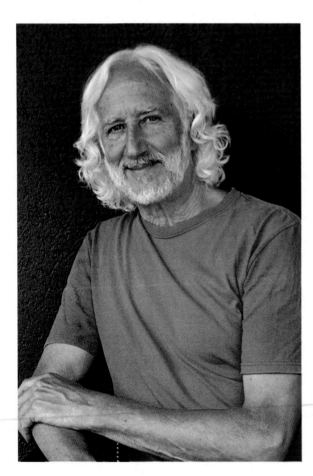

Dr. Phil Maffetone reports than an anaerobic workout—even a slightly anaerobic workout where your heart rate drifts out of the aerobic zone going up hills or sprinting for city limit signs—accelerates sugar burning at rest for up to seventy-two hours after the session. That's just enough time to recover and bang out another anaerobic workout and get round-the-clock service for sugar burning, sugar cravings, excess insulin production, suppressed immune function, and fat storage. If your goal is to perform well in endurance events, get leaner, be healthier, and delay the aging process, it's quite possible that your training sessions are promoting the exact opposite results of your goals.

*Dr. Phil Maffetone, the godfather of aerobic training, and balancing health in pursuit of fitness. Legendary exercise physiologist Dr. Tim Noakes says, "I'm clever, but Phil Maffetone is a genius. He saw through this [carbohydrate paradigm endurance training and eating] stuff 30 years ago."*

# HOW TO BUILD AN AEROBIC BASE

The most immediate triage response to escape the sugar-burning, fat-storing pattern is to *slow down* your workout pace into a heart rate zone that is predominantly aerobic, with little to no stimulation of the anaerobic system. When you hike, walk, jog, or pedal at a comfortable pace, you burn mostly fat for fuel. And since oxygen is required to burn fat, your comfortably paced training stimulates the development of additional mitochondria in your cells. These are the energy-producing "powerhouses" located in each cell that take in oxygen, along with fat, protein, and glucose, and convert them into energy in the form of ATP that fuels many cellular functions. Having mitochondrial density not only boosts performance in both endurance and explosive efforts, it supports general health by protecting you from stress-induced free radical damage.

Interestingly, your mitochondria have their own DNA, distinct from your cellular DNA. Mitochondrial DNA is inherited exclusively from your mother, which has made it valuable in tracing human ancestry and evolution. We know from the study of mitochondrial DNA that the first appearance of the genetically identical modern *Homo sapiens* was in East Africa around 160,000 years ago. This also means that whatever endurance gifts you have were inherited just from your mother (thanks, Mom!), not your father.

Science in this field from pioneers like physiologist John Holloszy in the 1960s showed that exercising aerobically for a long duration helped build more mitochondria. This helped validate the popularity of extreme long, slow distance training in those days. Science in the 1980s revealed that high-intensity workouts were also very effective in building more and better mitochondria.

## THE HEALTH AND PERFORMANCE BENEFITS OF MITOCHONDRIAL BIOGENESIS

Mitochondrial biogenesis describes the process of building new mitochondria, and increasing the efficiency of existing mitochondria, in response to the stimulation of both aerobic and anaerobic workouts. This is a fundamental element of the body's stress adaptation response. In the case of mitochondrial biogenesis, the stress is a depletion of cellular energy caused by the workout. Cellular depletion stimulates a metabolic regulator called AMPK (amp-activated protein kinase) that drives mitochondrial biogenesis.

High-intensity exercise increases mitochondrial density and oxidative enzyme activity by constructing completely different message-signaling pathways than those formed by aerobic endurance training. These pathways turn on a "master switch" called PGC-1Ð (pronounced "PGC-one-alpha") that triggers a favorable rise in mitochondrial density and oxidative enzyme activity. So, in order to develop the biggest, fastest, cleanest-burning engine, best results come from doing both aerobic and anaerobic workouts—in proper balance, of course, per the Primal Endurance guidelines.

Exercise not only increases the size and number of mitochondria, but also makes them more efficient by increasing the number of oxidative enzymes found in mitochondria. These enzymes improve metabolic function of your skeletal muscles, boosting fat and carbohydrate breakdown for fuel, and speeding energy formation from ATP. Having abundant oxidative enzymes improves exercise performance and provides greater protection against oxidative stress—a key marker of aging. Meanwhile, insufficient or poorly functioning mitochondria is one of the key contributors to accelerated aging.

Now, while the production of ATP is what makes us go—literally—free radicals are unfortunately created in the process. This is a fundamental element of being a living, breathing organism. If you have an ample amount of well-functioning mitochondria, they can successfully deal with the free radical load of ATP. It's all about spreading the load of energy production among enough mitochondria to absorb the free radicals before they do any damage—the more mitochondria you have, the better.

Interestingly, while both aerobic and anaerobic workouts help you optimize mitochondrial function, becoming fat-adapted in general is the best way to keep your mitochondrial energy production system functioning optimally. This means emphasizing aerobic workouts and following a primal-aligned eating pattern.

Mitochondria require oxygen to produce their energy, and thus play a central role in fat metabolism in the body, since fat requires oxygen in order to be metabolized. The amount of mitochondria increases when you train aerobically and become fat-adapted with your eating patterns. This increases the efficiency of oxygen processing throughout the body. In contrast, glucose metabolism can occur with (aerobically) or without (anaerobically) oxygen.

The exceptions are red blood cells, which lack mitochondria and thus must metabolize glucose anaerobically. When glucose metabolism occurs anaerobically, the by-product is lactic acid, the cause of the familiar "burn" in the muscles associated with strenuous exercise. In addition to their power plant role, mitochondria are responsible for a variety of other functions relating to cell growth, cell death, and respiration.

Mitochondria burn fatty acids (and ketones, which we'll discuss in detail later) much more cleanly than they burn carbohydrates. When mitochondria burn glucose, more free radicals are generated. Furthermore, since glucose burning can occur with or without oxygen, mitochondria are not mandatory when you are locked in carbohydrate dependency from a grain-based Standard American Diet and a chronic exercise pattern. When this is the case, your mitochondria can literally atrophy, making you inefficient at producing energy and more prone to oxidative damage in general. Chronic cardio and overtraining have been shown to cause gene mutations that damage mitochondria. This is known as mitochondrial myopathy.

Envision your body for a moment as a huge power plant, producing electricity for a small town. The contrasting examples of the dirty, inefficient, low-production coal plant versus the clean, efficient, high-production solar plant illustrates the importance of building a healthy system of capillaries and mitochondria, and becoming fat-adapted instead of carbohydrate dependent.

## Sugar-Burning Factory

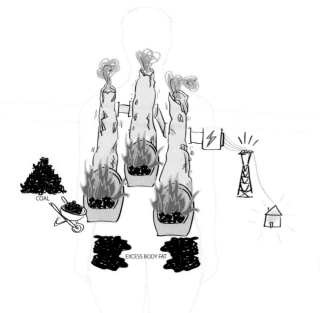

*Insufficient and inefficient furnaces (mitochondria) burn energy from a dirty energy source (carbs), causing pollution (oxidative damage) and low energy generation.*

## Fat-Burning Factory

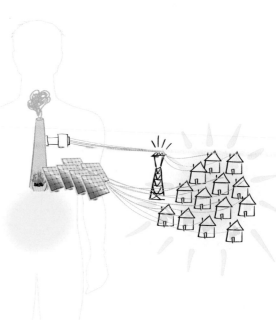

*Abundant, clean-burning solar panels (mitochondria, created/optimized through exercise) burn virtually limitless solar energy (stored and ingested fat), with no pollution. Even the occasionally used, more efficient smokestack burns coal (carbs) cleaner!*

The dilapidated smokestacks at the sugar-burning plant are burning coal—a dirty fuel source—and hence the pollution coming out the smokestack. Furthermore, while energy is plentiful, there aren't enough good smokestacks to operate at full capacity. This is a picture of a mitochondrially deficient, aerobically deficient sugar burner. The "coal" energy source is your ingested and stored fuel, mostly carbs since fat burning is deactivated by too much carb intake or insulin production. Carbs burn quickly and easily, generating lots of pollution—free radical production. The smokestacks are your mitochondria. Because you are unfit or over-trained/broken down, you have inefficient and insufficient furnaces. The coal piling up in surplus will be converted into fat and stored. You have an energy backlog (excess body fat) because your power plant sucks.

In contrast, look at the beautiful solar power plant, burning a virtually limitless source of clean energy. The solar panels are your mitochondria—abundant and highly efficient at burning the solar energy without free radical damage. The sun, your fuel source, is stored and ingested fat. The carbs you do burn are processed much more efficiently because your smokestacks (mitochondria) are robust and efficient.

Aerobic workouts have a significant impact on your metabolic function at rest, so comfortable training sessions up-regulate your fat-burning genes and down-regulate your sugar-burning genes around the clock. Slowing down your workouts helps stabilize mood, energy, and appetite throughout the day, optimizes your health, speeds recovery, and makes fat loss virtually effortless when you implement a primal-style eating pattern.

What's too hard? How much slower do you need to go? The answer is to conduct the vast majority of your endurance training sessions at or below what Dr. Maffetone calls your "maximum aerobic heart rate." This is defined as the point where *maximum aerobic benefits occur with a minimum amount of anaerobic stimulation.* At this intensity, best measured by heart rate, you are burning predominantly fat, feeling comfortable at all times, able to converse without running out of breath, and not stimulating significant stress hormone production or lactic acid accumulation in the muscles.

Maximum aerobic heart rate is the point where maximum aerobic benefits occur with a minimum amount of anaerobic stimulation.

In attempting to refine the Primal Blueprint position on this critically important heart rate value, we've reviewed plenty of studies and come to the conclusion that determining your maximum aerobic heart rate is not an exact science. Dr. Maffetone concurs with this, and touts his non-scientific but extremely well-field-tested "180 – age" formula—one with an assortment of subjective revision factors—as the best way to calculate your numbers.

Some endurance experts refer to this critical distinction point as the ventilatory threshold (VT), the point where an increase in effort would result in labored breathing and insufficient oxygen to perform comfortably. Exceeding this threshold causes ventilation rates to spike in a non-linear manner. You can identify your VT in a lab test, as it is believed to correspond with recruitment oxidative fast-twitch muscle fibers (known as Type IIa fast-twitch fibers; Type IIb fibers are glycolytic—reserved for maximum power efforts; Type I muscle fibers are slow-twitch and used for low intensity endurance efforts). Type IIa fibers are recruited when intensity switches from low (predominantly

Type I slow-twitch fibers) to moderate and higher intensities, and is also correlated with an activation of different brain cells connected to Type IIa fast-twitch muscle fiber use.

We want to deliver a comprehensive presentation of this matter here, so we'll also mention a couple of useful subjective tests to estimate where you transition from predominantly aerobic into anaerobic. Carl Foster, PhD, an exercise scientist at the University of Wisconsin-La-Crosse, and Stephen Seiler, an American exercise scientist teaching at Agder University College in Kristiansand, Norway, have co-authored several research studies on the effects of aerobic versus anaerobic exercise. Foster promotes a "talk test" that suggests that you can converse comfortably below your aerobic limit, but where an increase in pace would soon make reciting the Pledge of Allegiance, or telling a tall tale to your training partner, difficult to do without gasping.

Also helpful is an Eastern-philosophy-influenced suggestion detailed in John Douillard's book *Body, Mind, and Sport* that recommends breathing only through your nose to minimize the stress of a workout. If you are exercising in the aerobic heart rate zone, you should be able to obtain sufficient oxygen using only your nose, but you'll know you're exceeding that aerobic limit if you need to draw air through your mouth.

Furthermore, Douillard details how keeping your mouth closed facilitates taking deep diaphragmatic breaths, where you engage the oxygen-rich lower lobes of the lungs for maximum respiratory efficiency. Running or cycling along while taking deep, nose-only diaphragmatic breaths will reduce the stress level of your workout by stimulating the parasympathetic nervous system (calming, relaxing influence) as opposed to the more common stimulation of the sympathetic nervous system (fight-or-flight response) that occurs when you conduct even a moderately difficult workout.

Nose breathing also helps you filter pollutant particles, something of particular concern for urban athletes getting an unfiltered dose of car or industrial fumes through the mouth. Furthermore, nitric oxide—a potent vasodilator—is produced in the sinus cavity, so nose breathing increases nitric oxide levels, improving bloodflow and oxygen exchange throughout your cardiovascular system.

Nose breathing during a workout is simply taking a fundamental principle of yoga, meditation, Ayurvedic medicine, and other Eastern disciplines and applying it to a rah-rah Western pursuit of endurance training. It's true that pulling huge breaths through your nose during your workout is not the most natural or even fun thing to do, but it's a great thing to experiment with when you really want a relaxing, rejuve- nating, low-stress workout. If you tend to be stuffy or get annoyed by mucus interference, try applying a nasal strip, or just inflate your upper lip, your moustache area, and keep it puffed out. This helps the nostrils execute smoother inhalations and exhalations.

When it's time to conduct a true recovery workout, where you don't exceed 65 percent of your maximum heart rate, nose breathing is an excellent technique to commit to for the duration of the session. Another excellent subjective marker is that you should finish aerobic workouts with a stable energy level, mood, and appetite, and bounce back the next day without any lingering soreness or fatigue.

It's critical to be conservative and highly disciplined about staying aerobic. Using a heart rate monitor with an identified number as your aerobic maximum and setting a limit alarm is mandatory to ensure your success with aerobic training. It's just too difficult to maintain that level of concentration and focus on your intensity level during a casual ses- sion where your mind, and your pace, can easily wander. Besides, when we are presented with a hill, a headwind, an enthusiastic training part- ner increasing pace a bit, or a natural decline in efficiency that happens in the latter stages of any ordinary training session, our natural tendency is to just hang in there and allow our metabolic functions to adjust to the increased demands. That includes pulling even more aggressive breaths from your nose and achieving an undesirable acceleration in effort while still playing by the rules!

When you respect the importance of emphasizing aerobic devel- opment, workouts transition from a succession of mini-competitions (with your usual time on the route, with your training partners' pace, whatever) to actual training sessions with a specific metabolic focus that promotes your long-term development and protects your health. Instead of sticking to arbitrary and irrelevant goals like maintaining a certain pace per mile throughout the workout, you honor irrefutable biofeedback to keep your effort level consistent and get in the habit of slowing down in the latter stages of workouts. You also get into the habit of generally training at a much slower pace than usual. No doubt about it—it can get more than a little frustrating to stick with the aer- obic program, but the dividends are enormous and completely quantifi- able by results in a simple, repeatable sub-max performance test known as the MAF (Maximum Aerobic Function) test.

For many athletes, it's time to have a heart-to-heart (pun intended) in front of the mirror and consider how your daily behavior patterns align with your stated long-term goals. If you can't muster the focus or discipline to conduct a proper aerobic training session (because some wanker on a cruiser bike blew past you on the bike path and you just had to give chase, because your annoying training partner is subtly increasing the pace on every hill, or because of whatever superficial stimulation you react to), you should admit that you are behaving in a manner incongruent with any peak-performance-related goals—or, in the case of chronic or OCD training patterns, incongruent with your health. In summary, it's time to put aside your ego demands, set that beeper, and honor it by slowing down!

## AEROBIC VS. ANAEROBIC CONTRIBUTION RATIOS

The energy to produce an hour-long all-out effort comes 98 percent from the aerobic system. Even a two-hour race is 99 percent aerobic—not to mention anything longer than that. This might be hard to believe when you are hammering your brains out during an hour time trial, but as Dr. Maffetone reminds us, "These ratios come right out of exercise physiology textbooks, and while it refers to the whole aerobic system and the use of both fat and sugar, it's quite a complicated concept. Clearly, all endurance events are sub-max efforts. Ironman winners, for example, usually race around 70 percent of their max efforts; marathoners around 85 percent. So developing the sub-max mechanism—improving your MAF test results—is vital to performance success."

Granted, highly trained endurance athletes are able to maintain a heart rate well above aerobic maximum for an event that lasts only an hour, or even two hours. What this means is that the entire aerobic system is in use as the predominant metabolic source, burning both fat and glucose, but you are well beyond that important training heart rate where maximum aerobic benefits occur with minimal anaerobic stimulation.

Research published by Dr. Paul Gastin, senior lecturer at the Deakin University School of Exercise and Nutrition Sciences in Australia, quantifies the relative contribution of the aerobic and anaerobic energy systems during intense exercise. The results are quite surprising if you harbor the notion that aerobic equates with slow movement only. Gastin estimates that an all-out effort of around seventy-five seconds requires an equal contribution from the aerobic and the anaerobic energy systems. By comparison, a ten-second sprint is 94 percent anaerobic and 6 percent aerobic, and a six-minute all-out effort is 79 percent aerobic and 21 percent anaerobic. It seems hard to imagine that even an all-out time race of six minutes is mostly aerobic, but accepting these physiological realities can be helpful to recalibrate your attitude about the importance of building the aerobic system from the ground up, and having the patience and restraint to do so properly.

## DETERMINING YOUR MAXIMUM AEROBIC HEART RATE

There is an assortment of opinions about what exactly constitutes that heart rate where maximum aerobic benefits occur with a minimum amount of anaerobic stimulation, but where an increase in effort would cause a non-linear spike in ventilation, glucose metabolism, lactate accumulation, fight-or-flight hormones, activation of Type IIa muscle fibers and associated brain function, and so forth. Ventilatory threshold studies suggest that in well-trained athletes, VT is around 77 percent of maximum heart rate. However, it is believed that VT arrives at a lower percentage of max heart rate in unfit individuals. While attaching VT to aerobic max is encouraging, it implies that you have an accurate maximum heart rate value. This is no easy task to determine, as it's difficult to perform an effective test outside the lab, and the estimate calculations—while getting better than the dated and oversimplified "220 – [age]"—can still be imprecise.

Primal Endurance recommends that you use Dr. Maffetone's "180 – age" formula to establish your maximum aerobic heart rate. If you have a techie bent, know your maximum heart rate, and want to go by a percentage of maximum heart rate, we'll present the details on this calculation process too. Using either Maffetone or a percentage of maximum heart rate, you should get very similar numbers. If the numbers are disparate, we urge you to train at the *lower* of the two numbers!

Calculate your maximum aerobic heart rate with Dr. Maffetone's simple "180 – age" formula. Set that number as your beeper alarm, and stick with it!

Dr. Maffetone's formula entails subtracting your age from 180 and then using that number as your maximum aerobic heart rate. Or, add or subtract five beats according to Maffetone's adjustment factors relating to one's level of health and fitness (details below). Maffetone has time-tested this formula over decades of hands-on work (including, interestingly, a change in running gait that Maffetone believes tips your hand that you are drifting above aerobic maximum) and detailed recordkeeping with his clients.

Whatever number you adhere to, make a sincere effort to integrate subjective factors into your analysis. You should be able to converse comfortably or breathe through your nose only (okay, with a bit of practice to get used to it) at your designated aerobic max number. You should finish aerobic workouts feeling refreshed and energized, not slightly foggy, depleted, or craving calories. If things don't fall into place and you experience fatigue or sugar cravings in the hours after aerobic workouts, lower your numbers!

Maffetone 180 – age Formula Adjustment Factors: Here are the adjustment factors Dr. Maffetone offers in *The Big Book of Endurance Training and Racing*. Take 180 minus your age as your baseline number, and then adjust it accordingly if appropriate:

1. **Subtract 10:** Recovering from illness, surgery, disease, or taking regular medication.
2. **Subtract 5:** Recent injury or regression in training, get more than two colds/flu annually, allergies, asthma, inconsistent training, or recently returning to training.
3. **No Adjustment:** Training consistently (4x/week) for two years, free from aforementioned problems.
4. **Add 5:** Successful training for two years or more, success in competition.

Let's do some comparisons to validate the Maffetone formula against percentage of max heart rate calculations. First, let's take a forty-year-old who has had decent fitness progress in recent years. The new gold standard for estimating max heart rate is 208 – (.7 x age), giving a forty-year-old an estimated max of 180. Hitting VT at 77 percent of max would be 139 for an aerobic max. Using the Maffetone formula, the athlete would generate a result of 140—good matchup here. An unfit forty-year-old athlete (or one who has struggled a bit with injuries and illness) might hit VT at 75 percent of estimated max, or 135. Using the Maffetone formula, this athlete would take 140 and subtract 5 beats to get 135—again a good matchup. On the other hand, some athletes perform calculations where the numbers are significantly disparate. See sidebar "Ageless Wonder" for details.

As far as the confusing assortment of training "zones" out there are concerned, we'll tell you right now they are of minimal concern. All you need to worry about is staying below your maximum aerobic heart rate during aerobic workouts. Of course, if you are exercising below 55 percent of max heart rate or so, you aren't getting much of a training effect, but you're still moving! As we'll discuss further in Chapter 8, we need to become better about blurring the lines between training and sitting on our butts all day congratulating ourselves because we have a workout on the books.

All forms of movement, including five-minute breaks from your work desk and leisurely twenty-minute strolls around the block with the dog, contribute to your aerobic development, and deliver an assortment of immune, musculoskeletal, and cardiovascular benefits that can make a significant contribution to your fitness goals and greatly improve your overall health and well-being. But let's call a proper aerobic training session something that lands between 55 percent of max heart rate and your "180 – [age]" calculation upper limit.

## BEWARE OF THE BLACK HOLE

When you drift above maximum aerobic heart rate, glucose burning accelerates and fat burning gets pushed aside accordingly. Stress hormone production increases and a bit of lactic acid starts to accumulate in the muscles. Type IIa muscle fibers and brain cells start to kick into gear and get you into a bit of an intensity mode instead of an extremely comfortable aerobic mode. None of these metabolic shifts are easily discernable or at all debilitating. In fact, you may still feel quite comfortable as you extend your effort well beyond aerobic maximum heart rate. Psychologically, you might even gain a greater sense of satisfaction that you are actually "getting a workout" because of your slightly labored breathing pattern, elevated perspiration, and elevated perceived exertion in the brain.

Dr. Seiler coined the term "black hole" to describe the training zone just outside aerobic maximum and up to the anaerobic threshold. Anaerobic threshold (AT) is the intensity level where lactic acid is accumulating in the bloodstream faster than you can buffer it; hence the characterization of AT as the "burn" or the "red-line" pace. Obviously, you are not going to drift a routine training session into AT range without feeling the burn and slowing down.

On the other hand, the black hole has been confirmed by numerous studies as the default landing area for people relying solely upon perceived exertion to govern intensity level. It's a pace you can maintain for long duration without falling apart, feel like you are focused and working intently like a real athlete, and feel a sense of exhilaration and euphoria (from stress hormone production, a.k.a. the "endorphin buzz") after the session. "Vigorous" is a good word to describe a black-hole workout. Not "brutal," but certainly not entirely comfortable and nose-breathable like a proper aerobic session either.

While studying the training habits of elite endurance athletes in Nordic skiing, rowing, running, cycling, and triathlon, Seiler's team discovered that elite athletes spent around 80 percent of the time training at aerobic heart rates, and only 20 percent of workout time doing high-intensity workouts. With respected follow-up studies to strengthen the initial observations, Seiler and others observed that elite performers in a variety of endurance sports either go really easy (aerobic base training) or really hard with proper interval or other high-performance sessions.

Seiler says the reason that the black hole is an ineffective middle zone is that it's too slow to make you better, and too fast to allow for sufficient recovery. An astronomy buff, Seiler said that athletes drifting into this intensity level by default is akin to the gravitational pull caused by a black hole in space. Unfortunately, other studies have revealed that the average recreational competitor spends at least half of his or her total training time above the aerobic maximum and into black hole, anaerobic threshold, or maximum intensity heart rate zones. Fine-tuning the DumbCar!

As we consider different training philosophies, including diametrically opposing views, and try to make some sense of everything to dial in our own approach, please stay focused on the big picture. For example, one book referencing Seiler's research called *80/20 Running* promotes training aerobically 80 percent of the time and going fast 20 percent of the time. The book asserts that 80/20 models the habits of elite athletes across many endurance sports and has great science to back it up. It's surely a lot safer and more sensible than defaulting to a 50/50 pattern like most exercisers, but it's still making a blanket conclusion where none is warranted.

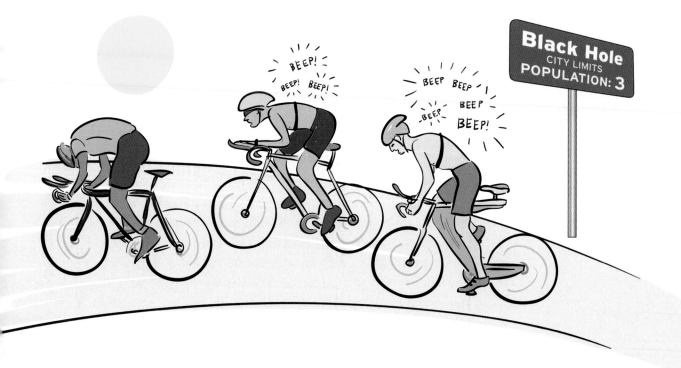

# COMFORTABLY PACED AEROBIC TRAINING BUILDS ENDURANCE WITHOUT INTERRUPTION FROM SETBACKS CAUSED BY HIGH-RISK, CHRONIC TRAINING IN THE BLACK HOLE.

Every bit of training strategy you are exposed to requires personal experimentation and fine-tuning. It's not as simple as following a magic formula, even one proven by elite athletes and respected studies. Furthermore, your training patterns and intensity ratios will vary widely over the course of a year with a periodized approach. During an aerobic base building period, you have to be in the aerobic zone 100 percent of the time. Going 80/20 during an aerobic period represents a dismal failure. During a high-intensity training period, you focus on maximum-effort sprints and strength-training sessions, and getting tons of rest between these explosive workouts. You drastically reduce aerobic training volume with lots of short, slow recovery workouts and far more rest days. Why worry at all about your ratios at those times?

The black hole is the default landing spot when you rely on perceived exertion alone to dictate intensity.

Phil Maffetone elaborates on the metabolic consequences of training in the black hole: "When you move out of the pure aerobics system, where 90 to 95 percent of an endurance athlete's energy comes from fat, to a black hole pace that burns more sugar, the first big downside is that you run out of fuel faster. The other is a big rise in your stress hormone levels. The black hole is really the first stage of overtraining—and it comes on fast. I've seen athletes train just a couple of heartbeats too high, and over time they become overtrained." Dr. Foster adds that, "We think there's a physiological tripwire. Slip into the black hole for a few minutes—or do an interval or two—and the body reads the whole workout as hard. It cancels the [aerobic session's] recovery effect."

Of course, it doesn't hurt to occasionally open up the throttle a bit and have some fun climbing a tough mountain or completing a group training run with faster folks. You can leave the heart watch at home for these sessions, as a similar training effect has been observed when you exercise anywhere from 10 percent below AT (black hole territory) to a couple of percentage points above AT. Whatever you want to call these sessions—tempo, fartlek, hill repeats, intervals, time trials—they should be considered breakthrough workouts that approximate competitive challenges and stimulate fitness improvement.

When you eat right and sleep like a primal champ, your body does a good job recovering and getting stronger from bouts of appropriate stress like an occasional tough workout. Indeed, that's what the fight-or-flight response is designed for—to briefly elevate your physical and cognitive function to deliver a peak performance effort, then settle back into a stress-balanced routine.

The problem comes when black-hole workouts become a pattern. The super hardcore competitors jamming through the streets in their pacelines or meeting at the track to drop the hammer every Tuesday evening are guilty of these chronic patterns, but so are the routine gym goers who show up to aerobic, Zumba, or Spinning classes several times per week and rock out to the blasting music. Invariably, these group workouts include lots of time spent above aerobic maximum for everyone in the class, except perhaps a super fit instructor. Ditto for group training programs like Team In Training or even a high school cross country team. When a training group of disparate abilities gathers for a long run intended to be aerobic, it's typically only aerobic for the select few folks at the front of the pack, like the top few runners on the varsity. For the majority of participants, it can easily turn into a destructive black-hole session.

Because it's so easy to drift above aerobic maximum into the black hole, we must repeat that using a wireless heart rate monitor to constrain your intensity inside the aerobic zone is absolutely mandatory. You don't necessarily need to pull a home equity loan for the latest $400 GPS or wattage meter gizmo, unless you are inspired and motivated by the techie elements of training. For proper aerobic base building, you simply need a monitor that will beep when you set a limit alarm. And you need to slow down when you hear the alarm. Training by perceived exertion alone just won't cut it. We know a few pros who claim they can train effectively by feel, but they're pros!

Get a simple heart rate monitor like a Polar FT1 (approximately $70) or another reliable brand, and use it every single time you train. Notice how your max aerobic heart rate correlates with maxing out on nose breathing, or losing your wind on the Pledge of Allegiance or in conversation with a training partner. Notice how easy it is to get pulled into the beeping zone by a small hill, an energetic song in your earbuds, or a wanker passing you on the bike trail, or just see your rate drift a bit higher at the same pace during the latter stages of the workout due to fatigue.

By the way, it's also really important to warm up gradually to avoid black-hole risks. When your body goes from a resting state into a workout too abruptly, this can kick you into a stress response and glucose metabolism that is hard to recalibrate into calm, fat-burning mode even when you maintain a disciplined aerobic pace. Spend the first five to ten minutes of your training sessions moving very slowly, to allow blood to transfer smoothly from your internal organs to your extremities. Ditto for a gradual cooldown to minimize the stress effects of going from active to sedentary too abruptly.

If you've spent many hours in a sedentary position before a training session, it makes sense to start out with just a walk for a few minutes, then break into light jog for a few more minutes (apply something comparative for whatever sport you are doing) before commencing a proper training session at or near maximum aerobic heart rate. You'll know you are fully warmed up when your skin becomes warm and moist, and your joints feel lubricated and fluid.

Regardless of your fitness level, your exercise intensity as a percentage of maximum heart rate has a similar metabolic effect on your body. In the aerobic zone, the effort feels easy, plenty of oxygen is available, and fat metabolism is emphasized. If you are an elite professional, you can run (relatively) incredibly fast at this comfortable heart rate, while a less fit person might have to alternate between slow jogging and walking to maintain aerobic heart rate levels.

Become skilled at staying comfortable during your entire workout and building upon this momentum over time with a natural increase in the pace you can sustain while still feeling comfortable. In essence, you are taking a sure-fire, low-risk approach to improvement, by methodically getting stronger and more efficient without interruption from setbacks caused by high-risk, chronic training in the black hole.

**DID YOU KNOW?**
*Your speed at aerobic maximum is relative to your fitness level. An unfit athlete might be walking at aerobic max, while an elite might be clicking off 6-minute miles.*

# GET THAT AEROBIC HEART RATE DIALED IN, OR ELSE!

The conventional approach to heart rate training zones works off percentage of maximum heart rate. Various authorities define an "aerobic zone" limit of 75 percent (unfit), 77 percent (fit), or 80 percent (elite). The Maffetone formula is easier and more accurate, because max heart rate calculations can be inaccurate for some (and the science is inexact anyway). For example, the aging former elite athlete authors deliver a much higher max than the age-predicted formula, possibly because decades of heavy training slow the "one beat per year" decline rate that the age formulas use.

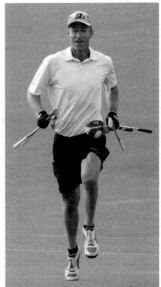

With Brad hitting the big 5-0 in 2015, a full twenty years removed from his days on the pro circuit, he can still generate a heart rate of 190 during his primal 400-meter time trials (check blogspot.bradkearns.com for "Running in the 50's [59 sec 400m] in my 50s")—17 beats higher than his predicted max with the 208 formula. This would deliver an aerobic max of 152 at 80 percent (hey, he's a former elite athlete!), or 146 using a more modest 77 percent calculation on account of his age.

After years of minimizing endurance workouts and emphasizing primal sprints and strength workouts, Brad decided to get back into some modest endurance running training to prepare for competitive Speedgolf tournaments ("modest" due to his extremely stressful job with an incredibly demanding boss...). In Speedgolf tournaments, you combine golf score with running time to produce a total Speedgolf score. At the 2014 World Speedgolf championships, Brad was the twentieth pro, playing the championship Bandon Dunes, OR course in fifty-one minutes and shooting an 83, for a Speedgolf score of 134 (he repeated his twentieth place finish at the 2015 World Championships in Chicago). There goes your "too busy to play golf" excuse!

As Brad attempted to build a good aerobic base at a heart rate of 145 or less over a period of several months, he started to experience declining performance and accumulated fatigue, most likely due to training at too elevated a heart rate and being out of serious training for twenty years. Despite feeling like he was moving really slowly and not running for long (under an hour) in comparison to his professional days, Brad had successfully entered the black hole.

In consultation with Dr. Maffetone for this book and about Brad's particulars, Maffetone asserted the significance of the "180 − [age]" formula as follows: "If an athlete is not progressing with their aerobic training, they are most likely training at too elevated a heart rate. In Brad's case, I urged him to use the 180 − [age] formula for a training heart rate of 130. And rather than using the 'add 5' adjustment factor on account of his historical training success that he requested, I said he might even subtract 5 due to his recent struggles." He wasn't joking.

As Brad faithfully set out at the even slower pace of 130 beats per minute or less, he regained his energy and experienced the steady progression in efficiency promised by aerobic base building. From having to basically transition into a walk upon any incline to stay under 130 bpm, a few months of uninterrupted success with aerobic runs now allows Brad to keep a respectable pace, even on hills. In a Speedgolf tournament, Brad and the other professionals run at anaerobic threshold heart rates (in Brad's case probably 175 bpm or higher), covering a distance of five miles over an eighteen-hole course in forty to fifty-five minutes. An all-out Speedgolf effort bears little resemblance to Brad's comfortable morning jogs or casual Speedgolf practice rounds at 130 or lower. However, Brad having the patience to condition aerobically translates directly into him being able to run faster during competition, and recover faster when it's time to take a swing.

Beyond the athletic arena, Brad's health improvements were validated by blood markers for the all-important testosterone: 6.8 free-T (clinically hypo) in April '15 during chronic training patterns, and 14.7 free-T (1,013 serum T) in October while training aerobically. That's legit for a high school dude, forget about a 50-year-old! *Note:* Brad's serum T values during his racing career ranged from 200-300, what with the extreme chronic stressors of pro racing, traveling, and constant schmoozing of sponsors and media.

As Brad explains, "We must admit that endurance athletes like to fudge numbers and make rationalizations that allow them to put in more work or go a little faster. In my case, when I tried to return to actual training after years of just goofing around, I honestly wanted to pick the right number to enable the building of an aerobic base. I felt comfortable at 145 beats per minute, because endurance athletes and their focused mindsets can talk themselves into feeling comfortable whenever they want to. As in, 'I've raced Kona seven times; now I feel comfortable on the lava fields...' You know what I'm talkin' about!"

Brad continues, "When I returned to significant aerobic training at a 145 heart rate, I responded very well for a couple months with rapid fitness progress. However, this was likely due to a chronic elevation of adaptive stress hormones like cortisol as my body tried valiantly to keep up with a work demand that was excessive. Eventually, I noticed fatigue accumulating and compromising my daily energy level, my recovery, and my performance (eventually, I had fodder for the sidebar in Chapter 10, see page 293). I couldn't believe I was going 'too fast,' at a heart rate of 145—I was only running perhaps a nine-minute mile pace. Meanwhile, my mentality was stuck in the old millennium. I applied a vision of my former pro triathlete self—a guy (now literally half my age!) who could float along for hours at 155 beats per minute and not break a sweat—into present-day behaviors. A lot of this was subconscious, but my experience of a bigger, better, badder-ass past definitely compromised my thinking and judgment of the here and now. It's probably how those fallen hedge fund guys feel when they have to fly business class now instead of private."

Dr. Maffetone goes to great lengths to urge endurance athletes to be conservative with their numbers; hence the admonition in this book to choose the *lower* of whichever formulas you play with. Furthermore, if you experience a regression in performance, lingering fatigue, or any illness or injury, this is a call to train at a lower heart rate. You certainly can't go wrong when being conservative with your aerobic development, and you can very easily go wrong when you creep just a bit above a healthy number, whether it be from calculation errors or lack of discipline during workouts. As Dr. Maffetone reminds us, "It all comes down to the MAF test. You should expect to see steady improvement, and if you don't, something is wrong and you need to change it."

## SLOWING DOWN REALLY WORKS!

Yes, it can be quite frustrating to your competitive nature to have to slow way down during your workouts in the name of getting leaner and fitter, but it's the absolute truth that this is the path to endurance greatness. This has been proven true by every elite athlete in every endurance sport for over fifty years, starting with the phenomenal success that New Zealand distance runners had under legendary coach Arthur Lydiard in the late 1950s.

Lydiard was the first coach to introduce overdistance training and periodization for middle- and long-distance runners. Prior to his era, distance runners essentially trained by running intervals around the track at high speeds until they collapsed. For example, Roger Bannister reported that he only trained for thirty minutes per day in preparation for the Olympics and his four-minute mile in 1954. Lydiard's revolutionary insight was that distance runners didn't need to develop more speed as much as they needed to develop more endurance to maintain a winning pace for as long as possible. He experimented on himself, running insane mileage (up to 240 miles per week!) and becoming the top Kiwi marathon runner in the late 1950s.

Lydiard rose to international prominence as a coach at the 1960 Olympics in Rome. He wasn't even part of the official New Zealand coaching staff, but two of his runners won gold: Peter Snell at 800 meters and Murray Hallberg at 5000 meters. Snell, who today is a respected human performance physiologist in Dallas, TX, is a remarkable example of the importance of aerobic development in even high-speed track events. Prior to bursting onto the world scene, Snell jogged comfortably for months and months in the sand dunes of New Zealand, building endurance, strength, and aerobic capacity—without interruption from injury or burnout so common with high-intensity track training (Lydiard was also big on scheduling flexibility and personalization of individual athletes' workloads and recovery times—what he called "feeling-based" training).

In 1962, Snell leveraged his hundred-mile training weeks and twenty-two-mile-long runs to shatter the world record at 800 meters with a time of 1m:44. This time is still world class today, and would have qualified him for every single Olympic and World Championship final since 1962. Amazingly, contention still exists about the value of aerobic development for middle-distance athletes. Even endurance and ultra-endurance athletes are captivated by increasing their "speed" through track workouts, hill repeats, and strenuous swimming interval sessions, when in reality the aerobic system is supplying almost all of the energy during competitive efforts. In a 2003 interview, Snell revealed his exasperation—here are some choice excerpts:

> Even in New Zealand the feeling today is that Lydiard's ideas are passé. I can't believe it! I still hold the New Zealand 800 meter record—it's [53!] years old. Most physiologists are trained on the idea of specificity and simply can't understand that slow training makes you faster. I attended a USA Track and Field conference where the sentiment was, "We're disturbed about the fact that we're not getting any medals in middle-distance and distance running at the Olympics, and why is this?" And someone concluded, when they looked at the Olympics, American runners are getting buried in the last lap. Therefore, we need to teach them how to sprint. So that's unbelievable. [laughs] There's not a lack of speed—they're just running out of gas, and so everyone else is cruising because of the superior endurance, is what that boils down to.

> Just about every scientist I know cannot understand why slow running works. It just doesn't seem to fit their—I suppose they're brought up on the concept of specificity—if you're going to be a middle-distance runner, you need to be doing something that's related to the demands of your event. These are sort of cornerstones of coaching and so on. And then, why would you run slowly? And I've seen some very derogatory statements by scientists about long, slow running. Very derogatory. And I'm trying to be equally derogatory back.

The reason that emphasizing aerobic training works and that chronic cardio sucks is as follows: When workout intensity drifts out of the aerobic zone, you start burning an ever-greater percentage of glucose (the preferred fuel choice when oxygen is insufficient) and stimulate the release of stress hormones and lactic acid into your bloodstream. While it's beneficial to simulate high-intensity competitive efforts in training once in a while, it's destructive to simulate scaled-down competitive efforts all the time. When you drift above your aerobic max and into the black hole at 82, 85, or 90 percent of max heart rate, it's not as hard as an all-out race, but it's hard enough to compromise your fitness progress and challenge your health.

Lydiard's legacy has been honored by astute modern-day coaches like Maffetone, who was the first guy to bring aerobic training into the limelight through his association with the 80s- and 90s-era top triathletes Mark Allen, Mike Pigg, and Tim DeBoom. Allen's story is particularly compelling because we are talking about a guy who, early in his career, earned the nickname "Grip," as in Grip of Death. This referred to how one held the handlebars when trying to hang with Allen on training rides, as he was known for pushing brutally hard virtually every time out in his early years in the sport. As many swimmers schooled in high-volume, high-intensity training patterns have discovered, this all-out, all the time approach didn't work very well out of the water. Allen was forced to reconsider his strategy and rein in his competitive intensity due to recurring injuries in his early years on the circuit.

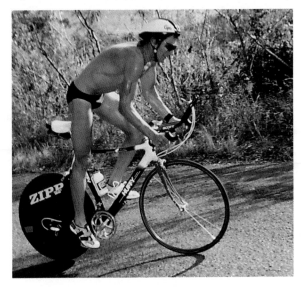

*Mark Allen, "The Grip," the greatest triathlete in history and an early adopter of aerobic heart rate training, climbs the infamous "Beast" on St. Croix, a 1,000' ascent in one mile. He remained aerobic for the entire climb...NOT!*

In consultation with Maffetone, Allen addressed his metabolic condition of aerobic deficiency and anaerobic excess by patiently conducting all workouts at or below his maximum aerobic heart rate of 150 beats per minute for several months. At first, the experience was almost laughable. Allen had trained at such a high intensity for so long that he found he had to slow to a walk during routine training runs to avoid the dreaded beeping of the watch.

Grip was a fine-tuned, world champion *anaerobic* machine, but he could not even break eight minutes per mile pace when training *aerobically*. Allen stayed the course and built the biggest, most efficient engine ever seen in the triathlon world. His aerobic pace, measured in regular Maximum Aerobic Function (MAF) tests we'll describe shortly, steadily dropped from the eights down to a phenomenal 5m:10 per mile for a five-mile test at the same heart rate—150 beats per minute.

Naturally, Allen's progress came without the injury, illness, and burnout land mines that come from an anaerobic-based program, and dramatically improved his performance in the ultradistance events where the ability to burn fat and spare glycogen is even more relevant than in a two-hour Olympic distance triathlon. In Allen's famed "Ironwar" duel with Dave Scott at the 1989 Hawaii Ironman, he recorded an astounding 2h:40 marathon split en route to his first of six victories. This is after swimming 2.4 miles, cycling 112 miles, and then running in the oppressive afternoon heat of the lava fields of Kona. Allen's marathon split remains the race record a quarter of a century later.

Because Allen was able to preserve his health with a lower stress aerobic-style training approach, he was able to extend his career and go out on top at age thirty-seven. In his very last race, the 1995 Ironman, Allen came back from 13.5 minutes behind on the marathon, the biggest deficit in Ironman history, to beat twenty-six-year-old German rival Thomas Hellriegel for his sixth Hawaii world title.

# AEROBIC TRAINING IS PRIMAL ALIGNED!

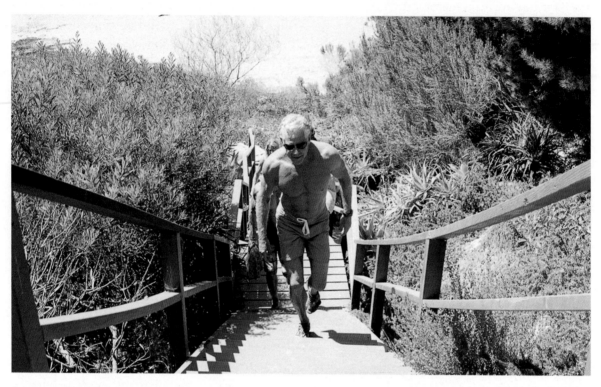

To put a little plug in for primal here, we must realize that our human genes are hardwired to respond to fight-or-flight environmental stressors that are brief, life or death matters that end quickly and are balanced by extensive rest and recovery. We are simply not adapted to grind away day after day, calling upon the fight-or-flight response too often for too long until exhaustion ensues.

Exercising in your aerobic zone of 180 minus age or below allows you to hone your fat-burning skills even further, and to develop a strong fitness base without the breakdown and burnout caused by chronic cardio. There is a time and place to push yourself really hard and achieve fitness breakthroughs, but casual and serious exercisers alike can benefit from moderating their workout pace, and reducing overall training volume of both aerobic and high-intensity sessions. You can make your difficult "breakthrough" workouts less frequent—and of higher quality—when you harness your resources on a day-to-day basis.

Comfortably paced aerobic workouts do not burn the mega-calories that chronic exercise burns, but eating primally predominates over caloric expenditure concerns when it comes to weight management. Exercise is not about the calories burned: it's about the movement—building a solid foundation of cardiovascular and musculoskeletal fitness, and enjoying the psychological benefits of being active.

# THE SEVEN HABITS OF HIGHLY EFFECTIVE PRIMAL ENDURANCE ATHLETES

Here, at a glance, are seven key elements that summarize the Primal Endurance approach:

**1. Sleep:** Yes, sleep is number one—the next frontier of performance breakthroughs in all sports, especially endurance sports. Your athletic pursuits require you to sleep significantly more than if you weren't training. Reject conventional wisdom's "eight hours" recommendation and individualize your approach, honoring these two maxims: minimize artificial light and digital stimulation after dark; and awaken each morning, without an alarm, refreshed and energized. If you are training more, sleep more. If you can't honor the aforementioned maxims, stop training until you can. If you fall short of optimal sleep one day, take a nap the following day—instead of your workout! More on this topic in Chapter 8.

**2. Stress/Rest Balance:** Primal-style endurance training allows you to reach for higher highs (breakthrough workouts) and observe lower lows (more rest, shorter, easier recovery workouts, and staying below aerobic maximum heart rate at the vast majority of workouts). This appeals to your competitive intensity by focusing on peak performance and recovery, instead of focusing on the flawed notion of "consistency" in this context. Furthermore, realize that virtually all athletes, from novice to elite, do too much training and not enough rest. Consider backing off on both your mileage and your intensity, and adding more sleep, recovery, and complementary practices.

**3. Intuitive and Personalized:** Your training schedule is sensible, intuitive, flexible, and even spontaneous instead of regimented and pre-ordained. Respect your daily life circumstances, motivation levels, stress levels, energy levels, immune function, and moods. This means backing off when tired, but also pursuing breakthrough workouts when you feel great! Experimentation is necessary to dial in the best approach that works for you, and entails some trial and error. Also, what worked for you last year may not work in the future, so be open to flexibility. The top priority is to enjoy your program and feel confident that it works well for you.

**4. Aerobic Emphasis:** Endurance success is primarily dependent on aerobic efficiency. Aerobic base building delivers by far your best return on investment, and is best achieved by strictly limiting heart rate to aerobic max or lower during defined aerobic workouts and training periods. Stay out of the black hole, and don't venture into high-intensity training blocks before you have a strong base.

**5. Intensity Structure:** Intensity can deliver exceptional results for endurance athletes, when a strong base is present, when workouts are brief in duration and really intense, when they are conducted only when you are highly motivated and energized, and during defined periods that are short in duration and always followed by a rest period and preceded by an aerobic period.

**6. Complementary practices:** Increased general daily movement, spontaneous, unstructured play sessions, mobility work such as technique drills and dynamic stretching, movement practices like yoga and Pilates, and high-intensity strength training are essential for success, because we live sedentary lives of extreme physical ease. Remember, in endurance competitions, you have to "endure." Cranking out your daily hour-long workout and then sitting at a desk, in a car, and on a couch the rest of the day is not preparing you to endure anything except perhaps a beatdown on the race course at the hands of a more well-rounded athlete! Expand your perspective to embrace total fitness and an active, energetic lifestyle.

**7. Periodization:** An annual program always commences with an aerobic base period (minimum eight weeks). With success, high-intensity periods can follow, with a maximum duration of four weeks. Intensity periods are followed by micro periods of rest, followed by aerobic, followed by a return to intensity/competition. The annual program always ends with an extended rest period or off-season, followed by a new macro aerobic base period to commence a new annual program. This overview offers plenty of flexibility, but you have to respect the need to engage in blocks of specific training focus as an immutable law of endurance training.

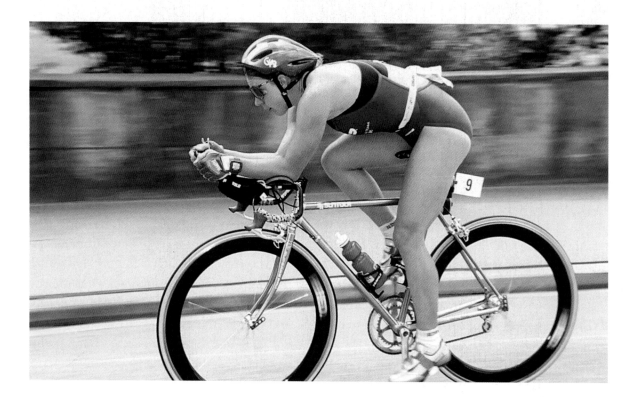

# CHAPTER SUMMARY

- Ditch chronic cardio
- Be flexible and intuitive
- Build a base at HR of (180 – age)
- Beware the black hole

The conventional approach to endurance training has athletes addicted to the endorphin high to the detriment of their long-term health and aerobic development. The delicate fight-or-flight response hardwired into our genes is being abused today by unrelenting stress, especially chronic endurance training patterns.

Successful endurance training is not as simple as the "quantity vs. quality" debate; rather, it's an intuitive and personalized approach that respects the fundamental laws of exercise physiology, while allowing for plenty of flexibility.

The prevailing **chronic cardio training patterns promote chronic inflammation, elevate cardiovascular disease risk, and promote hormonal abnormalities** that lead to compromised endurance, strength, explosive power, cognitive function, sexual function, and immune function. The ultimate result of chronic cardio is burnout. Even a workout that is slightly too difficult can alter metabolic function to inhibit fat metabolism and promote carbohydrate dependency—not just during the workout, but for hours afterward.

Building an aerobic base is the key to success in endurance sports, and this is achieved by exercising for a sustained period of time—at least two months to begin each season—at or below maximum aerobic heart rate. Primal Endurance recommends **Dr. Maffetone's 180 – age formula to identify maximum aerobic heart rate**. You can try the talk test or nose breathing test to remain aerobic, but a wireless heart rate monitor with a beeper alarm will keep you most compliant.

Compliance with staying below aerobic maximum is essential for aerobic development and protection against burnout, but many highly motivated athletes have difficulty training at much slower speeds than they are accustomed to. **The black hole is that zone above aerobic maximum and below anaerobic threshold** that is not hard enough to quality as a proper high-intensity session, and too hard to easily recover from. Elite athletes avoid this zone, but casual exercisers default into the black hole frequently, as perceived exertion confirms you are "getting a good workout."

**The seven habits of highly effective Primal Endurance athletes are: getting adequate sleep, expertly balancing stress and rest (in workout patterns and in life), implementing an intuitive and personalized approach to training, emphasizing aerobic development, carefully structuring high-intensity workouts and training blocks, engaging in complementary movement and mobility practices, and following an annual periodization program.**

# CHAPTER 2

# BALANCE OUT, CHILL OUT

*Following the fundamentals of periodization*

*with a flexible, primal approach*

**2**

Endurance athletes typically adopt a driven and methodical approach to training that fails to properly balance stress and rest. An intuitive approach that respects an assortment of other life variables and stress factors will deliver more favorable results. Workout difficulty should be aligned with daily level of energy, motivation, and health.

Periodization entails focusing on different types of training during specific blocks of time over a calendar year. The big picture annual periodization strategy involves an aerobic-base-building period to start the year; sequences of mini-periods where you introduce intensity, followed by rest and aerobic periods—repeated over the course of the year in alignment with your progress and your competitive goals; and finally a lengthy rest period to end the competitive season.

It is essential to be highly intuitive and flexible with your training patterns, while adhering to the foundational principles of periodization. The importance of "consistency" in the context of endurance training is a flawed notion that can easily lead to mediocrity, chronic patterns, and burnout. The ideal training pattern is fractal, flexible, subject to change on the fly, and ultimately your responsibility.

· · · · · · · · · · · ·

**PERHAPS YOU HAVE HAD SOME** exposure to the musclehead crowd and the hilarious "bro-science" that pervades that scene? Their ethos is always worth a laugh or two amidst a group of high-minded endurance folks, once they leave the gym parking lot, reach the trails, and are out of earshot. Time to sober you up a bit and realize that these dudes have us beat in the balancing stress and rest department. That's right, the readership of triathlon magazines, who have an *average* college education of 4.3 years (!), are put to shame on the simplest of training concepts by the average shaved-down, yoked-up musclehead from the nearest gold (or even silver…) gym.

You see, anyone who has been able to achieve muscle hypertrophy, to inflate their body to cartoon-level (or at least NFL-level) proportions, has successfully optimized the delicate balance between stress and rest. There is simply no other way to get huge guns. If a bro were overzealous in his quest to blow up and drifted into a chronic training pattern, muscle catabolism would result and his T-shirt would not stretch till the words "Sun's Out, Guns Out" became illegible.

Bodybuilders honor the simple, common-sense principle of challenging muscles to their maximum capability, then affording generous time periods for rest, nourishment, and repair (okay, and the injection of foreign substances, but that doesn't weaken the argument here at all!) so that the muscles come back stronger and larger. Meanwhile, endurance athletes challenge their muscles, cardiovascular systems, hormonal systems, and immune systems to maximum capability, then drag their butts out the next day to perform more work at the expense of rest. "Dude, what's your problem?!" the bros say in response.

We're having a little fun here at the expense of the proud endurance community, but we want you to take this revelation seriously. The cerebral, analytical, regimented, methodically driven approach to getting fit simply doesn't work as well as a simple, intuitive, spontaneous, sporadic approach. It's a tough pill to swallow, because our Type-A personalities and keen intellects crave a methodical approach. Furthermore, modern life rewards and reinforces the "to-do list" approach as the path to success. Write down specific measurable goals, establish checkpoints along the way, make yourself accountable, apply your exceptional discipline and willpower to stay the course no matter what, and you shall [fill in the blank: graduate college, pass the bar exam, reach your quarterly sales quota, get your startup ready for an IPO, and, uh, win your age group in a triathlon].

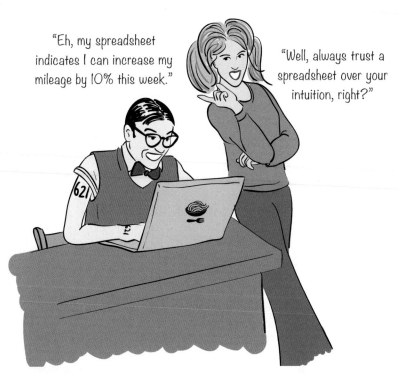

THE CEREBRAL, ANALYTICAL, REGIMENTED, METHODICALLY DRIVEN APPROACH TO GETTING FIT SIMPLY DOESN'T WORK AS WELL AS A SIMPLE, INTUITIVE, SPONTANEOUS, SPORADIC APPROACH.

Unfortunately, the human body doesn't get fit in a linear manner. The process of fitness is dynamic—subject to dozens of important variables far beyond your workout choices. Sleep patterns, eating habits, other forms of life stress, your emotional state, and your physical environment are just a few factors that influence your fitness progress and whether or not it syncs with your health. You can try your best to create a scientifically sound, methodical training schedule designed to get you onto the podium, but it must always be subject to revision at a moment's notice if your workout choices are not in alignment with your general state of health and your subjective level of energy and motivation at the time of your training session.

If you feel intimidated at the daunting task of balancing stress and rest in an intuitive manner instead of relying on regimented patterns like "hard day–easy day," or lengthy schedules created by an expert coach, rest assured that you are already an expert in this department. Deep down, you know the correct workout decision to make each day to optimally balance stress and rest. Unfortunately, what typically happens is your intuitive voice gets snuffed out by the demands of your ego, your insecurities, and your obsessive/compulsive behavior tendencies.

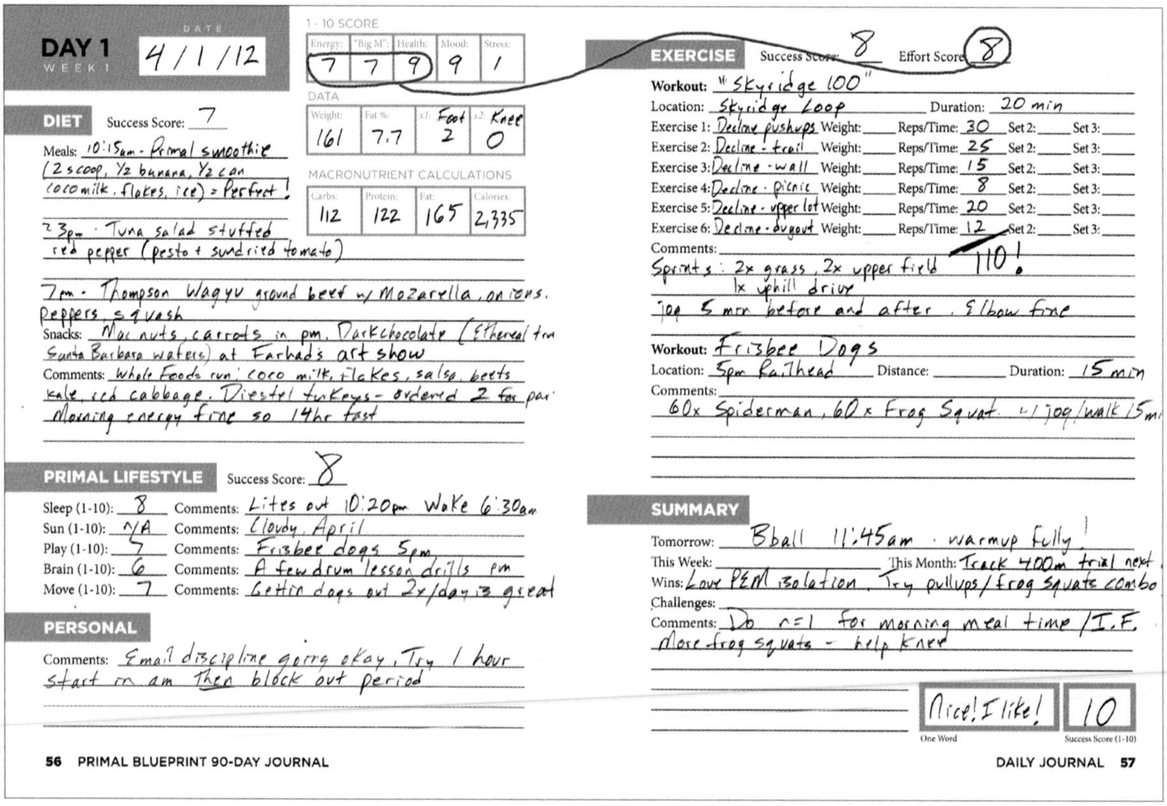

Balancing stress and rest can be a complex topic to fill an entire book on its own, so let's make things simple here: **align the difficulty of your workouts with your daily level of energy, motivation, and health**. Make a quick assessment each day and give yourself a 1–10 score in each of these three categories. *The Primal Blueprint 90-Day Journal* has daily journal pages designed for this purpose if you want to really get focused. Or, just jot your daily scores into a ninety-nine-cent spiral notebook or digital device.

*Journaling can help you get into the rhythm of aligning workout difficulty with subjective levels of energy, motivation, and health.*

Journal form, Day 1, handwritten entries.

If you wake up feeling refreshed and energized, with perfect immune function and a strong desire to get out and hit the road, you might give yourself a score of 8, 9, or 10. If you are amidst a stressful work deadline, experiencing family or relationship struggles, feeling fatigued upon waking up, have stiff or sore muscles, have a scratchy throat, feel a bit hot, or simply don't feel like working out on a certain day, you might give yourself scores of 2 or 3 in energy, motivation, and health.

## DEEP DOWN, YOU KNOW THE CORRECT WORKOUT DECISION TO MAKE EACH DAY TO OPTIMALLY BALANCE STRESS AND REST.

The trick is to conduct a workout with a similar 1–10 score in degree of difficulty—the degree that the workout stresses your body. A score of one or two would be an easy recovery session, while a ten would be a competitive race or other maximum effort performance. When you establish a pattern of aligning your subjective scores with the difficulty of your workouts, you are on your way to huge guns…or rather, on your way to an endurance career that is rewarding and successful, and supports your health instead of compromising it.

### PERIODIZATION — HOW TO PROPERLY BALANCE AEROBIC TRAINING, HIGH-INTENSITY WORKOUTS, AND REST

You may not be totally comfortable with a suggestion to be 100 percent airy-fairy with your workout decisions and just train how you feel each day. Please appreciate the opening comments of this chapter as an attempt to get your mind right and to break free once and for all from any sort of obsessive/compulsive influences in your training decisions.

With a healthy respect established for the importance of an intuitive approach to training, we'll proceed to add some broad general guidelines in the form of an annual periodization template. Periodization is simply periods of time—over the course of a calendar year, for example—characterized by different types of training emphasis.

These are not rigidly prescribed periods of a specific duration leading to a single date where you peak in an important competition. That approach might be relevant for an Olympic athlete with tremendous control over life variables and all the marbles riding on a single day when they give out the gold medal. For our purposes, we are going to adhere to the philosophical guidelines of periodized training, but allow for plenty of flexibility and adjustment along the way based on real-life variables.

*Periodization* means periods of time characterized by different types of training emphasis, but with plenty of opportunity for flexibility and adjustment along the way.

There seems to be a huge percentage of endurance athletes whose behaviors suggest they are opposed to periodization. Instead, they try to train an assortment of energy systems and sport-specific skills every single week, are reluctant to complete a strict aerobic period and create a proper base, and seem to skimp on a proper off-season of drastically reduced training. Consequently, they aspire to be at or very near peak racing shape virtually year-round—including winter endurance events in many cases.

As with the other admonitions and spicy talk in this book, we're not trying to tell you how to live your life; we're just strongly suggesting an approach that will deliver the most competitive success, the most enjoyment, and the least offense to your general health. If you want to realize your peak performance potential, it is imperative you engage in precisely defined and focused periods of training. We don't know why this is so difficult to embrace—we get amped up just talking about it, like Pete Snell in Chapter 1. We have decades of time-tested success from elite athletes practicing periodization, but if you flip open a random magazine or download a random podcast, you are likely to hear about "balanced" training programs where you have overdistance, tempo, intervals, and resistance training on the docket week in and week out. This is not balanced; this is *imbalanced,* with too much stress and not enough specificity!

The most important and probably least respected aspect of periodization is the rest component. It's indisputable that every serious athlete can benefit from an extended rest period annually. Usually this coincides with the end of a long season and the onset of winter, where less daylight and colder temperatures offer great excuses to back off. Giving your body a physical break from devoted fitness pursuits and giving your mind a break from the struggle of balancing workouts with other life responsibilities, as well as the mental energy expended worrying about compelling athletic goals, is tremendously refreshing and restorative.

Similarly, every endurance athlete, from world-class racer to novice, can benefit from a lengthy period of exclusively aerobic base building prior to the start of the competitive season. Here, you can develop your fat-burning systems without the metabolic interference and increased risk of breakdown associated with high-intensity workouts. Finally, virtually everyone will experience best results with intensity when it is performed in short-duration time blocks, with dramatically reduced overall training volume or concern with aerobic development. Intensity periods are always followed by a rest period of an appropriate duration and a mini aerobic base-rebuilding period before introducing another intensity block.

## "BALANCED" TRAINING WEEKS WITH OVERDISTANCE, TEMPO, RESISTANCE TRAINING, AND BACK-BREAKING INTERVALS ARE NOT BALANCED: THEY ARE IMBALANCED, WITH TOO MUCH STRESS!

These guidelines are purposely generalized, because the periodization philosophy does not warrant a cookie-cutter approach, but rather an adherence to philosophical guidelines with plenty of flexibility and customization. Unfortunately, with today's popular internet-based coach/athlete model, intricate and lengthy programs are designed to culminate with a peak performance at a distant goal event. One elite reportedly engaged in a *thirty-eight-week build* to the big event of the season (which did not go well, by the way). This is periodization at its worst—or at least we can call it high-risk periodization. Catch a little cold or a minor injury, perform poorly at some workouts somewhere along the way, and the whole algorithm is blown. What a joke, and what a heartbreak for an athlete putting his or her heart and soul into following an expert-designed program to the letter.

What's cool with the Primal Endurance approach to periodization is that the duration of all of your periods and mini-periods is flexible and subject to your intuitive evaluation of what works best for you. When you suffer a setback like an illness or injury, you just shuffle the deck instead of completely invalidating your previous hard work. When you experience declines in energy, motivation, or immune function, you adjust your ambitions and embark upon a short or lengthy rest period. When you find yourself in peak condition and succeeding on the racecourse, you can keep the magic going for perhaps a little longer than planned, and build in a longer rest period accordingly. Why not capitalize on your hard work? Everything you do is aligned with your intuition, while still respecting the fundamental principles of periodized training.

In essence, what we want to strongly argue against here is the misguided notion of "consistency" when it comes to your training schedule. Consistency in this context is simply a consistent application of a similar type of stress to the body week after week, month after month. This diminishes your potential to excel during peak competitive periods and comes with an extreme risk of burnout. Worst of all is trying to continually train all of your energy pathways, with a weekly schedule that includes overdistance aerobic sessions, high-intensity workouts, strength-training sessions (especially "blended" sessions that have both strength and endurance components—more on this in Chapter 5), and pre-programmed rest days. This type of approach will make you consistently mediocre at very best, and more likely consistently burnt out.

Unfortunately, this is exactly what many misguided endurance athletes are doing in the name of consistency, and with a nagging fear in the back of their minds that they might get out of shape (or at least lose their endurance, lose their speed, or lose their feel for the water) or fat (not knowing that 80 percent of body composition results are dictated by diet, specifically carb intake) if they deliver a week with any deficiencies from their normal pattern.

Consistency in the context of endurance training is simply a consistent application of stress, and a higher risk of mediocre performance and burnout.

We're assuming that you are a serious athlete with distinct performance goals, along with a desire to protect your health, delay aging, be a positive role model for your kids, and all that other good stuff. If you absolutely must get out of the house or the office and push yourself to

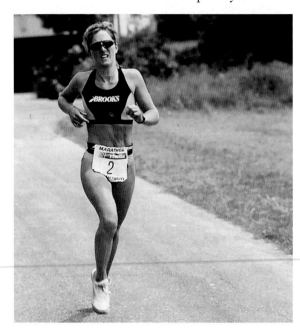

reach a sweaty, depleted state to cope with the stress of hectic daily life, this is the wrong book for you. Granted, getting out there and working hard with the "jack of all trades, all the time" approach is still a huge step up from being a couch potato. But the more time and energy you devote to training, and the deeper your commitment to peak performance, the more you must respect the principles of periodization. After all, the average weekend warrior who plays hoops at lunch on Tuesday, does a gym session with his trainer on Thursday, and runs a 5K on the weekend is not dealing with the hormonal irregularities, overstretched right ventricles, and overtraining issues that serious endurance athletes traffic in.

## PERIODIZATION IN PRACTICE

Honoring the KISS mission stated at the beginning of the book, this chapter presents a simplified view of an annual training and competitive season filled with both major periods and mini-periods that respect the three fundamental training elements required for success in endurance sports: aerobic development, high-intensity workouts, and rest and recovery.

Here's what an optimal annual training pattern will look like: A strict **aerobic base building period** to begin an annual training cycle; **brief periods of high-intensity workouts** (including competitions) with greatly reduced aerobic work and overall training volume; **mini-cycles** where you rest after an intensity period, rebuild base briefly, and reintroduce an intensity period; and finally an **extended rest period/ off-season** of minimal exercise and zero high-intensity sessions. This completes an annual training cycle, and you would resume a new season with an extended aerobic base building period.

An annual periodization pattern consists of an initial aerobic base period, brief, high-intensity periods always followed by rest and aerobic rebuilding, and an extended rest/off-season period.

This approach allows you to achieve and maintain peak condition at numerous times during the season, and to be super-flexible throughout the season to both balance other forms of stress in your life and strike when the iron is hot. Following are more details about the composition of the major training periods.

# TRAIN EASY, WIN BIG—LIKE PIGG

The remarkable success Mike Pigg experienced working with Dr. Maffetone that we glimpsed in the sidebar in the Introduction deserves a second look. While Pigg made headlines blowing up bike courses and opponents all over the globe throughout the late 1980s, his success was coming at a cost, and he was hanging on by a thread. "By the end of 1989, I was completely burnt out," remembers Pigg. "I'd raced like crazy for several years all over the globe. I had pushed myself extremely hard with high-mileage, high-intensity workouts, often alone in Arcata, CA [his hometown]. I had contracted the stomach ailment *Giardia* swimming in dirty water somewhere on the planet, and couldn't shake it. It really affected me at long-distance races, where I could no longer compete with the best. I really thought my career was nearing an end because I simply could not push anymore."

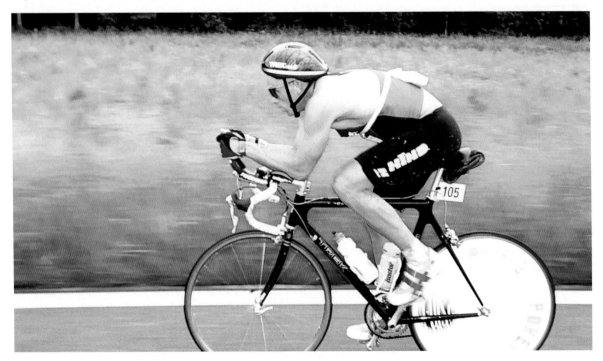

Dr. Maffetone gave Pigg some "doctor's orders" to start the new decade training indefinitely at strictly aerobic heart rates. Despite the pressures and expectations that come with being an elite performer, Pigg mustered the courage to blow off speed workouts for months on end, building his aerobic engine at 155 beats per minute or less. After several months of strictly aerobic workouts, Pigg started to feel his health and energy normalize, as it was finally liberated from the unrelenting stress of high-intensity workouts.

Pigg remained aerobic all the way up to the starting line of the first big event on the calendar, the America's Paradise Triathlon in St. Croix in April. Wanna guess what happened? Typically behind after the swim and known for catching and passing the field on the bike, Pigg was so far ahead of the pack after the swim that he rode off unseen by the pack.

They waited all day for him to catch up and when he never appeared, they assumed he had crashed out...until they saw him heading home while they were still outbound toward the run turnaround—leading the race by a mile, literally!

With no preparatory speed workouts at all, Pigg delivered a world-class performance in St. Croix, and at the next race, and the next, and the next, and so on through two full triathlon seasons where he won almost every race and every award in sight. During this period of time in the early 90s, Pigg's races were his speed workouts, while his training focused on aerobic development and stress management. Granted, Pigg had lots of high intensity races and workouts in his legs prior to 1990, but there is no discounting the fact that even the fastest guy in the world improved significantly when he slowed down and emphasized aerobic training—not just for the minimum of eight weeks, but for virtually two full calendar years, followed by many more years at the top of the sport with a drastically less intense, less stressful training program.

When Pigg did go hard in training, it was typically on a whim. "I would naturally decide to go hard about two to three times per month," explains Pigg. "Once in a while I just needed to see what I had, but it was hard to predict when those days would be. It was all based on intuition. I wish I had discovered these methods earlier in my career. Switching to aerobic emphasis literally added *seven years* to the length of my career."

**Aerobic Base Period:** Train at strictly aerobic heart rates for a minimum of eight weeks to begin your annual season. While there is some difference of opinion on the matter, we favor Dr. Phil Maffetone's admonition to complete a strict base-building period of aerobic activity only. That means taking a break from any kind of strength training (which is anaerobic by nature), Sunday night adult pickup basketball, and any other activities requiring anaerobic efforts. If you do rehabilitative/preventative strength routines for joint or imbalance issues, that's fine. But don't take the base period to go crazy with the weights or extracurriculars—something that, shockingly, is advocated by several leading endurance coaches.

The group of professional triathletes Mark used to coach in Los Angeles, including Brad, welcomed the winter months as a chance to get off the roads and have some fun in the mud with loosely structured mountain bike rides. Mountain biking in the wintertime offered a great mental break from the routine routes, timed climbs, and heart rate constraints of road riding, but when Mark joined them once for a mud fest, he realized a huge problem: mountain bike riding is tough! With everyone leaving their chest straps at home, there was no alerting the group that heart rates were going through the roof on steep hills or dismount/remount areas over challenging terrain. This was especially so when ringers joined the group—mountain bike specialists champing at the bit to put the hammer down on the season-weary triathletes.

A proper base period entails comfortably paced workouts that are relaxing, easy to recover from, don't make you want to ransack the nearest convenience store for a Hostess pie at the end, and don't leave you feeling stiff and sore the next day. However, a weekly overdistance breakthrough workout and the general accumulation of substantial hourly volume can still be taxing, so rest days, easy days, and easy weeks are still important during the base-building period. It's also imperative to be strict and disciplined about never exceeding your maximum aerobic heart rate—no excuses!

A friendly sprint to the city limit sign to break the monotony of a long aerobic bike ride may seem inconsequential, but it's not. Drifting out of the aerobic zone even briefly can cause a bit of lactate to accumulate in the bloodstream, a bit of fight-or-flight hormonal response, and a bit of acceleration in glucose metabolism to the detriment of fat metabolism. When you slow back down, these anaerobic processes obviously normalize a bit, but not completely. A few ill-advised or inattentive pace escalations lasting only minutes in total can significantly compromise the intended benefits of a fully aerobic two-hour run or four-hour ride.

## DRIFTING OUT OF THE AEROBIC ZONE, EVEN BRIEFLY, DURING A LONG WORKOUT CAN COMPROMISE THE INTENDED BENEFITS OF THE WORKOUT AND PROMOTE SUGAR DEPENDENCY INSTEAD OF FAT ADAPTATION.

Granted, this is really hard to believe, hard to accept, and not as much fun as unleashing your competitive intensity at a moment's notice. But the base period is a great time to reflect on your priorities, how well you behave in congruence with your stated goals, and how ego demands might get in the way of the fitness benefits (not to mention the positive character attributes) that accrue in an athlete who exhibits discipline and restraint when it's called for. Dr. Phil Maffetone does an exceptional job detailing the negative metabolic consequences of being undisciplined with your aerobic limits, so read *The Big Book of Endurance Training and Racing* if you are particularly vulnerable or need more support here.

It's important to respect that eight weeks is the *minimum* time required for a base period. Reflecting on the list of ambitious goals to achieve during the base period (no setbacks, numerous breakthrough overdistance sessions, improvement in Maximum Aerobic Function test results), it's a lot to accomplish in a short time. In many cases, spending more time in base-building mode results in further aerobic development, as evidence by a continued improvement in MAF test results. This means you are building a bigger and bigger engine, and that aerobic sessions continue to be the best return on investment of any kind of training.

## WHEN SHOULD I INTRODUCE INTENSITY?

Many athletes, and coaches, unwisely apply a regimented formula to this delicate and highly individualized question. For the unfit, it's pretty obvious you don't need to worry much about your next session of 400-meter repeats if your MAF test pace is 14-minutes per mile. For those ready to open up the throttle, keep the big picture goals in mind of moderating your stress levels and protecting your general health.

Here's a checklist that might help you determine the time to transition from aerobic base to an intensity phase:

- Complete a minimum of eight weeks of strictly aerobic training
- Steady improvement in MAF times (at least three tests)
- No illness, injury, or training interruptions during base period
- Optimal sleep habits where you awaken most mornings without an alarm clock, feeling refreshed and energized
- Steady energy levels and appetite at rest, throughout the entire day
- Strong motivation to introduce some intense sessions

These bullet points aren't lighthearted blather. You are better off staying aerobic indefinitely until you attain this exalted state of feeling fresh, energetic, smooth, and strong over even the longest workouts. Your greatest return on investment as an endurance athlete, by far, will come from improving your aerobic capacity.

As you continue to progress with your aerobic development, you may reach a true plateau in your MAF test results. This isn't in the bullet list because we don't want it misconstrued by an eager intensity hound who is aerobically deficient, not seeing MAF improvement, and declares this a "plateau." Remember, a plateau is defined as "an area of relatively level *high* ground"! So, if you've had a nice steady improvement in MAF and then a couple/few tests where you stagnate, introducing a high-intensity phase can stimulate further fitness progress.

**Intensity/Competition Period:** Enter this period if and only if you have completed a successful aerobic period of at least eight weeks, quite possibly more, and are fully rested and energized to start going fast and doing explosive strength-training sessions. We're talking about eight weeks or more of actual aerobic training, so unfortunately you can't start the clock with your winter snowboarding trip or the two weeks you were laid up with a cold. That's part of the Rest period!

The intensity/competition period lasts for a *maximum* of four weeks. Dr. Maffetone suggests that best results come from anaerobic periods lasting just two to three weeks, and that only the fittest, most experienced athletes can benefit from going as long as four weeks. A maximum edict on the intensity period bookends nicely with the eight-week minimum requirement of the aerobic base period. When you've hit four weeks of intensity, a couple or a few weeks of rest are due, followed by a couple or a few weeks of rebuilding your aerobic base. After you rest and rebuild, you can introduce another intensity/competition period. We discuss these micro-cycles of the major season periods below.

When it's time for the intensity/competition period, you have to make a concerted effort to put your obsession with volume, mileage, and consistency aside and focus on delivering high-end peak performance efforts, and successfully resting and recovering from these sessions. While any endurance athlete can recite the gospel of the importance of a rest day every week, Primal Endurance ups the ante here big time and suggests that three or four days of your week will involve either total rest or short, easy recovery sessions. Spend your free time off the roads and on family time, catching up on your reading and digital entertainment, yoga classes, foam-rolling sessions, and massage therapy appointments.

> During intensity/competition periods, three or four days of your week will involve either total rest or short, easy recovery sessions.

Science suggests very strongly that you will not lose any fitness when you cut your volume significantly during an intensity period. Dr. David Costill of the highly regarded Human Performance Laboratory at Ball State University in Indiana is one of the pioneers in studying and promoting the benefits of tapering for peak performance. In one study, collegiate swimmers reduced their training volume by 66 percent (dropping from 10,000 yards per day down to 3,200 yards per day) for fifteen days before a performance test. They delivered an outstanding 4 percent improvement in performance (ask any swimmer about dropping from 1m:00 in the 100 meters to a 57s:6!) and a 25 percent increase in muscular power. Another Japanese study with runners revealed that cutting back mileage by *90 percent* and doing only race-pace intervals for a week produced substantial improvements in 5K race times.

Numerous other studies suggest that just maintaining a small fraction of your normal training routine for weeks on end will not compromise fitness or peak performance. One study summarized that tapering between 60 to 90 percent of normal volume for anywhere from four to twenty-eight days will deliver excellent results. That said, it must be respected that an optimal taper entails conducting regular high-intensity workouts while reducing volume. De-training is another matter entirely. If you get sick or otherwise completely cease exercising, you will lose heaps of your fitness very quickly. But fear not, you can also get your fitness back quickly when you return to normal training.

## DETRAINING AND RETRAINING: A ONE-TO-ONE CURRENCY EXCHANGE RATE

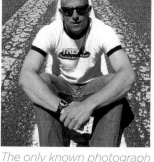

*The only known photograph in existence of Mike Pigg sitting still.*

While this is very hard to quantify, there seems to be plenty of anecdotal evidence to suggest that a detraining period of a certain duration requires around an *equal duration of retraining* to get back to the fitness level you were at when you stopped or cut back dramatically. If you get the flu and can't do much of anything for three weeks, it will likely take you three weeks of steadily rebuilding your fitness when healthy to get back to where you were before the flu hit. If you take six months off to have a kid or work crazy hours to ascend to partner in the firm, you may require six months of buildup to return to your previous form.

Doesn't this one-to-one concept feel incredibly reassuring and empowering?! It seems many athletes harbor an assortment of dark fears and anxieties about the mysterious and sinister issue of detraining, despite repeated personal experiences of getting back into form quickly after a cold or a bout of heavy travel. When real life throws a curve into your normal training routine, you can relax and let the process play out, knowing your body will respond magnificently when you build back to your typical workload.

Furthermore, as the tapering studies assert, even maintaining a fraction of your normal production will greatly minimize the detraining effect. If you go from an aggressive ten- to fifteen-hour-per-week triathlon training schedule to jogging a few days per week and pedaling casually for a couple hours on the weekend, even for as long as two or three months, you will lose very little fitness.

It may be hard to believe, but countless anecdotes support this. Recall Peter Snell coming right out of jogging the sand dunes to step on the track and set an 800-meter world record. Similarly, many endurance enthusiasts report coming right out of base training and setting PRs in the swimming pool or on a time trial hill climb. Yes indeed, your first anaerobic effort in months can turn out to be your best ever. And if you carry on with an intensity/competition period lasting longer than four weeks, as is routine in the endurance community, you will often see a gradual decline in performance ending in burnout, illness, or injury—your body's emphatic way of telling your stubborn ego to take a break.

While moderate training can preserve fitness for a long time, and base training can deliver competitive PRs right out of the gate, a true detraining period—where you fail to provide any stimulation to your muscles or cardiovascular system—will lead to a quick nosedive in your fitness capacity by any measure. Most serious old-time runners can relate with horror those first couple runs after returning from a four-week or six-week injury break back in the days before the advent of cross training. It felt like you'd never run a step before in your life! Those previously lean, ripped thighs would get chafed after a mile of shuffling, and you'd wake up stiff and sore from arches up to traps the following day—from an effort that amounted to a simple cooldown during normal training periods. Fortunately, a careful review of the big-picture calendar usually revealed that after four weeks, or six weeks, one was almost always back running at peak form.

These days, there is really no excuse to be deliberately sedentary for extended periods, so you should have minimal concern about lengthy detraining periods. If your worst case arises, where you can't exercise for a month or two due to illness, injury, or unique life circumstances, rest assured that you will get everything back and more in due time—one-to-one with your downtime—as you patiently progress back to your normal workload.

**Rest Period:** At the conclusion of the season, you will turn off your brain and body for a *minimum of four weeks* and focus on the neglected other areas of your life and your personality. It's essential to take time away from exercise as well as *thinking about exercise* to properly refresh and restore your batteries. In the example of the previously mentioned mountain-biking triathletes in Los Angeles, they enjoyed a bit of a mental break with the different dynamics of unstructured mountain biking, but they failed to achieve a proper physical or mental break from high-caliber endurance training.

As much as you love to train, to balance the sedentary elements of daily life with exercise, to linger with the boys at the pool or the gals at the trailhead, unplugging for a while will inject some critical balance and expanded perspective into your life each year. It's no secret that endurance sports, especially the time-consuming, all-consuming ultradistance variety, can easily place a strain on romantic, family, and personal relationships. Don't be one of those endurance athletes with blinders on, running away from a balanced lifestyle, from little faces calling out for more quality time, from gentle, well-intended reminders from a partner or other loved ones to slow down, reflect, and regain some balance and perspective.

When you make the commitment to observe a proper rest period, what often happens is that you gain a greater appreciation for living a stress-balanced life, for cutting loose and having a little

# THE OFF-SEASON REST PERIOD MEANS TIME AWAY FROM EXERCISE AND FROM *THINKING ABOUT EXERCISE.*

fun once in a while, for consuming food and drink that's off your usual training table (and not stressing about it!), for hanging with interesting people who may not live and breathe your sport, and for a taking a leisurely hike on your favorite running trail, instead of a run! Don't worry, odds are that you won't drift into a life of slothfulness and decadence if you take a month away from early-alarm swims or headlamp-running sessions after a long day at the office.

When you give yourself true mental and physical restoration, you might even feel more sleepy, sluggish, and stiff for a while when you stop training. What's happening here is you are finally giving your stress hormone production a break and allowing yourself to actually process fatigue in an authentic manner. Yes, this sounds weird, but certainly you can relate to going into vacation mode. You know, when you escape your normal hectic routine and spend a week sleeping in and lying on the beach all day, and only then gain the epiphany that you really needed a week of sleeping in and lying on the beach all day.

Similarly, even if your go-getter brain has no problem rising for that morning swim workout or that rainy, snowy evening run, taking time off from these schedule fixtures will demonstrate to you how badass you really are in real life, and how pleasant it can be to grab an extra ninety minutes of sleep in the morning or leisure time in the evening.

True restoration entails not just fewer weekly heartbeats, but a relief from the constant time pressures endurance athletes face—not just from measuring workouts, but from squeezing those workouts into a time-stressed society. You have to give yourself permission to feel comfortable being lazy for however long your mind and body need to be lazy for, and allow for a steady building of inspiration and excitement about your eventual return to training, your future goals, and getting back into an enjoyable routine.

# GIVE YOURSELF PERMISSION TO BE LAZY FOR AS LONG AS YOU NEED; RETURN TO TRAINING WHEN YOU FEEL REFRESHED AND RE-ENERGIZED TO GET OUT THERE AGAIN!

In fact, that's a good benchmark for how long your break should last: when you feel the bubbling of an underground geyser that's about to burst if you don't get out there and start training again. As with the aerobic base period, this means that you might tremendously benefit from a rest period lasting longer than the minimum four weeks.

We already discussed the folly of comparing your training approach to that of the world's elite athletes, and it's worth emphasizing here that professionals have a virtual absence of a working or family person's time pressures and responsibility-juggling pressures. Picture for a moment, instead of having your actual job, you have a job as a professional athlete in your chosen sport. You always have time for your job no matter what, right? Ah, the luxury of knowing without question that you can exercise for as long as you want every single day, that you can sleep for as long as you want every single day, and that once you get your sleep and do your workout, there are minimal other pressures on your free time or demands on your cognitive function. Of course you will recover faster and perform better!

While it's true that exercise is a great "stress release" from the pressures of work and a great balance to the many sedentary forces of modern life, you must also recognize that exercise is merely another form of stress to the body—it lands on the same side of the balance scale as a daily commute in traffic, arguing with your teenager, or facing deadline pressures at work. The term "stress" might more accurately be described as "stimulation." Your fight-or-flight hormones make no distinction, no matter whether you consider the stimulation enjoyable (a workout) or unpleasant (your commute).

Exercise may be a great release from other forms of stress, but it's piled on the same side of the balance scale as working, commuting, arguing, and the rest of hectic modern life.

That's why even the psychic energy you spend on your endurance passion must be earmarked for a rest period. That's right, you aren't even allowed to surf the internet and look at race splits or workout ideas during your rest period. Put everything aside for at least a month so you will really get pumped when you return to action.

# DON'T SWEAT THE DETAILS, OR THE WEATHER...

Maybe you've seen books or articles with fancier and more descriptive periodization terms like the "pre-competitive tiered sub-threshold buildup phase" or whatever. We have to scoff a bit at the complexity and regimentation often applied to the simple concept of periodization. While today's coaches are, for the most part, presenting concepts that are steeped in science and common sense, this hairsplitting with a sub-elite athlete might be akin to rearranging the deck chairs on the *Titanic* if the big-picture, stress-balanced lifestyle elements are deficient.

Even if an athlete has his or her act together and is primed to conduct highly specific and scientific workouts, it's worth reflecting on the profound statement from Dr. Phil Maffetone that all forms of anaerobic workouts have a similar training effect on the body. You can do descending sets in the pool, ascending sets on the track, alternate gearing hill repeats on the bike, or alternate gradient treadmill workouts indoors. If you are looking for an edge over the competition in this area, rest assured that the specifics of your high intensity workouts *really don't matter.* You are better off closing whatever magazine, book, or email you are reading about this stuff and getting more sleep. Go hard when it's time to go hard, doing whatever kind of workouts seem the most fun and interesting. You can mix things up with a different session each time, or you can do the exact same speed workout for years and years (like several world champions we know) and fare just fine.

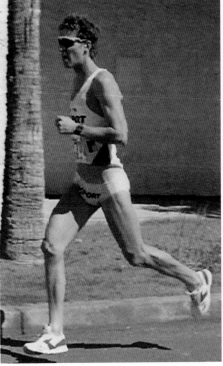

*Triathlon legend Andrew MacNaughton, the best pure climber ever in triathlon, let his moods dictate his workout decisions—a sage approach that took him to the top of the sport.*

Just as there are many roads to burnout, there are many different routes you can take to the podium. What top athletes seem to have in common are not the mechanical elements of their training schedules, but a deep conviction that what they are doing works for them and a great enjoyment of their particular workout patterns and training environment. During the days that Mark traveled the pro triathlon circuit with Brad and his teammates that he coached, top performers came in all shapes and sizes (okay, they were all lean, but a muscular 5'8", 175-lb swim specialist could often be seen competing side-by-side with a 6'4", 175-lb run specialist), from all corners of the globe, and with tremendously disparate training approaches. Guys who lived in Florida or the Midwest would often be seen going off the front on hilly rides. Guys from cold climates would often thrive in hot-weather races, not because they were genetic freaks but more likely because they were well-trained, rested, and happy with their training circumstances.

At one early season event in steamy St. Croix, U.S. Virgin Islands, the top finishing spots were dominated by athletes from the Foxcatcher training enclave in Pennsylvania (yep, that Foxcatcher, sponsored by the infamous late John E. DuPont). These guys had just endured an extremely snowy winter with zero outdoor bike riding, but they disposed of the more numerous and similarly highly ranked warm weather athletes—likely because they weren't overtrained from a winter of festive daily hammer sessions in sunny San Diego.

During the buildup to the 1984 Olympic marathon in Los Angeles, athletes from around the world were deeply concerned about the predictable heat and smog forecast for the race's August afternoon start time. American Alberto Salazar, the world's top-ranked marathoner at the time, was concerned enough to uproot from his Oregon training base and relocate to the oppressive humidity of Atlanta—the better to prepare for the Olympic run. He even underwent extensive testing in a human performance lab to analyze his sweat rate and dial in the best hydration strategies. Salazar showed up on the starting line in LA with his beautiful USA uniform cut to shreds—the better to dissipate heat. In summary, he spent a lot of time and energy and logistics preparing for and likely stressing about the heat.

Ever run in Atlanta in the summer? Right, not many people have! It's plausible that Salazar experienced an extreme and highly stressful disruption of the routine that made him the fittest runner in the world, and that his warm weather acclimation efforts actually compromised his readiness for the Olympics—likely chipping away at his reserve as well as his resolve. In going human guinea pig with the lab testing, he discovered that he had a super-high sweat rate that put him at a decided disadvantage in hot-weather races. So he had that weighing on his mind, while training in the highest sweat-producing environment he could find. Ouch!

On race day in Los Angeles, which we were both lucky enough to witness up close with NBC-TV credentials as official "spotters," we "spotted" Salazar all right—looking exhausted as he finished in a dismal fifteenth place. It actually turned out to be an unseasonably pleasant day in Los Angeles, free from the predicted brown haze, with temperatures at the 5:00 p.m. start by the beach in the 70s, and topping out in the mid-80s at the inland downtown Los Angeles finish line. Still far less than ideal conditions for a marathon, but no one was dropping like flies from the heat.

As Salazar plugged along behind the leaders, a lightly regarded thirty-seven-year-old, Carlos Lopes of Portugal, floated along, quietly tucked into the lead pack and obscured from clear television view. At around mile 20, Lopes rocketed to the front and won the gold easily. His time of 2h:09:24 was astonishing for the warm conditions, and stood as the Olympic record for twenty-four years. The most unlikely winner had attempted only three marathons prior to the Games, and finished only one of those. Furthermore, Lopes was still nursing minor injuries from being hit by a car (rolling over the hood and crashing his elbow through the windshield) fifteen days before the marathon.

After the race, the oldest Olympic marathon gold medalist in history was asked in an interview how he was able to outlast both the weather and the competition. He explained that he did not concern himself with the heat; he preferred to train in his temperate seaside home in Portugal and build his fitness to the highest level possible.

While you can dig up science that suggests physiological benefits conferred by acclimating to warm weather, high altitude, hilly terrain, or even the time of day that you race, the science fails to account for stress caused by disruptions to familiar routine and environment. If your efforts to acclimate to competitive conditions are more stressful (physically and/or emotionally) and less enjoyable, you may be better off sticking to your familiar routine, like Carlos Lopes. Furthermore, no matter how well acclimated you are to extreme conditions like heat or altitude, the fact is you still have to slow down when conditions are tough.

**Mini-Periods:** So you know to start every season with an extended aerobic base period, followed by your first intensity/competition period. After that first bout of competition or high-intensity training, you will take a short rest period, and cycle into an assortment of mini-periods to carry you through the season, and eventually observe a season-ending rest period. The pattern and duration of these mini-periods is highly individual and customizable, but you must adhere to the general principles presented here: start your season with a minimum of eight weeks of base, never exceed four weeks of intensity without a break, and always take a hearty off-season break of four weeks minimum.

Here are some more rules and guidelines for the mini-periods. First, each intensity/competition period must be followed by a *period of nearly equal duration* that involves rest and then strictly aerobic exercise. If you indeed complete a maximum duration four-week intensity/competition period, take at least four weeks (maybe more) that are composed of rest and aerobic rebuilding before introducing another intensity period.

If you complete a three-week block of racing and/or high-intensity workouts, you can follow that with three weeks of a mix of rest and aero-

THE TRAINING PATTERNS OF THE WORLD'S ELITE ATHLETES FEATURE A STRONG INTUITIVE COMPONENT AND TONS OF FLEXIBILITY.

bic. Again, an even trade for mini-intensity periods and mini-rest/aerobic periods presents a *minimum* rest/aerobic period. It's likely that you might have a four-week intensity period that leaves you pretty fatigued, or unlucky with an illness or injury to deal with. You may need to rest for two, three, or four weeks until you feel healthy and energetic enough during everyday life to even consider returning to aerobic base training. Then, you might need to train aerobically for another two, three, or four weeks until you experience a progression in MAF test results and are full of energy and enthusiasm to return to the race course or high-intensity workouts.

While your periodization details are flexible and customizable, it's not a good idea to ignore the minimum rules or disregard the spirit of the rules. The odds are that you will crash and burn if you do. For example, if you take a lengthy mid-season rest period of several weeks, spend a few more weeks going at low heart rates, and still feel stiff, sore, tired, burnt out, or sport a lingering cough or crusty iliotibial band, you are not going to benefit from introducing high-intensity workouts. You can proclaim that it's "time" by manipulating or misinterpreting these rules, but it simply won't work.

The training patterns of the world's elite athletes all feature a strong intuitive component and tons of flexibility. This is so even though they take great pains to control all other life variables and mitigate all other potential life stressors. If a top athlete doesn't feel right, he or she will not open up the throttle. Yet droves of amateur athletes are obsessed with opening the throttle as often as possible in a dogged quest for competitive success. Take a step back and realize the folly of this approach, embrace the simple rules presented here, and accept the friendly edict to take what your body gives you each day and nothing more.

THE ESSENCE OF INTUITIVE, SENSIBLE, PRIMAL TRAINING IS TO TAKE WHAT YOUR BODY GIVES YOU EACH DAY AND NOTHING MORE.

Something wonderful will happen when you relax, harness your dogged competitive intensity and work ethic, honor your inner voice, and respect the scientifically validated principles of successful endurance training: *You will get faster!* It's hard to say it any more plainly than that. The path to going faster requires that you balance out and chill out.

## WEEKLY SCHEDULES ARE WEAK!

With a solid understanding of the annual periodization plan and mini-period strategies, the next question many endurance athletes have is, "what should my week look like?" Here, our hackles get raised a bit at the mere mention of the word "week." A week is an arbitrary block of time (okay, not totally arbitrary; the Babylonian astrologers took a bit of inspiration from lunar cycles to start the tradition of seven-day weeks) that has no relevance to the dynamic process of getting fit or balancing stress and rest. Weekdays and weekends have tons of relevance to our orderly modern society, but it's better, safer, and more fun for you to reject the conventional approach of orchestrating a perfect training week on paper and then trying to duplicate it over and over on cue. Your analytical brain may be balking right now, but we cannot stress enough the importance of freewheeling when it comes to your workout patterns.

MAKING OPTIMAL DECISIONS IN TRAINING IS NOT THAT COMPLEX. YOU DON'T HAVE TO ADHERE TO A PREDETERMINED SCHEDULE OR "HARD DAY–EASY DAY" GUIDELINES. LET INTUITION BE YOUR ULTIMATE GUIDE.

Even a seemingly sensible concept like following a hard day–easy day pattern is guilty of being regimented and disconnected from the dynamic process of getting fit and balancing your health while doing so. Consequently, magazine articles and books on workout scheduling may very well be scientifically sound, eminently sensible, highly strategic, extremely well thought out, and likely of minimal help to you personally.

Next we were about to say, "scheduling is not that simple," but we really mean to say, "it's not that complex!" There is no justification for adhering to any predetermined workout schedule or guidelines like "take a day off every week" (that could be too few!), "never increase mileage by more than 10 percent a week" (why not? A healthy, stress-balanced, aerobically strong body can certainly handle, and benefit from, an occasional temporary spike in volume), and so on. These and other maxims are merely ancient stopgap measures designed to guard against unbridled obsessive work and insufficient rest. Remember, endurance

sports originated from the rudimentary ethos of "that which does not kill you makes you stronger." Today, with all that we in the endurance community know and have learned, your intuition should be your ultimate guide. This means that your ideal training pattern will be fractal, flexible, subject to change on the fly at any time (including revising a planned workout in the middle of it), and—no matter how many highly paid training experts are in your entourage—ultimately *your* responsibility.

> The ideal training pattern is fractal, flexible, subject to change on the fly, and ultimately *your* responsibility.

Unless you are living in a vacuum (or an altitude tent) at the Olympic training center, with your entire life totally dedicated to being present and perky for every single intended workout in your carefully designed schedule, you are going to have to accept that fractal workout patterns align much better with your other life responsibilities. As mentioned at the outset, taking the simple step of aligning your workout difficulty with your level of energy, motivation, and health each day is a great way to recalibrate your approach away from robot and toward healthy and balanced. Remember, in *Rocky IV*, the robotic, laboratory-trained Soviet boxer Drago lost to Rocky and his free-spirited methods anyway.

## THE STRESS-FREE APPROACH OF OLYMPIAN NICK WILLIS

If some part of you deep down bristles at the suggestion that being loosey-goosey and carefree can actually be more effective than being grim and regimented, you might be interested in some perspective offered by one of the fastest runners on the planet, New Zealander Nick Willis. Nick was the Olympic silver medalist in the 1500 meters at the 2008 Beijing Games, and the New Zealand record holder at 3m:29. He has had a long and consistent career at the top level of the extremely competitive middle-distance track circuit.

Nick calls his approach Simply Running, and delivers some memorable insights on a couple of blog posts at theteamwillis.wordpress.com. "The point of my Simply Running approach is not to find the ultimate schedule that maximizes all

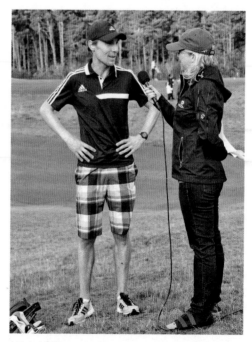

*Nick Willis representing nicely in Kiwi colors at the World Speedgolf Championships. Nick's offbeat competitive interest is a testament to his balanced approach to elite middle distance running.*

energy systems in my body, but to find a schedule that frees me of any stress, and allows me to enjoy what I do, which seems to produce better, more sustainable performances anyway," Nick says.

As Nick describes his simple, minimalist training week, it's hard to comprehend that we are talking about an Olympic silver medalist! But here's his description, time-tested under the most competitive circumstances imaginable: "I run once a day, and take one day off a week. I have removed the two to three thirty-minute secondary runs I used to do in order to top up my weekly mileage, and this has greatly opened my days to enjoying family, balancing other interests, studying full-time for a Master's degree, competing in professional Speedgolf tournaments, and enjoying an overall higher quality of life."

*"The Simply Running approach is not about finding the ultimate schedule that maximizes all energy systems in my body, but to find a schedule that frees me of any stress, and allows me to enjoy what I do."*
—Nick Willis

Nick continues, "I have also removed gym work (my least enjoyable aspect of training). To offset this, I run hill sprints once a week, and do five minutes of plyometric drills three to five times a week. I do believe weight training is an important part of many training programs, but for me, the benefits [of replacing weight training with shorter, more enjoyable workouts] are far outweighed by the negatives [of eliminating weight workouts]. Five minutes of plyos is a far less invasive time commitment than a sixty- to ninety- minute trip to the gym." For you aficionados, here is a typical weekly Nick Willis schedule:

**Monday** – Day off
**Tuesday** – Run 2h:00, 10–12 miles.
**Wednesday** – 1h:00 easy jogging (7 min/mile pace)
**Thursday** – Run 1h:15 (6 min/mile pace) + drills and 4 x 70-meter hill sprints.
**Friday** – Run 2h:00, 10–12 miles.
**Saturday** – Run 2h:00 (17–18 miles at 6m:30/mile pace)
**Sunday** – Run 0h:45 + plyo drills and 5 x 100-meter sprints

Nick's rationale for his simple, shall we say casual, approach to elite running is high-minded, but it is also incredibly practical: "When you place sport as an important but not all-encompassing component of your life, it allows you to cope with success and failure with much more stable emotional maturity. This takes a lot of pressure off of performances, and so when you toe the line in races, there is much greater opportunity to maximize your ability, as you are not weighed down by pressure or expectation."

# *IN*CONSISTENCY IS KEY! BRAD'S CASE STUDY

Furthering this theme of fractal and intuitive training patterns, it's not out of the question to stack hard days together to enable longer rest periods. When Mark coached Brad in the early 90s, they implemented a bold adjustment to the typical approach of spacing out hard workouts over a week. Instead, Brad experimented with stacking his long, hard Tuesday run next to a long, hard ride on Wednesday. This was followed by four days of minimal training, including two days of total rest.

We decided to try this approach because Brad was struggling with inadequate recovery. Trying to repeat the seemingly sensible "Before" weekly pattern detailed shortly (you'll notice the strategic interspersing of hard days and easy days, the obligatory one rest day a week, all the usual

recommended behaviors) was catching up to him. Race results started to suffer and he was far too inconsistent. He was still a world-ranked athlete, but we knew that more potential was possible with some tweaks to his approach. We realized that if Brad could deliver two elite-level efforts on his two big days, the rest of the week was basically just fill-in—do what he could comfortably do while ensuring a full recovery for the next cycle of back-to-back hard sessions.

Let's compare the following before/after presentation of Brad's late 1980s typical weekly training pattern versus his 1990–1991 training pattern. See which one you think involves less risk of drifting into chronic pattern/overtraining and more potential for peak performance on race day:

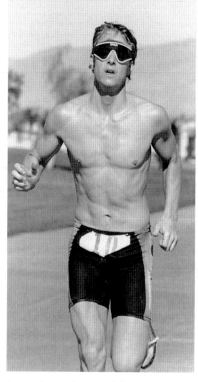

Long-lost photo of the surprise winner of the 1986 Desert Princess World Championship Series Duathlon race #1. No clothes, no sponsors, no competition—at least on this day in the desert.

BEFORE (1987-1989)

**Monday** – Swim 3,500 yards, bike 1h:30 aerobic, run 0h:30 easy
**Tuesday** – Bike 5h:00 in mountains (5,000–7,000' of vertical gain), run 0h:20 easy, swim 1,000 easy
**Wednesday** – Run 0h:40 easy, swim 2,000 easy
**Thursday** – Run hard 1h:20 (12-mile AT session in mountains, including 6 x 3 min @ AT with thirty-second rest intervals), bike 2h:30 aerobic (to trailhead and back)
**Friday** – Bike 1h:30 aerobic, run 1h:10 aerobic, swim 3,500
**Saturday** – Bike 3h:00 aerobic, swim 1,500 easy
**Sunday** – Rest day

**Weekly Totals**
**Swim (5):** 11,500 yards
**Bike (5):** 13h:30
**Run (5):** 4h:00
**Sessions:** 15
**Hours:** 21:30

## AFTER (1990)

**Monday** – Swim 2,500, bike 1h:00 easy
**Tuesday** – Run hard 1h:20 (12-mile AT session in mountains, including 6 x 3 min @ AT with thirty-second rest intervals), swim 1,000 easy
**Wednesday** – Bike 7h:00 in the mountains with 7,000–12,000' of vertical gain
**Thursday** – Sleep in until 10:30 a.m., massage, swim 1,000 easy, watch movies all afternoon and evening
**Friday** – Run 0h:40 easy, swim 1,500
**Saturday** – Run 1h:00 aerobic, bike 2h:00 aerobic, swim 3,000
**Sunday** – Rest day

### Weekly Totals
**Swim (5):** 9,000 yards
**Bike (3):** 10h:00
**Run (3):** 3h:00
**Sessions:** 11
**Hours:** 16

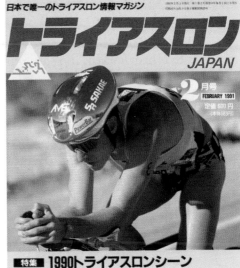

*Behold the chrome dome, and the eighth habit of highly effective endurance athletes: call attention to yourself with flashy equipment...*

The "Before" strategy looks suspiciously like an attempt to max out weekly mileage and deliver the requisite number of workouts in each sport, so as not to lose any fitness if a couple of days go by without getting wet or clipping into the pedals—the typical endurance athlete's "volume and consistency" approach.

There are a couple of important takeaways from the "After" strategy. First, you'll notice higher highs (the difficulty of the already long, mountainous weekly bike ride increased from five to seven hours, and on harder climbs) and lower lows (two days of near total rest each week, two other days considered "easy"). Essentially, what Brad did was deliver a Tuesday run and a Wednesday bike that were comparable to the big workouts his competitors did. However, due to Brad's increased sensitivity to overtraining,

he produced significantly lower total training volumes than the other top pros on the circuit, many of whom routinely delivered superhuman mileage totals such as 25,000 yards swimming, 300 miles cycling, and 50 miles running (probably taking about thirty-five hours to complete) in a typical week.

Brad's schedule modification worked quite well, as he won six races in 1990 and delivered numerous other top-three finishes in big races. However, he still had some spotty performances, including a handful of DNFs to go with his wins. Realizing that tweaking of conventional wisdom's volume and consistency approach delivered results, we took things a few giant leaps further away from triathlon norms leading into 1991, his best season on the circuit.

In discussing 1991 and beyond, it's hard to even offer up a weekly training pattern like the "Before" and "After" examples presented. Instead, we totally rejected the idea of delivering a nice, tidy weekly training package and stopped even discussing the concept of weekly schedules. We looked at the big picture of Brad's season goals, his strengths and weaknesses, and the training methods that had worked, and those that didn't work. Packing his stress into two consecutive days was much better than continually having a hard workout looming around the corner, and the success of this strategy helped us realize that, at least in Brad's case, *everything was negotiable* when it came to scheduling. By this time in his career, Brad had already built a high level of fitness, so we just extended our training time frames out to a big-picture season view, instead of the "what's the best weekly schedule?" view.

Brad describes the continued modification of his approach:

The first major change in 1991 was to train alone, coinciding with a move from Los Angeles to Northern California. This enabled me to pace myself according to my daily energy levels, and avoid the large pack rides and swims in Los Angeles that were fun and fitness-building, but could easily wear me down. Secondly, I relied almost entirely on intuition every single day to choose my workouts. Mark and I would plan and plot strategy as usual, but it was outside the crucible of weekly scheduling.

Third, I didn't even purchase a new training log for 1991. We all know how training logs can develop a sinister little voice of their own, luring you into overtraining patterns. Instead, I picked up a ninety-nine-cent spiral notebook and filled it with free-form thoughts about my daily training and general life. I learned this from Mike Pigg, as he offered me a glimpse of his "training log" one night in a shared hotel room. I opened up the spiral binder expecting to see badass split times and other juicy workout particulars, but instead it read like a free-form personal diary. All his workouts were faithfully logged, but the details were sparse. You'd see entries like, "Did Bridgeville-Kneeland loop—chilly. Then swam 3,000 with 15 x 100 yards on 1m:10. Still stressed about that clothing deal coming through. Right shoulder a bit looser, but better take it easy for one more week and do the stretching exercises every night."

"Did the Bridgeville-Kneeland loop—chilly." Ho-hum, sounds like one lap around Central Park. Actually, this is an absolutely epic hundred-mile ride deep into the Shasta-Trinity National Forest in extreme Northern California. First, you head south for fifty miles on flat roads, then start climbing and descending on crazy dirt logging roads for thirty-three miles before rejoining pavement near your starting point. Magnificent views of the Pacific coast are afforded en route, but my favorite view when I did the route with Pigg was a huge cloud of dust at the bottom of one of the dirt descents. It was Pigg sailing off the road after trying to take a corner too hard. No wonder he was perhaps the best descender ever in the sport; he practiced on *dirt roads*!

## AFTER-AFTER (1991)

**Swimming:** Knowing this was Brad's weakest event and that it is less stressful physically than running or cycling, Brad did his best to get to the pool as often as he could—usually four days a week. Instead of hammering intervals in group workouts, he swam alone at a comfortable pace, focusing on improving stroke mechanics and aerobic conditioning.

**Typical swimming week:**
- 1–3 days of recovery swims of 1,000–1,500 yards. Focus on stretching and rejuvenating after races, travel, or hard days.
- 1–3 proper training sessions of 3,000–5,000 yards. Emphasis on stroke mechanics, often in a small nearby lake.

**Cycling:** The centerpiece of Brad's entire training program was an incredibly challenging "Death Ride" that he attempted once a week, a 107-mile loop into the High Sierra with 12,700 feet of climbing out of very steep river canyons—some steeper than anything seen in the Tour de France. After so many years on the circuit, we realized that Brad's success came down to being fresh and fast on the run. Running more mileage or more speed workouts in training is very risky, so we figured that building his strength with extreme overdistance cycling on unbelievably challenging terrain, while always maintaining an aerobic heart rate, would not only help his cycling but also his ability to run off the bike.

Brad fondly remembers his Death Ride days:

> After I moved out of LA, I didn't do intervals, time trials, hill repeats, or pack rides. I could always rally for the crazy pack rides in Los Angeles, but they made me feel hot and tired in the days following. The tour through the Sierras at a comfortable pace was no easy feat, but it was fun, social, and scenic. I also discovered that I could recover from it easier than fast riding.
>
> I did my best to be sure I was fresh and rested for the Tuesday Death Ride, but I would routinely abort the mission when I wasn't feeling my best. In these cases, I would ride the first ninety minutes, all uphill, to a gas station—the final refreshment opportunity for the next four hours of travel on old logging and mining roads deep in the Sierra. If my legs didn't feel good-to-great on that initial climb, I would turn around and pedal back down the mountain, using the free time that I'd allotted for the ride to watch videos and sleep. I'd hand the map to training partners I'd invited along (and were counting on me to lead the route!) and wish them luck. That's not a friendly tour guide, but our group dynamics were to prioritize what was best for the individual athlete, every day and in every workout. We commonly flaked on each other with no repercussions or bad feelings.

# "I FINALLY LEARNED TO TAKE WHAT MY BODY GAVE ME EACH DAY AND NOTHING MORE." —BRAD

Even with all my instrument dials pointing in the direction of succeeding on that one ride—sleeping like a champ and carefully moderating exercise stress during the lead-in days—it was still aborted 25 to 33 percent of the time! All the strategic planning and periodization is great, but things don't always go according to plan, even for a dedicated professional athlete. With my competitive nature, I was willing to work as hard as possible to succeed as a pro, but I finally learned to take what my body gave me each day and nothing more. By only completing the Death Ride when I felt "strong, to quite strong" (as Ben Stiller would say in *Meet The Parents*), the body of work I accumulated was a bunch of epic all-day aerobic rides where my legs and body felt great and I became stronger and stronger over time—on the bike *and* on the run.

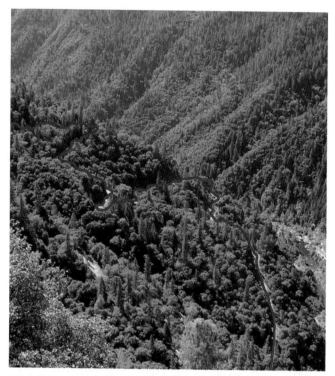

*Behold the notorious Corkscrew Wall in California's High Sierra. The climb ascends 2,200' in 3.5 miles out of the Rubicon River, and comes midway through Brad's "Death Ride" loop.*

**Typical cycling week:**
- 1–3 aerobic/recovery rides of 1h:00–2h:30. Hilly terrain but heart rate typically only 100–120 bpm (aerobic max was 155 bpm).
- 1 Death Ride of 7h:00. 107 miles in high Sierra, 12,700' climbing. All aerobic except climbing the Corkscrew Wall (2,200' in 3.5 miles), where it was impossible to stay aerobic. Doing this made his 40K time trial + 10K run feel like a breeze.

**Running**: Brad was racing and traveling a ton during his peak years on the circuit, so instead of trying to make big fitness gains in training, Brad focused on feeling comfortable at all workouts. Sometimes this meant going very slowly and other times it meant flying along the Auburn State Park trails at an impressive speed while remaining aerobic. We avoided the high-risk track workouts he had done in the early years of his career (alert: sore throats and sore calves ahead!). When he went hard, it was on long-duration hill climbs where he'd go 6 x 3 minutes at 10K race pace with thirty-second rest intervals. Triathletes are primarily training to run well with fatigued legs, so this session emphasized strength more than building raw speed on the track.

**Average over an entire year:**
- 1–3 recovery jogs of 0h:20–0h:45 (He had a calf problem and was sore for three days after every race where he couldn't run a step, so his weekly mileage was in the teens or twenties).
- 1 run of 10–12 miles (1h:30), including 6 x 3 min with thirty-second rest (when not racing)

**Summary:**
- One day of no exercise each week
- 1–2 other days of one hour or less of total exercise
- 2–4 days of entirely aerobic workouts, 3–4 hours total exercise
- 1–2 days of long duration/multiple workouts (e.g., Death Ride)
- Sleep 10 hours per night and 1–2 hour nap every afternoon (i.e., during his nine years on the circuit, half of his life was spent asleep!)

As you can discern from this trip down memory lane, and all the science and real-life experience that's happened in the endurance scene in the ensuing twenty-five years, we grew to despise the concept of schedules in general, and in particular using the completely arbitrary time period of a week on which to base one's schedule. The periodization guidelines in this chapter should be adhered to for best results, but there is plenty of opportunity for renegotiation along the way.

All this talk about adopting an intuitive and unstructured approach might have your analytical mind feeling a little frazzled right now. Understand there is nothing inherently damaging about having a techie bent or preferring a methodical, data-driven decision-making style, but you will very likely be better served by always blending subjective factors with whatever objective, precise, high-tech tools you enjoy training with.

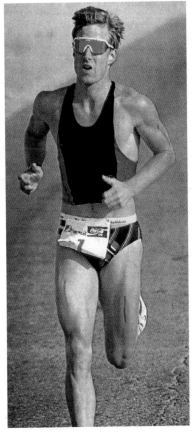

*Departing from the structured weekly schedule approach paid big dividends for Brad (pictured here, winning in Eilat, Israel, in 1991) on the racecourse. He had fifteen victories over the 1990–1991 seasons, including a national sprint championship, national series/Coke Grand Prix championship and No. 3 world-ranking in 1991, with a seven-race win streak to end that season.*

# CHAPTER SUMMARY

- Sporadic, intuitive, periodized training schedule
- Align workouts with energy, motivation, health
- Periods of base, intensity, rest & mini-periods
- *Inconsistency is key!*

The highly motivated, goal-oriented qualities of endurance athletes often lead them into overtraining patterns. A methodical, regimented approach with a scientifically validated, carefully contemplated workout schedule can easily be rendered ineffective and irrelevant by other life variables and stress factors. Training plans should be subject to revision on the fly, with the athlete always having final approval and veto power over whatever expert guidance they receive with workout planning. **The intuitive voice that has a great sense of balance and stress management** should always be respected over the demands of the ego and the compulsion to attain instant gratification.

A simple strategy to become more intuitive and balanced in training is to **align workout difficulty with daily level of energy, motivation, and health or immune function**. You can assign a 1–10 score to each of these markers and journal your results to get workouts aligned with subjective factors over time.

**Periodization entails devoting specified periods of time over the calendar year to emphasizing different types of workouts, the three major ones being: aerobic base building, high-intensity workouts and competitions, and rest/recovery periods.** Primal Endurance allows for extensive flexibility and adjustment, provided you adhere to the philosophical guidelines of periodized training. The first fundamental of an annual periodization calendar entails an **aerobic base building period of at least eight weeks** (and quite possibly longer) to begin the annual training cycle. During this period, all workouts are conducted at or below maximum aerobic heart rate. Subject to success with Maximum Aerobic Function tests, freedom from injury or illness, and good sleep, energy, and motivation, one can introduce a period of high-intensity workouts and competitions.

During these **intensity periods (lasting a maximum of four weeks before rest is introduced)**, volume is dramatically reduced in favor of high-intensity strength and sprint sessions, recovery sessions, and more rest. **A mandatory rest period of at least four weeks** (and quite possibly longer) should be observed at the end of each competitive season. The rest period involves a physical and mental break from the stimulation of endurance training.

After the base period and initial intensity/competition period, a sequence of **mini-periods** can be implemented over the course of the season. The general pattern is to **match the duration of intensity periods with a nearly equal duration of rest and aerobic**, with the ratio of rest to aerobic being flexible. For example, a competitive period of four weeks, followed by two weeks of rest, two weeks of aerobic (or three weeks rest, one week aerobic), tees up a new intensity/competition period.

Striving for consistency or adhering to a regimented, pre-determined periodization schedule is ill-advised; best results come from being flexible and adaptive based upon how your body responds to training and other life stress variables. Along those lines, the concept of designing an ideal weekly schedule is illogical, since a week is an arbitrary time block and repeating a seven-day sequence of workouts may not correlate with fitness progress. Instead, the **ideal training pattern is fractal, flexible, subject to change** on the fly, and ultimately *your* responsibility. For example, doing two hard days in a row in trade for an extended rest period can be an effective, if unusual, approach.

As demonstrated by the evolution of Brad Kearns's training approach over the years, the highest level of sophistication in training is not repeating a consistent pattern of workouts, but becoming more intuitive and adopting a longer-term view of the process of getting fit. Align workout difficulty with daily energy, motivation, and health, respect the general principles of periodization, and take what your body gives you each day and nothing more.

# THE PRIMAL BLUEPRINT
# EATING STRATEGY

*Escape carbohydrate dependency*
*and become a fat-burning beast!*

3

## IN THIS CHAPTER

Time to integrate primal-style eating into your endurance training goals and become a fat-burning beast! This chapter will detail how to transition from a traditional grain-based, high-carbohydrate diet into a primal-style approach centered on natural, wholesome foods that are deeply satisfying and highly nutritious. Going primal will enable you to finally shed stubborn excess body fat, improve endurance performance, minimize the oxidative stress of endurance training, and lessen your reliance on external calorie sources for energy.

Going primal entails first ditching the three most offensive foods in the modern diet: sugars, grains, and highly refined polyunsaturated vegetable oils. Sugars and grains promote carbohydrate dependency and fat-storage patterns. Industrial oils inflict oxidative damage directly upon our cells, accelerating aging and increasing disease risk.

Next, create new habits that emphasize the nutritious and deeply satisfying primal foods: meat, fish, fowl, eggs, vegetables, fruits, nuts, and seeds. Far from a regimented diet, primal-style eating is driven by personal preference, flexibility, fractal eating patterns, and most of all maximum enjoyment of one of the greatest pleasures in life.

Optimal carb intake depends on whether you carry excess body fat or not. Restrict carb intake according to the Primal Blueprint Carbohydrate Curve until you attain ideal body composition, then optimize carb intake by personal preference to ensure recovery from training.

Becoming fat-adapted entails a twenty-one-day transition period where you train strictly at aerobic heart rates and eliminate refined carbohydrates. Be diligent to ensure that you don't succumb to the addictive properties of sugar and grains. Once you are fat-adapted, try waiting until you get hungry before eating your first meal of the day. This will optimize your fat-burning genes and help you drop excess body fat quickly.

· · · · · · · · · · · · ·

**WE'VE DISCUSSED AT LENGTH** the benefits of improving your aerobic efficiency during endurance exercise—which is essentially your ability to burn more fat and less glucose at sub-maximum exercise intensities. Obviously, transitioning away from chronic patterns to emphasize aerobic training will help you become a better fat burner, but you may be pleased to know that your dietary habits can also make a huge contribution to your performance.

Adopting a primal-style eating pattern, where you eliminate heavily processed carbohydrates like grains and sugars in favor of wholesome, nutrient-dense plant and animal foods, will help you escape carbohydrate dependency and become a fat-burning beast. First and foremost, you will finally be able to deal with excess body fat issues swiftly and decisively. All other things being equal, improving your body composition will save you huge chunks (pun alert!) of time on the racecourse. Secondly, you will recover faster because you are obtaining more nutrients and more antioxidants, and generating less inflammation and free radicals when you choose primal foods. Finally, you will reprogram your genes to prefer fat for fuel, both during workouts and around the clock. This delivers substantial benefits to endurance performance, as well as assorted health and anti-aging benefits.

## EATING PRIMALLY ENABLES YOU TO ESCAPE CARBOHYDRATE DEPENDENCY AND BECOME A FAT-BURNING BEAST!

With the primal approach to fat loss, there is no need to engage in the folly of caloric restriction combined with chronic training. As you may realize already, this doesn't work long-term—and it's no fun, either. Instead, when you moderate your dietary insulin production and transition from a carbohydrate-based diet to one where fat provides most of your energy and much more satiety, you will experience a more stable appetite, diminished sugar cravings, and an up-regulation of your fat-burning genes so the fat will melt away without you even paying attention.

Alas, breaking free from the grain-and-sugar-dominant Standard American Diet is not easy. Dr. Maffetone makes an excellent point by assigning some blame to the performance nutrition companies for keeping the endurance culture entrenched in a dated paradigm, convincing athletes that they are dependent upon energy drinks, bars, gels, and other high-performance fuels in order to go long. Phinney and Volek also relate in their writings how performance nutrition companies fund research and influence conclusions that support the dispensation of their products to athletes. Who can forget the somber narrator's opening line on that classic Gatorade commercial: "When you sweat, you lose more than water. You also lose critical electrolytes…!" And there's the excellent parody from the classic movie *Idiocracy*: "Brawndo: It's got…electrolytes!" The same dynamic plays out in the world of Big Pharma—objectionable study conclusions feed the beast.

Though the powerful advertising forces convincing us that we need sugar before, during, and after exercise or we might collapse in a heap deserve scrutiny, the truth is that they are right—*if* you operate in the carbohydrate paradigm: eating the standard American grain-based diet and training in a chronic pattern. If you've ever bonked during a tough workout, you'll concur.

Oh, if you don't know what bonking is, don't Google it or you'll get the British slang for intercourse. In the endurance community, bonking is something much less pleasant: it's when blood glucose supplies run dry and your brain and body immediately shut down. We're talking about running along at a steady pace, totally focused on your performance and perhaps staying in the pack with your competitors, and then seconds later being completely trashed: brain completely unfocused on your effort and only able to process a single simple thought—likely related to the immediate ingestion of something sweet; your limbs unwilling and unable to generate forward propulsion; and even numbness, hallucinations, and serious confusion about which direction you are supposed to go to make it back home or to the finish line. Bonking is an absolutely precipitous occurrence that comes on with very little warning, unlike the fuel warning light on your car's gas gauge. As anyone who's been there knows, it's downright scary.

Skip one meal or forget your gels on a long run and your brain gets really pissed at you and shuts down external operations. And if you fail to take advantage of the highly touted "window of opportunity" for recovery—where you are advised to slam down carb and protein calories immediately after exercise (since that's when the muscles are most receptive to glycogen reloading), you may indeed compromise your recovery. It's true that a high-carb eating and burning pattern makes you highly dependent on a constant ingestion of low octane, quick-burning fuel that by the way has a very small storage tank in your body compared to your virtually unlimited fat stores.

Carbohydrate scarcity is a lucrative truth for those in the powder/gel/bar game, and it's a hassle for the athletes trying to manage constant depletion of that glucose tank. If the DumbCar versus Tesla analogy isn't bad enough, now imagine your DumbCar only has a two-gallon tank. Commuting and errands are annoying enough, but how about having to stop for gas a couple of times every day!

Becoming fat-adapted moderates inflammation, buffers lactate in working muscles, preserves lean muscle mass, and dramatically speeds recovery.

Meanwhile, evidence mounts about the extraordinary benefits of becoming fat- and keto-adapted: you improve your ability to regulate inflammation, slow the rate of lactate buildup in working muscles, preserve lean muscle mass—since you don't have to engage in emergency gluconeogenesis anytime you skip a meal or run low on blood sugar during a long workout—and dramatically speed recovery (because burning fat and ketones generates much less oxidative stress, i.e., free radicals, than burning glucose). See Timothy Olson's story in Chapter 7 on how he went from a month's recovery time after running the Western States 100 to feeling better in a *week* after switching to a primal-style eating pattern.

When it comes to matters of the physique, primal-aligned eating gets you so good at burning fat that your body adapts to your training and dietary patterns by burning off excess body fat effortlessly, twenty-four hours a day, until you reach your ideal composition for your particular genetics and level of training. This means that even if your genetics predispose to you to being a little softer than magazine cover subjects, you will nevertheless be easily able to attain your *personal* ideal body composition in short order when you train and eat primally.

Even lean endurance athletes are not immune to the extra oxidative damage caused by a carb dependent lifestyle.

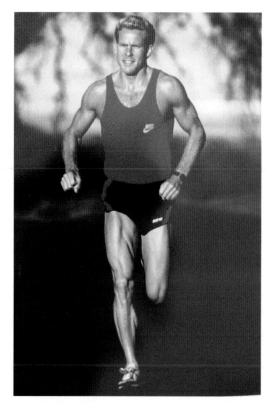

In contrast, as stated at the outset, today's carb-dependent, SAD-eating endurance athletes are plagued by excess body fat despite impressive training volume and disciplined portion control. Okay, a certain minority of today's carb-dependent, SAD-eating endurance athletes are actually pretty ripped, thanks to favorable genetics that leave them less inclined to fat storage. However, even the most veined specimens on the start line are absolutely not immune to the extra oxidative damage caused by a carb dependency lifestyle, not to mention the fragility of relying on a successful assimilation of carbs to make it to the finish line.

What's most unfair here is that the disparate levels of body fat you see on the triathlon or marathon starting line today are largely determined by the roulette wheel of genetics. You can devotedly train side-by-side with your training partners and eat the same meals, but still carry more spare cargo because you are more genetically predisposed to storing fat. Primal-style eating and training greatly minimize the importance of any genetic predispositions to storing excess body fat by getting you really good at burning fat all day long. That said, your personal ideal might fall short of the genetic outliers like the occasional female sporting an impressive six-pack, but you likely won't be too disappointed to look and feel your personal best—perhaps looking as good or better than you did a decade or two or three ago as a teenager.

One thing we haven't discussed much is how primal-style eating can actually protect you against the

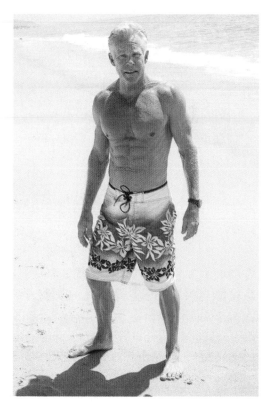

*Mark trained twenty hours a week to maintain his athletic physique back in the 1980s. Today, at age 62 in 2015, he works out an embarrassingly little amount and has no problem maintaining a similar level of body fat to his days as a high-volume elite athlete.*

negative effects of extreme endurance training, namely the oxidative and hormonal stresses on your system that literally accelerate the aging process. You may think those hours of exercise are adding years to your life, and when you train sensibly instead of chronically, and eat a nutrient-dense diet instead of a diet high in refined carbohydrates, this can be true. Unfortunately, a vast number of devoted endurance athletes are basically walking, talking, living, breathing examples of inflammation and stress hormones gone wild. They compound the pro-inflammatory effects of chronic training with a pro-inflammatory high-carbohydrate diet.

Emphasizing aerobic workouts and expertly balancing stress and rest with a periodized program can mitigate much of the inherently damaging effects of chronic exercise, but the fact remains that being a serious endurance athlete can severely challenge your health and easily accelerate the aging process. The longer you go, the more you race, the less you rest, and the more years your toes are on the start line, the greater your risk for breakdown, burnout, accelerated aging, and disease. But perhaps the greatest health challenge of all is a high-carbohydrate diet that goes hand-in-hand with endurance training. This chapter will detail a compelling alternative to the prevailing carbohydrate dependency approach, by helping you integrate primal-style eating and training to become a fat-burning beast, and perhaps eventually a ketone-burning beast (more in Chapter 4).

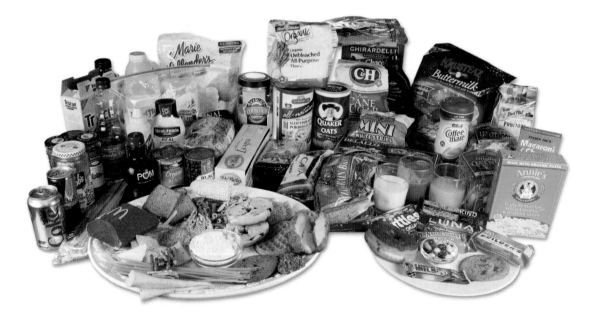

## GOING PRIMAL STEP 1: DITCHING SUGARS, GRAINS, AND INDUSTRIAL OILS

When you break free from sugar dependency, you can actually focus on consuming highly nutritious, delicious food instead of constantly having to fill your gas tank with low-octane, heavily processed carbohydrate fuel. This is what primal eating is all about. You may have heard primal/paleo eating described as "low-carb" or "high-fat" and been scared off accordingly. While these characterizations are true in comparison to the egregiously high intake of nutrient-deficient processed carbs in the Standard American Diet (SAD), the Primal Blueprint eating style is highly flexible and customizable. You emphasize the foods you enjoy and that help you to perform at your best, while honoring the simple evolutionary principle that we consume foods that humans have evolved over millions of years to thrive on.

Concurrently, we avoid the assorted heavily processed modern foods—SAD centerpieces—that we are not genetically adapted to consume and that destroy our health accordingly. In general, this means ditching sugars, grains, and industrial oils, three of the biggest caloric contributors in the SAD diet and three things that will quite possibly kill you if you eat them for a lifetime.

## THE PRIMAL BLUEPRINT EATING STYLE IS HIGHLY FLEXIBLE AND CUSTOMIZABLE. BY COMPARISON TO THE UNHEALTHY SAD DIET, IT'S HIGH FAT, MODERATE PROTEIN, AND APPROPRIATELY LOW CARB.

**Sugar**: We are building some pretty nice momentum lately for the undisputed concept that sugars—sweetened beverages, snacks, treats, and, yep, even performance fuels made for endurance athletes—are bad for you. Sure, sugar can be less problematic if you are burning a ton of calories every day, but sugar consumption still has a pro-inflammatory effect on your body, so it can hamper your health, delay your recovery from exercise, and promote the oxidation and inflammation process in the bloodstream that is the true cause of heart disease—even if you are a lean, mean endurance machine.

If you do happen to carry any excess body fat, reducing sugar consumption is the single biggest change you can make to break through plateaus and generate quick results. Know this from the Primal Blueprint scripture: *Sugar drives insulin production drives fat storage*. The more sugar you consume in your diet, the more likely you are to store excess body fat. And the more likely you are to become addicted to additional feedings of sugar, because of the way that sugar stimulates excess insulin production, disturbs your appetite hormones, and activates the stress response in your body. Sugar gives you an immediate high followed by a crash, cravings, crankiness, inflammation, and suppressed immune function.

## FAMILIAL GENES VS. *HOMO SAPIENS* GENES

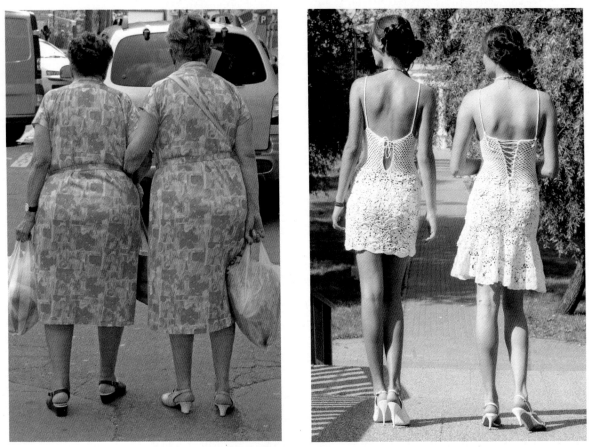

Now, you may notice tremendous variation in body fat percentages between individuals who have similar lifestyle patterns. Familial genetics dictate how lucky or unlucky you might be with your current set point and body composition, as well as your frame shape, your height, and so forth. Some people are predisposed to storing fat more easily and having more difficulty taking it off, and some people can be sugar-hounds and stay lean, even when they train at much less volume than you.

Them's the breaks that Mom and Dad gave you, and you can't do a whole lot to alter predispositions. But when you consider the literal meaning of the term predisposition, you will realize that nothing happens until you introduce the triggering environmental signals—

in this case, your food choices—to actualize them. You are predisposed to storing excess body fat if and only if you eat the Standard American Diet, and genes have no effect until they are expressed.

*Genes have no effect until they are expressed* is worth reflecting upon for a moment. If you don't eat a high-carbohydrate, high-insulin-producing diet, you will not over-activate those fat storage genes that Mom and Dad bestowed upon you. Similarly, you might possess the most exceptional set of endurance genes on the planet, but if you don't train, you will never realize your potential. You might be genetically predisposed to lung cancer or alcoholism, but if you don't smoke or drink, these predispositions won't matter a lick. We can go on and on here, but you get the point, and it's an extremely empowering and liberating point to get. You are not at the mercy of your familial genetic predispositions, and instead can focus on sending the right signals to your *Homo sapiens* genes to experience your own personal peak performance potential, ideal body composition, and maximum longevity.

> Genes have no effect until they are expressed; they require environmental signals (food choices, exercise habits, lifestyle behaviors) to switch on or switch off.

That said, realize that your genetic particulars mandate that you focus on your *personal* peak performance potential, rather than get caught up in comparison to magazine cover models, elite professional competitors, or even your training partners, for that matter. When you modify your current routine to eat and train primally, you can expect a steady reduction in excess body fat, improved competitive performance, better recovery and stress management, and improvement in many other aspects of health. You may or may not land on the podium accordingly, because genetic factors definitely play a strong role in the finishing order, especially as the level of competition gets higher.

What we are concerned about on this journey is you looking and feeling your best, period. Don't forget, we all share an identical set of *Homo sapiens* genes, and we all respond positively to lifestyle behaviors that are in alignment with our genetic expectations for health—behaviors that have been framed by the longest and most severely scrutinized scientific study in history, known as human evolution.

We are who we are today as a result of millions of years of withering, life-or-death selection pressure. We survived unimaginably harsh environmental challenges and rose to the top of the food chain by eating certain foods, engaging in certain lifestyle behaviors like getting appropriate exercise and sufficient sleep and sun exposure, and so on. Every suggestion in this book is validated by modern epigenetics and evolutionary biology as supporting human health and fitness progress, and avoiding the breakdown caused by overly stressful modern lifestyle practices, chronic exercise patterns, and unhealthy modern eating habits.

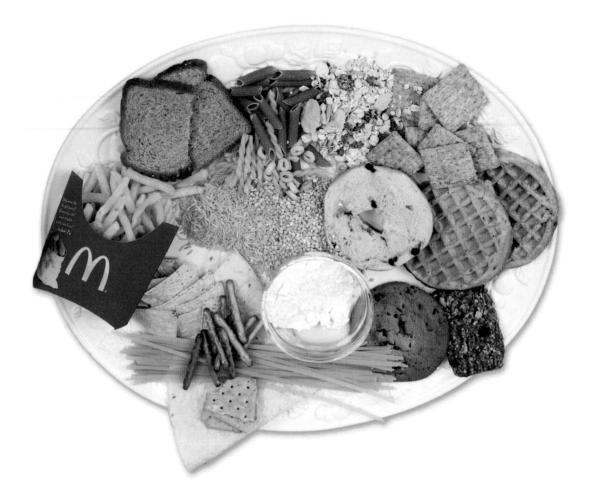

**Grains**: Sorry to break it to you, but grains are not part of the primal plan, and could actually be the most health-compromising thing you eat if you carry excess body fat, and/or are sensitive to gluten and other objectionable anti-nutrients contained in them. First of all, understand that any carbohydrate you ingest is immediately converted into glucose. So when we say that "sugar" is the catalyst for fat storage, we really mean all forms of carbohydrate, when you consume carbohydrate in excess. Whether you scarf a two-hundred-calorie bowl of brown rice or a two-hundred-calorie handful of Skittles after your workout, the net effect on your body composition goals and total insulin production for that day is similar. Yes, you can argue that slower-burning whole grains are more healthful and less offensive than refined grains and sugary foods and drinks, but we must set the record straight: All of these processed carbohydrate foods offer minimal nutritional value, contribute to excess insulin production, and can disturb immune and digestive function in sensitive people. Dr. Phil Maffetone relates that of all the carbs you can consume, from sodas to sweet potatoes, 40–50 percent of them are converted into fat.

Grains are merely cheap sources of calories that are easy to store and sell at high profit to the SAD consumer. Mark coined a catchy nickname for grain foods: "beige glop," because that's what they are. Breads, cereals, pasta, rice, corn, pancakes, rolls, crackers, muffins, cooking grains, and so forth form the foundation of All-American breakfast, lunch, and dinner offerings, but they are essentially empty calories that cause an insulin spike and lock you into a fat-storage pattern.

GRAINS ARE "BEIGE GLOP"—EMPTY CALORIES DESIGNED TO PROVIDE QUICK ENERGY, BUT CAUSING AN INSULIN SPIKE AND LOCKING YOU INTO A FAT-STORAGE PATTERN.

Granted, grains were the catalyst for the advent of civilization and the great transition of the human race from a hunter-gatherer existence to civilized society. While I'm not arguing that we ditch the comforts of modern civilization and return to primitive hunter-gatherer lifestyles, we must recognize the importance of honoring our hunter-gatherer *Homo sapiens* genes when it comes to food choices.

Grains make us tired, sick, and fat, because we are not genetically adapted to successfully process the massive loads of carbohydrates that we ingest at every grain-based meal (especially when you add sweetened beverages, snacks, and treats into the picture). The insulin-processing system in humans and all other animals is extremely delicate and sensitive. We are capable of processing only a moderate amount of glucose, burning it for energy immediately, and storing any excess as fat. This is a great evolutionary adaptation; in primal times we likely ate fresh berries in the summertime and fattened up a bit in preparation for the fall and winter months of less abundant food. But we slam our bodies with grain-based meals three times a day for years and decades, we overstress the delicate hormonal mechanisms that regulate energy levels, mood, appetite, and body composition, and end up tired, sick, and fat.

Over the last several decades, conventional wisdom has pounded the idea into our brains that grains are healthy, and that whole grains are more nutritious than the refined grains that have been stripped of their fiber (bran) and oil (germ) components to leave only the starch (endosperm). While it's true that refined grains spike blood sugar more quickly and have less nutritional value than whole grains, it's important to realize that all grain foods have minimal nutritional value in comparison to primal foods like vegetables, fruits, meat, fish, fowl, eggs, nuts, and seeds.

> All grain foods, even whole grains, have minimal nutritional value in comparison to primal foods.

Furthermore, whole grains contain higher levels of objectionable "anti-nutrients" (components of foods that compromise your health instead of supporting it) in the form of lectins, gluten, and phytates. Lectins are natural plant toxins that damage the delicate lining of the small intestine, allowing undigested foreign protein particles to enter the bloodstream and trigger an autoimmune response. This condition is commonly known as "leaky gut syndrome."

Gluten, found mainly in wheat, is a highly allergenic type of lectin. Gluten ingestion causes a mild to severe inflammatory response in the body (depending on the individual), compromising digestive and immune function. Phytates bind with nutrients in the digestive tract in a manner similar to that of fiber. While phytates offer some nutritional benefits when consumed in moderation, excess consumption of phytates can lead to nutrient deficiency. This is common when following a grain-based diet.

Knowledge and awareness about gluten sensitivity and leaky gut are increasing, and while the highly sensitive know full well where they stand, the Primal Blueprint position is that *every one of us* is mildly sensitive to these agents that we have not had time to adapt to genetically. Mark details his personal experience with departing from a grain-based diet and going primal, a transition that was completed in the early 2000s:

> It wasn't until I experimented with a total elimination of grains from my diet that I realized just how much they were compromising my health. The stomach bloating and gas after meals, the bowel irritability every morning, the fatigue I experienced after a high-carb pasta feeding—I attributed these symptoms to the stress of training or a busy workday, failing to recognize that I was slamming my digestive tract with foods that poked holes in my intestinal lining and allowed

shit to enter my bloodstream (the undigested and oversized foreign proteins leaking into the bloodstream through a damaged intestinal tract are literally categorized as fecal matter) and interfere with critical structural proteins in organs and systems throughout my body.

Even the arthritis that I was alarmed to notice in my forties when gripping a golf club (sadly, one of the reasons that I didn't make it to the Champions Tour in golf; another reason was playing each hole one to two strokes worse than a pro player...) was largely caused by a mild system-wide inflammatory reaction to gluten ingestion. All of these mild but annoying symptoms I'd chalked up to normal life, stress, and the aging process completely vanished in a matter of weeks when I went off grains. There is simply no good reason to ever eat grains, and many reasons to avoid them.

Every one of us is sensitive at some level to gluten and other anti-nutrients.

## BUT WHAT ABOUT CONVENTIONAL WISDOM?

This stance on grains is where the primal/paleo/evolutionary health movement contrasts sharply with the conventional wisdom's low-fat diet emphasizing whole grains and shunning fat. At least everyone agrees that a so-called "plant-based diet" is a winner. But primal/paleo eating emphasizes plants along with nutrient-dense animal foods such as high quality meat, fish, fowl, and eggs, and other primal-approved foods like nuts, seeds, high-fat dairy products, and high-fat plant foods like avocadoes, olives and olive oil, and coconut products.

When you factor all these primal foods together, including heaping servings of vegetables, responsible consumption of fresh fruits, and a strict limitation on grains and sugars, what you have—by conventional standards—is a high-fat, low-carbohydrate diet. This is the exact opposite of the traditional endurance athlete's high-carbohydrate, low-fat, whole-grain-based, glycogen-packing diet.

It can be confusing and disturbing to process conflicting information, especially when your training partners are religiously slamming high-carb, moderate-protein recovery concoctions within thirty minutes of finishing workouts, when your doctor is warning you about the evils of cholesterol and saturated fat, and headline stories warn that eating red meat (uh, including hot dogs, bologna, and other processed crap, if you read the fine print) increases cancer risk. We encourage you to read *Primal Blueprint* or another popular paleo diet book (*The Paleo Diet, The Paleo Solution, Practical Paleo,* etc.) for more details about the evolutionary health dietary rationale.

For our purposes here, realize that health care professionals are in agreement that metabolic syndrome is the number one health epidemic facing modern society, and that this catch-all term to convey diet-related conditions like excess body fat, high triglycerides, and other heart disease risk factors is strongly driven by excess insulin production, which is strongly driven by excess carbohydrate intake. Mainstream health and medical professionals do not dispute these characterizations.

Furthermore, the long-held conventional wisdom that consuming foods high in saturated fat and cholesterol will elevate disease risk is now being disproven by respected studies like the Framingham Heart Study, the longest and most comprehensive epidemiological study (study of how diet and lifestyle practices affect health, tracking residents of Framingham, MA, since 1948) ever conducted. Saturated fat and cholesterol only become problematic in the presence of excess carbohydrates and excess insulin.

As Gary Taubes explains wonderfully in his book *Why We Get Fat*, there has never been a single study published to indicate that saturated fat is unhealthy in and of itself. Only when it's paired with wildly excessive carb intake (and other inflammatory circumstances are present, like high-stress lifestyle behaviors) does it become potentially problematic. Saturated fat is a clean-burning energy source for the body and it's what composes the membrane of our cells.

Humans evolved for 2.5 million years with fat as a dietary centerpiece. In fact, evolutionary biologists believe that the consumption of nutrient-dense animal foods (particularly omega-3 fatty acids found in marine life, land animals, and eggs) was a strong catalyst for humans to branch out from our predominantly vegetarian ape cousins and evolve the large and complex brain that enabled us to rise to the top of the food chain. In contrast, gorillas, with whom we share 98 percent of our DNA, still spend fourteen hours a day feeding and foraging for stems, shoots, fruits, and ants!

> *"There has never been a single study published to indicate that saturated fat is unhealthy in and of itself."* —Gary Taubes

When it comes to cholesterol, the purported evils have been widely misrepresented. Cholesterol is critical to numerous metabolic functions, including the production of vitamin D and testosterone. Everyone agrees that HDL cholesterol is healthy—it scavenges the bloodstream for oxidized LDL molecules and other waste products and returns them to the liver for repair and recycling. Meanwhile, LDL—the so-called "bad" cholesterol—only becomes problematic when other disease risk factors are present. These risk factors of oxidation and inflammation in the bloodstream (high triglycerides can reveal this problem) are driven strongly by a diet of excess carbs and excess insulin production.

Furthermore, the Framingham Study and other respected health studies have shown no correlation between dietary cholesterol intake and blood cholesterol levels. The body needs cholesterol, and if you make a misguided attempt to avoid eating it, you will simply manufacture more internally to provide for your critical metabolic needs. If you take statin drugs hoping to magically and effortlessly minimize your risk factors, you won't be directly addressing the true catalysts of oxidation and inflammation, and you'll be suppressing HDL—potentially elevating your risk profile in the process.

*"The direct damaging effect on the body from consuming oxidized polyunsaturated vegetable oils is literally no different than eating radiation."*
—Dr. Cate Shanahan

**Industrial Oils:** It's common knowledge that chemically altered trans and partially hydrogenated fats, present in highly processed junk foods and cheap fast foods, damage your cells at the DNA level immediately upon ingestion and are directly linked to hundreds of thousands of cancer deaths annually.

We must also recognize the dangers of the prevalent vegetable oils that we have been falsely told are healthy for decades: canola, corn, soybean, sunflower, and other vegetable oils, buttery spreads and sprays, and the many, many packaged or frozen food-like products that contain these oils.

Dr. Cate Shanahan, author of *Deep Nutrition* and *Food Rules*, nutrition director for the Los Angeles Lakers, PrimalCon presenter, Primal Blueprint Podcast recurring guest, and family physician in Denver, CO, who specializes in medically supervised weight loss through primal-style eating, explains that heavily processed polyunsaturated vegetable oils are essentially free radicals in a bottle; they inflict oxidative damage to the body immediately upon ingestion. They accelerate aging, are directly linked to assorted cancers, hamper immune and cardiovascular function, and can severely compromise your ability to remove excess body fat. Dr. Cate explains that the direct and immediate damage that industrial oils inflict at the cellular level makes them "literally no different than eating radiation." Ouch. If you have any vegetable or seed oils in your home, toss them in the garbage can now.

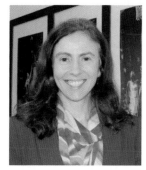

*Dr. Cate Shanahan, a family physician in Denver, CO, specializes in medically supervised fat loss using a primal-style eating approach. She also supervises the Los Angeles Lakers' nutritional program to keep players well nourished and steering clear of junk food.*

Once you take the easy step of tossing out the canola oil and the butter-like oily spreads, go deeper and examine the labels of the packaged snacks, salad dressings, powdered meal replacements, and other hidden sources that might be lurking in your diet. Even healthy-sounding products like "Newman's Own Red Wine Vinegar and Olive Oil" features soybean and/or canola oil as a prominent ingredient. Seriously, it says "and/or" on the bottle, so perhaps Paul throws in whatever surplus product from the oil factory is cheaper at the time of production. Muscle Milk recovery fuel is laden with pro-inflammatory sunflower oil, canola oil, and sugar too. Just what you don't want after a workout!

## GOING PRIMAL STEP 2: EMPHASIZE PRIMAL FOODS

On the heels of the best-selling *Primal Blueprint* book (released in 2009), we published the *Primal Blueprint 21-Day Total Body Transformation*, which details a step-by-step process to overhaul your diet and commence a smooth transition to primal eating over a twenty-one-day period. Here, we're going to cut to the chase and give you the specific instructions to transition to a Primal Blueprint eating style. If you want further details and rationale for the hows and whys, you can always grab the book or enroll in our online 21-Day Transformation course at primalblueprint.com.

The thing is, it's pretty simple—you must ditch offensive SAD foods and start enjoying these primal foods: meat, fish, fowl, eggs, vegetables, fruits, nuts, seeds, highly nutritious supplemental carbs (sweet potatoes, wild rice, quinoa), assorted other approved modern foods like high-fat dairy products, and an occasional sensible indulgence of dark chocolate. The particulars are left up to you, with the ultimate goal of maximum enjoyment of your diet. Don't like fish but love hamburger and steak? Hate broccoli but love blueberries? No problem! Love omelets but hate bacon? Well, you might not be human, so we can't help you there…just kidding. We primal/paleo folks like to gush about how fun, easy, and satisfying it is to eat according to Primal Blueprint principles. If you imagine a day of eating a delicious spinach, mushroom, and cheese omelet for breakfast, a big-ass turkey, bacon, and avocado salad for lunch, and a dinner of steak and steamed vegetables slathered in butter, it's hard to argue that there is any deprivation involved.

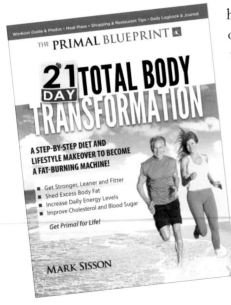

GOING PRIMAL IS PRETTY SIMPLE: DITCH TOXIC
MODERN FOODS AND EMPHASIZE THE NUTRIENT-DENSE
NATURAL FOODS THAT FUELED HUMAN EVOLUTION.

Transitioning to a primal-style eating pattern does not entail any suffering, struggling, or regimentation. You have to follow those important basic laws of avoiding sugars, grains, and industrial oils and choosing fresh, nutritious, whole foods from the "hunter-gatherer" list described. If you're a foodie, you'll find dozens of cookbooks to explore with primal/paleo aligned meals. And if you like things simple and habitual, you can make your omelet or your salad every single day and get into a nice groove.

Simple and flexible as the rules may be, you could experience some difficulty when you begin your transition out of the grain-based, sugar-burning dietary pattern. After years and decades of slamming high-carbohydrate meals at the appointed times with nary an hour's delay (come on, when's the last time you skipped a meal, or two in a row? Primal folks do it all the time, often without even noticing), your body has become physically dependent upon carbs as its primary fuel source. So even though you fully satisfy yourself with that morning omelet and snack on macadamia nuts till your heart's content, you still might experience visions of bagels, scones, and Arizona iced teas when you first go primal.

Some of the most chronically trained, sugar-addicted folks will report feeling sluggish in the afternoons and craving sugar in the evenings in the initial weeks of their primal transition, signs that the body is literally detoxing from a lifetime of abusing sugar consumption and insulin production. Take comfort in knowing that it takes about twenty-one days to reprogram your genes to prefer fat for fuel—to up-regulate fat-burning genes and down-regulate sugar-burning genes.

You will assist with your primal dietary transition by ceasing any anaerobic exercise during the first few weeks in favor of comfortably paced workouts that teach your body to prefer fat for fuel at rest. In tandem, you will achieve the critical goal of *moderating dietary insulin production* by ditching sugars, grains, and industrial oils. This will help you avoid the sugar highs and insulin crashes that perpetuate the sugar-burning, sugar-craving cycle. Instead, you will transition into what is effectively a high-fat, moderate-protein, appropriately low-carb diet—consuming appropriate levels of carbs to ensure you recover from workouts, but avoiding the processed junk and obsessive refeeding that happens in carbohydrate dependency. Yep, fat will become your primary source of caloric energy because it's extremely satiating, offers an excellent, long-lasting source of energy to your body, and doesn't elevate blood sugar or stimulate insulin. This is the energy source that has fueled human evolution for 2.5 million years.

## HOW DIET CAN IMPROVE YOUR ENDURANCE

While backing off the chronic cardio will help you kick sugar dependency because you won't be constantly depleted and doing an excessive number of glycolytic (glucose burning) workouts, the most impactful way to reprogram your genes and become a fat-burning beast is actually through diet. We wanted to set you up with a new training mindset in the first couple of chapters before even addressing the subject of diet, but transitioning to a primal eating pattern could just as easily be argued as the first step in your evolution from sugar-burning, fat-storing, underperforming endurance athlete to the fat-burning, PR-setting beast you deserve to be.

In any case, you can begin your dietary transition concurrently with your base-building period, or start eating primally for three weeks without even worrying about exercise, like during the off-season. One thing you don't want to do is start eating primally while training in a chronic pattern or during an intensity training phase. You absolutely need to

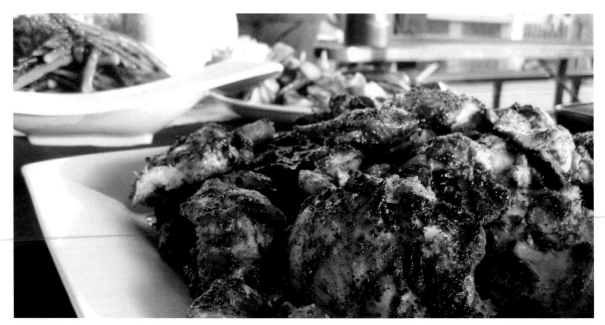

focus on improving fat metabolism and eliminating sugar dependency, and intense workouts will make this transition extremely difficult, if not impossible.

However, if you reprogram your genes with a prolonged period of primal eating, and build a huge aerobic engine during a strict base-building period of at least eight weeks, you will be able to excel at high-intensity workouts when you commence that period. You will have better endocrine function and hormone balance for giving your fight-or-flight system a needed break. You will have less system-wide inflammation from eliminating the pro-inflammatory sugars, grains, and refined oils from your diet, and ditching inflammatory training patterns (chronic cardio). You will have improved immune function from moderating stress hormones and improving your gut health by eliminating gluten and other lectins.

It's completely acceptable to increase intake of high-nutrient-value carbs during those distinct training phases when carb requirements are higher.

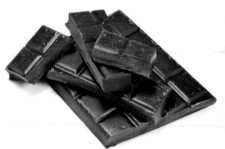

When it's time to go hard, you will absorb and benefit from these high-intensity workouts instead of breaking down. And since you took the time to build a Tesla engine (and fuel it with the highest-octane, cleanest-burning fuel, instead of the sugar you dump in the DumbCar), you will experience amazing breakthroughs in your fitness level, and your body fat percentage, in a very short time. Be patient, knowing that you will be able to sport a six-pack and throw down the hammer like never before if you follow the process correctly.

With the Primal Endurance approach, it's completely acceptable to increase your carbohydrate intake during high-intensity periods to ensure muscle glycogen is completely restocked and recovery optimized after these highly glycolytic (glucose-burning) workouts. It's not that hard to restock glycogen as a primal athlete, and furthermore many athletes notice that their glucose needs are significantly reduced during and after these workouts when they become fully fat-adapted. Basically, we're talking about keeping the primal dietary centerpieces intact, and enjoying more generous servings of nutritious carbs like fresh fruit, sweet potatoes and other starchy tubers, quinoa, wild rice, and dark chocolate (75 percent cacao or higher) during those distinct training phases where you might need more carbs.

## DIALING IN CARB INTAKE AS A PRIMAL ENDURANCE ATHLETE

Time to pose the big question: What is the optimal amount of carbs to consume as a primal athlete? Let's leave the ketogenic training strategy, which requires a strict adherence to an extremely minimal level of dietary carbohydrates, aside for a moment. When you are simply trying to escape carb dependency and become fat-adapted, your optimal carb intake will vary according to an assortment of variables, such as your current body composition, what training period you are in, and your sex and personal genetic particulars. Following is a logical strategy of sequential questions and answers that you can apply to accurately dial in optimal carb intake for your particulars. This topic will resurface many times throughout the book, but we want to give you a simple and memorable overview right now to quell the uncertainties that might accumulate as you ponder your real-life decision-making.

TO DIAL IN CARB INTAKE, START BY ASKING YOURSELF THIS: ARE YOU CARRYING EXCESS BODY FAT OR NOT?

The process of dialing in carb intake starts with this question, which will determine on which path you will proceed: Are you currently carrying excess body fat? If your answer is **yes**, restricting carb intake is the predominant variable for enabling effortless reduction of excess body fat. You can get really strict and shed the pounds quickly, or proceed more gradually if you struggle with an abrupt and significant dietary modification. Getting carb intake down into the fat-burning or ketogenic zone entails ditching chronic exercise and making high-intensity workouts really brief so you don't stimulate carbohydrate cravings from depletion workouts. The Primal Blueprint Carbohydrate Curve offers a sensible guide to achieving body composition success at various levels of average daily carbohydrate intake.

One thing is for certain—you absolutely want to maximize the nutritional value of your diet by emphasizing primal foods and eliminating the aforementioned sugars, grains, and industrial oils. Even if you are a lean, mean machine, there is no rationale or free pass for storming the root beer float counter—even after an epic twenty-mile run or century ride. This will compromise your performance by suppressing fat burning, promoting carbohydrate dependency, and delivering calories that have zero nutritional value to someone with extreme nutritional requirements. Sugar binging, steady dripping from snacking habits, or otherwise wavering in your commitment to avoiding this dietary poison will promote a pro-inflammatory condition in the body and inflict oxidative damage upon your cells—exacerbating the oxidative damage that occurs from strenuous training.

Sorry to be a root beer float party pooper, but excellence in endurance athletics simply does not sync with pounding sugary foods and drinks, or basing meals upon mountainous heaps of pasta, rice, cereal, and bread. Of course, you may want to enjoy occasional indulgences—grandma's oatmeal cookies right out of the oven, or a slice of homemade cheesecake at your daughter's sweet sixteen—without feeling guilty or getting a scolding on our podcast. It's totally okay to enjoy your life. What we're talking about here is departing from the disastrous path of obsessive carbohydrate fueling and refueling (especially in the name of athletic performance) and grain-based meal patterns in day-to-day life.

This departure from carbohydrate dependency also entails skipping the safety-valve strategy of stuffing seven gel packets and a Ziploc of energy drink powder into your jersey or fuel belt for long rides or runs (uh, and littering the trail or roadside with the used packets). Instead, consider experimenting with high-fat nourishment during long training sessions (e.g., avocados, coconut butter, or almond butter), or even cutting-edge products like the high-molecular-weight, slow-burning-carbohydrate formulation UCAN SuperStarch.

> Excellence in endurance athletics does not sync with pounding sugary foods and drinks, or basing meals upon mountainous heaps of pasta, rice, cereal, and bread.

Please don't misconstrue these comments as edicts. If you are out there training and you need sugar, you need sugar. So you grab whatever you can and slam it down so you can make it back home, or back to the trailhead, without having to dial 911. The insulin response is muted during exercise, so you won't have the same negative metabolic repercussions you would experience when slamming sugar during a slow afternoon in your cubicle at work. Timothy Olson, two-time champion of the Western States 100-mile Endurance Run and one of the world's top ultramarathon runners, relates that he follows a primal-aligned, low-carbohydrate eating pattern in daily life, but when it comes to race day he has no qualms about utilizing quick-energy carbohydrates to help him get to the finish line.

Again, we are talking about recalibrating big-picture patterns. Instead of using long rides as an opportunity to sample the new à la mode offerings from the pie shop located at mile sixty-two on the route, try to teach your body to become fat-adapted and metabolically efficient by taking only the carbs you need to maintain your desired level of energy output and focus. Over time, your body will require less carbohydrate energy upon awakening, during sustained workouts, and during the recovery period immediately after workouts. Don't forget Dr. Maffetone's assertion in Chapter 1 that fat oxidation is suppressed for days after slamming a big load of carbs, not just over the couple hours where insulin is elevated. Phinney and Volek back this up with irrefutable data from the laboratory.

## CHOOSING FATS INSTEAD OF CARBS AFTER WORKOUTS WILL REWIRE YOUR APPETITE HORMONES.

As Dr. Shanahan details in the remarkable sidebar story about Speedgolfer Rob Hogan in Chapter 4, eschewing a heavy carb refeeding after long training sessions can help "violently" recalibrate ghrelin and other appetite hormones to promote fat-adaptation. If you arrive home and feel like you deserve to indulge in celebration of your awesome athletic feat, consider reaching for some high-fat treats. One triathlete in our training group from the old days showed up for a Super Bowl party (after we all banged out a hundred-mile bike ride the morning of the game) with a bag of chips and a huge bowl of guacamole made from nine avocados. Oh no, this was not his potluck contribution; the bowl remained cradled in his lap for the duration of the game, and no one dared even make eye contact with the delectable offering.

# THE PRIMAL BLUEPRINT CARBOHYDRATE CURVE

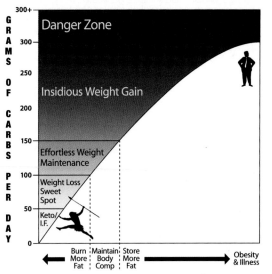

**0 to 50 grams per day:** *Ketosis and Accelerated Fat Burning*

Excellent catalyst for quick reduction of excess body fat. For new adopters, only minimal exercise is advised when going this low, and at low-intensity heart rates. Experienced ketogenic athletes can perform great endurance feats eating in this zone!

**50 to 100 grams per day:** *Primal Sweet Spot for Effortless Weight Loss*

Minimizes insulin production and accelerates fat metabolism. By meeting average daily protein requirements, eating nutritious vegetables and fruits, and staying satisfied with delicious high-fat foods (meat, fish, eggs, nuts, seeds, coconut, avocado), you can lose one to two pounds of body fat per week in the "sweet spot."

**100 to 150 grams per day:** *Primal Blueprint Maintenance Range*

Allows for genetically optimal fat burning, muscle development, and effortless weight maintenance. Allows abundant consumption of vegetables, selective fruits, and incidental carbs from nuts, seeds, starchy tubers, and dark chocolate. Refined grains, sugars, and sweetened beverages are eliminated.

**150 to 300 grams per day:** *Steady, Insidious Weight Gain*

Chronically excessive insulin production inhibits efficient fat metabolism and contributes to numerous health challenges. Chronic exercisers, active, growing youth, and those with physically strenuous jobs may eat at this level for an extended period without gaining fat, but eventually fat storage and/or metabolic problems are highly probable.

This "insidious" zone is easy to drift into, even for health-conscious eaters, when grains are a dietary centerpiece, sweetened beverages or snacks leak into the picture here and there, and obligatory fruits and vegetables are added to the total.

**300 or more grams per day:** *Danger Zone!*

Zone of the average American's diet, and in excess of official USDA dietary guidelines (which suggest you eat 45 percent to 65 percent of calories from carbs), thanks to stuff like soda tipping the scales over. Also the default zone for a hard-training endurance athlete eating a high-carb, high-calorie diet, including fueling extended workouts with refined-carbohydrate performance fuels.

Eating danger-zone-level carbs is the primary catalyst for the obesity and type 2 diabetes epidemics, as well as numerous other significant health problems. Even if you burn off most of the calories with extreme training, you are not immune to the oxidation and inflammation driven by high-carb eating. Immediate and dramatic reduction of grains and other processed carbs is critical.

**Carb Curve variables for endurance athletes:** The fifty-gram or two-hundred-calorie variation within each range on the curve attempts to account for individual energy disparities: a light, moderately active female will ascribe to the low end of the range, while a heavy, active male might operate on the high end.

Endurance athletes can consume higher amounts of well-chosen, nutrient-dense carbs and experience similar fat-loss benefits because of their extra energy expenditures. While this "endurance allowance" is highly individual, you can experiment with allowing a hundred additional grams of carbs for each hour of medium- to high-intensity exercise you conduct on a certain day, and perhaps fifty grams for each hour of aerobic exercise you conduct on a certain day.

"Experiment with carb intake" means first tracking your carb intake against body fat reduction, and secondarily making sure that your workout recovery is adequate. People like to get obsessed with the nuances of carb intake, but you don't need to worry much about this. Your appetite will direct you fairly well to the foods and macronutrient ratios you need without much conscious effort or recordkeeping necessary. Yes, you might feel like consuming more carbs during high-intensity periods, or even during the off-season—for even the most methodical, balanced, and primal-aligned athlete will still be depleted after a long, hard racing season.

Experimenting with carb intake is mainly about tracking your body fat reduction, and secondarily ensuring adequate recovery.

If you are eating and training primally, excess fat will work its way off your body in a matter of weeks or months, depending upon where you started. If you are not losing body fat as you desire, dial back on the carb intake for a while and make sure you don't overeat in general, and you will turbocharge fat reduction. If you really struggle here, take the next step to journal your food intake, input the data into an online calculator like fitday.com, and get an accurate representation of your carb intake. Compare that with the predicted results on the Carbohydrate Curve and proceed accordingly to ensure success with your body composition goals.

If you have a perception that you are losing a bit of high-end power during time trials or intense strength sessions, notice your body fat dropping too low, or feel like it takes longer to recover from high-intensity sessions, you can consider increasing your intake of high-nutrient-value carbohydrates and total calories. There might not be too many readers nodding heads about these issues. Generally, your brain and your hormonal processes that control appetite do an excellent job ensuring that you obtain adequate calories (stomach growling, etc.), but some of the more devoted primal enthusiasts might find themselves occasionally coming up short on energy requirements, and delaying recovery accordingly.

The ideal sources of supplemental carbohydrates for endurance athletes (assuming a primal-style starting point of abundant vegetable intake, selective fruit intake, and additional carbs from nuts, seeds, starchy tubers, and 75 percent cacao or higher dark chocolate) would be increased intake of fruit, increased intake of starchy tubers like sweet potatoes and yams, integrating foods like wild rice and quinoa into meals, and possibly adding beans if no anti-nutrient sensitivities to legumes are detected.

# FEMALE ENDURANCE ATHLETES: BALANCING BODY FAT, HORMONES, HEALTH, AND SANITY

The genetic factory setting for female *Homo sapiens* is to promote reproductive fitness, and carrying bare minimum body fat is at odds with this hard-wired goal, period. Female endurance competitors who sport ultra-low body-fat levels may have a good chance of getting onto the podium, but they are particularly susceptible to a disruption in normal hormone and metabolic function from low-carbohydrate diets combined with extreme endurance training. Furthermore, it's no secret that eating disorders are extremely common among elite female endurance competitors.

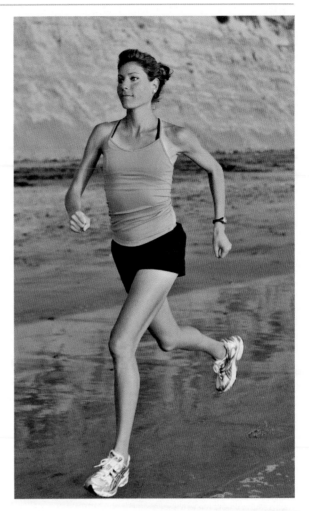

When push comes to shove, it's likely best to err on the side of health and balance. If this means you carry a couple of pounds of extra body fat but have optimal hormone function, you may find yourself passing the greyhounds on the race course—or making the start line instead of the injury/illness list. The greyhound approach of being totally fixated on competitive success, racking up a high training workload, and minimizing body fat is more likely to lead to illness, injury, and nutrient deficiency than it is to the podium anyway.

While we'll leave the eating disorder commentary to the experts, we'll assert that going primal can liberate you from the destructive mentality of associating body composition with caloric intake and caloric expenditure. When you understand that achieving and maintaining ideal body composition is more about insulin moderation and hormone optimization than it is a stressful, obsessive numbers game, you may be able to relax a bit, and in the process alleviate a common cause of unhealthy and disordered eating—obsession with calories eaten and calories burned. When you realize that you aren't utterly reliant on calories for energy, that your body can do just fine on fractal eating patterns (this also means you can chow down on occasion without causing a direct increase in body fat), you set an excellent foundation from which to cultivate a healthier relationship with food.

Achieving and maintaining ideal body composition is more about insulin moderation and hormone optimization than it is a stressful, obsessive, calories in/calories out numbers game.

It's likely that many dedicated endurance athletes land somewhere along the continuum of expressing unhealthy behaviors and attitudes toward eating. If you've ever binged due to emotional stress, or felt anxious, guilty, or frustrated about your eating habits, you might be able to relate to the goal of cultivating a healthier relationship with food.

Emily Deans, MD, is a psychiatrist who teaches at Harvard Medical School, and writes for *Psychology Today.* She is known for her evolutionary-health-based approach to treating eating disorders and other psychiatric conditions. She expresses enthusiasm for a primal-style diet helping to improve eating disorders, while offering a responsible caveat from her perspective as a physician.

Deans explains, "I've had success with patients following a primal-style diet that limits sugar and other heavily processed foods. By hormonally, psychologically, and metabolically disengaging from processed-food dependency, those who struggle with food issues can lose the cravings and the love/hate relationship with their bodies that can lead to disordered eating. A way of eating that keeps you healthy, provides all the nutrition you need, and overall helps you think less about food and body image is likely the healthiest diet for you, and offers a better chance to heal from the psychological factors that contribute to your condition. However, it's very important that you know yourself before you embark on a significant dietary transition, especially a structured program. If you have a history of a serious eating disorder, having a trusted counselor in your corner is advised."

As with the other major tenets of the Primal Endurance philosophy, a relaxed, intuitive, process-oriented mindset is advised here. We face so many cultural pressures to look, behave, and perform according to arbitrary standards set by society. It's easy to get caught up in the race times, mileage totals, and subtle six-pack competition at the Master's swim workout to the extent that this judgmental noise leaks into your pure, unadulterated enjoyment of nourishing foods and relaxing, deeply satisfying meals.

If you are disappointed that you carry excess body fat, why not bypass the lip service rationalizations, or behaving in a manner that is not in alignment with your stated goals and do something about it? But don't be fueled by anger, anxiety, or cultural pressures. And if you detect that your relationship with food is a little, or a lot, less than ideal, take the necessary steps to address the issue. Walk your talk by adhering to the primal philosophy of not just food choices, but the big-picture goal of placing enjoyment of life above all else. If you have trouble getting into that "enjoyment" realm with your eating habits, or otherwise struggle in a way that's really compromising your happiness, self-esteem, and stress management, by all means obtain professional guidance.

**What if I don't have excess body fat?:** If you answer a big skinny "no" to the excess body fat question, your primary carb intake parameter will be to ensure maximum dietary nutritional value, adequate recovery from exercise—especially intense exercise—and improve fat adaptation for performance and health benefits. If you go from a good weight to adding some extra body fat (as often happens to carb-dependent athletes in the wintertime), this indicates you are eating a little more carbohydrate than you need to enjoy the aforementioned benefits. Cut back until you return to your ideal body composition.

If you experience lingering fatigue (especially from high-intensity workouts) or delayed recovery, or drop too much body fat, it could be an indication to increase carb intake, especially in conjunction with high-intensity workouts. This is pretty rare, but it can happen to disciplined athletes who take primal eating to heart, perform high-intensity, glucose-burning workouts, and then don't quite refuel completely in the hours and days afterward.

Note that your metabolism is highly calibrated toward homeostasis, and there are assorted internal mechanisms that promote the status quo instead of assisting with your efforts to lose fat. Frustrating as it may seem when you are trying to shed a few extra pounds, our homeostatic drive is obviously another hard-wired survival mechanism to keep us going when caloric intake fluctuates.

## GET EXCESS BODY FAT HANDLED ONCE AND FOR ALL BY DITCHING TOXIC MODERN FOODS AND CHRONIC EXERCISE.

So, worrying about the nitty-gritty of caloric intake versus caloric expenditure is folly. Focus on simply ditching toxic modern foods—especially sugars, grains, and industrial oils—emphasize nutrient-dense primal foods of your personal preference, and rely on your natural appetite as a guide for how much fuel you need every day, including after tough workouts. The only caveat here relates to the excess body fat that you would like to eliminate once and for all without delay. Get that handled by ditching grains, sugars, and chronic exercise, and then proceed to focusing on pure enjoyment of delicious foods, and honoring your natural appetite and satiety levels so you don't overeat.

## WHY BEING FAT-ADAPTED IS A HUGE PERFORMANCE ADVANTAGE

For decades, endurance exercise science has asserted that the single biggest limiting factor in endurance performance is the relatively tiny amount of glycogen (the storage form of carbohydrate) that can be packed in the liver and muscles and used to fuel exercising muscles. We are only able to store four to five hundred grams, or sixteen hundred to two thousand calories (highly trained athletes can teach their bodies to store a bit more than the average person) of glycogen in our liver and muscle tissue, and there's only around five grams of glucose in our bloodstream at any given time.

As we burn energy during exercise, we carefully release glucose into the bloodstream (from glycogen storage depots or from ingested calories) in order to maintain that optimal glucose level. Amazingly, that's just a few drops circulating in the entire blood volume of our body, which is around 5 liters or 5.3 quarts. If we mess with this delicate balance just a bit, say by going too fast for too long and burning through glycogen stores while not ingesting enough supplemental fuel during a long effort, we bonk royally in short order.

Hence, the goal is to become more aerobically efficient through training, so that at any given pace you have enough oxygen available to burn a greater percentage of fat and spare glucose. As you get fitter, more efficient, or faster, you need less glucose at any given pace and can carry on comfortably while a lesser opponent runs out of resources. The reason the great African marathoners can run a marathon in two hours and change is because they have plenty of oxygen available to maintain aerobic metabolism even at the incredible sub-five-minute-per-mile speeds they maintain for twenty-six consecutive miles.

The reason you can only hang with these guys for the first couple of minutes of their two-hour journey, or only ride the first five or ten miles of a 112-mile Ironman triathlon bike ride at the leader's pace, is because you immediately go anaerobic at the speeds of the elite performer. Fat oxidation shuts off and you start burning heaps of glucose. Forget "your days are numbered"—your *minutes* are numbered!

No matter who you are, you will most assuredly bonk at some point if you go too hard for too long. The practice of refueling with drinks and gels during exercise is to stave off the bonk, not prevent it. In contrast to the incredibly delicate and temperamental nature of our glucose fueling system, we have a virtually unlimited supply of body fat to access and burn for energy. Even the skinniest elite runner—say a 5'11",

AS YOU BECOME MORE AEROBICALLY EFFICIENT—*FITTER!*—YOU NEED LESS GLUCOSE AT ANY GIVEN PACE AND CAN CARRY ON COMFORTABLY WHILE A LESSER OPPONENT RUNS OUT OF RESOURCES.

137-pound elf with 5 percent body fat—has at least twenty thousand calories of stored energy in the form of fat.

So we have ten to twenty times more fat energy than we do glucose, but we live in a carbohydrate paradigm where we are utterly dependent upon a constant supply of glucose to fuel our daily activities—not just for sustained workout performance, but also just sitting at our work desk or driving for hours on the highway. Consider what happens when the Standard American Diet eater skips a single meal: he or she quickly becomes tired, cranky, and unfocused, and craves quick-energy carbohydrates. Due to the disastrous effects of a high-insulin-producing diet, bonking occurs every afternoon in cubicles across the land—just not as dramatically as an athlete out on the road.

## GETTING STARTED AS A PRIMAL ENDURANCE ATHLETE

To this point in the book, we've covered a ton of strategy and philosophy, so let's get focused with a plan of action to transition out of carbohydrate dependency and become a fat-burning beast. The starting point is simple: dedicate twenty-one days to facilitating the reprogramming of your genes away from carbohydrate dependency and into a fat-adapted state. You achieve this in two main ways:

1. **Slow Down:** Conduct all workouts at or below maximum aerobic heart rate, so you burn predominantly fat during workouts, minimize glycogen depletion and resultant sugar cravings, and accelerate the gene reprogramming process through the stimulation of aerobic exercise—burning fat at a rate of up to ten times your resting rate. Once you become fat-adapted through a sustained period of aerobic training and primal-aligned eating, you can introduce some high-intensity workouts, but not now.

2. **Ditch Processed Carbs:** Eliminate sugars, sweets, sweetened beverages, grains (bread, rice, pasta, cereal, baked goods, breakfast foods, performance fuels, etc.) and also industrial vegetable/seed oils. Ditching your assortment of lifelong go-to foods won't be easy, but no one is saying you gotta go hungry. In fact, it's critical to make the transition as easy as possible by enjoying liberal servings of highly satisfying, nutritionally rich primal foods, like meat, fish, fowl, eggs, vegetables, fruits, nuts, seeds, and high cacao percentage dark chocolate.

Maintain a sincere commitment for twenty-one days to make a smooth and permanent transition into the world of fat burning. Most importantly, don't make a half-hearted attempt to reduce sugar intake, allow "cheat" days on weekends, or any other such nonsense. If you allow a little sugar to leak into the picture here and there as you attempt to transform out of carbohydrate dependency, you will most assuredly get sucked back into a hormonal state where you prefer burning glucose to fat, and crave more dietary carbs accordingly.

## THE TIERED PROCESS OF BECOMING FAT-ADAPTED AND THEN EFFORTLESSLY SHEDDING EXCESS BODY FAT

While we've talked extensively about losing excess body fat when transitioning to primal eating, you really shouldn't worry much about that in the first twenty-one days. If you experience lethargy or pangs for carbohydrate comfort foods during your transition, go ahead and indulge in generous high-fat snacks and meals, even if this means you are getting most all of your energy from meals and leaving your fat stores untapped for a while. Starting your primal day with a giant omelet with avocado slices on top and three slices of bacon on the side will help ease your longings for the usual oatmeal, toast, and orange juice. If you get the midafternoon blues and lustily eye that Iced Gingerbread Clif Bar (yes, that's a real flavor!) for a boost, perhaps a heaping handful of macadamia nuts, some celery sticks smothered with almond butter, a couple of slices of beef jerky and a few squares of dark chocolate will ease your pain—as will visualizing the big juicy steak and steamed veggies bathed in butter that are on tap for the evening meal.

The primary goal of your initial twenty-one-day transition is to reprogram your genes to prefer fat instead of sugar. If this entails burning mostly ingested fats instead of tapping into stored body fat for energy, that's just fine. Once you become fat-adapted, you can easily drop excess body fat by simply paying attention to your natural appetite and eating sensible, high-nutrient-value whole foods. Your high-fat, high-satiety eating patterns will soon normalize your appetite and fat-storage hormones like ghrelin and leptin—possibly for the first time in decades of riding on the carb train. Consequently, you'll have stored body fat (and glycogen and ketones) readily available at all times to burn. And you'll drift effortlessly in the direction of your ideal body composition respective to your lifestyle. If you are a devoted endurance athlete, you will start to look like someone adapted to cover twenty-six miles on foot.

*The challenge of optimizing body composition must be viewed as calories burned versus calories stored, which is distinctly different from calories burned versus calories consumed.*

To be clear, you must do whatever it takes to escape carbohydrate dependency and become fat-adapted, then allow fat reduction to happen naturally as a consequence of hormone optimization, instead of the disastrously flawed and ill-fated calorie-counting approach of trying to burn more than you eat.

The challenge of optimizing body composition must be viewed as calories burned versus calories *stored*, which is distinctly different from calories burned versus calories *consumed*. When your insulin production is moderated, your appetite hormones like leptin and ghrelin work optimally, and you naturally consume the exact amount of calories you need to sustain energy, preserve and repair muscle, and eventually optimize body composition by burning off any excess body fat as a consequence of your healthy, active lifestyle.

Gene reprogramming is serious business requiring serious commitment. Experts assert that sugar and grains are addictive at the same level as illicit drugs. In the bestselling book *Wheat Belly*, author Dr. William Davis discusses how *gliadin*, the most abundant protein in our genetically modified modern-day wheat crop, has profound appetite-stimulating effects to the extent that wheat eaters are prompted to consume an average of four hundred additional calories per day. When gliadin is ingested, it degrades in the gastrointestinal tract into opioid polypeptides called exorphins. These exorphins cross the blood-brain barrier and bind to opioid receptors in the brain, causing significant appetite stimulation, behavior changes (such as aggravation of ADHD or manic illnesses), allergic responses, and impairment in normal immune and neurological function. Dr. Davis believes that when food manufacturers discovered, some twenty-five years ago, just how strongly gliadin stimulates appetite, they made a concerted effort to include some wheat in all manner of processed foods.

The drug-like properties of sugar are widely acknowledged, and include the drug addiction hallmarks of binging (propensity to consume large quantities at one time), withdrawal (causing anxiety and behavioral depression), craving (enhanced neurochemical motivation to consume), and cross-sensitization (increased locomotor response to other substances, such as alcohol or nicotine). Sugar ingestion results in changes in dopamine and opioid-receptor binding in the brain similar to taking serious drugs, though to a less severe degree. So sugar *dependency* is a more accurate description than sugar addiction.

# BECOMING FAT-ADAPTED TRANSFORMS YOUR POLLUTION-SPEWING, CARB-FUELED DumbCar INTO A SQUEAKY-CLEAN, FAT-BURNING TESLA.

Due to the physical dependencies and health disturbances caused by the consumption of sugar and wheat, eliminating these foods from your diet can result in some unpleasant initial side effects as your body literally detoxes from decades of chronically excessive consumption of refined carbohydrates. Some of the wheat withdrawal symptoms cited by Dr. Davis include headaches, fatigue, nausea, depression, and cravings for the missing foods. If you have been way deep into the carb-dependency lifestyle for many years or decades, your primal transition might involve some struggle, but pacifying yourself with liberal consumption of high-satiety primal foods will make the transition easier. Each day you avoid these dependency foods and moderate insulin production will create momentum to enable you to stay the course with less and less discomfort over time.

## HOW WILL I KNOW IF I'M FAT-ADAPTED?

So you've done your best for twenty-one days—moderating exercise intensity to be completely aerobic, ditching grains, sugars, and bad oils, and enjoying primal foods that deeply satisfy while moderating insulin production to up-regulate fat-burning genes and down-regulate sugar-burning genes. Consequently, you should start to feel more stable appetite and energy levels, and diminished cravings for quick energy carbohydrates. You should be better able to skip or delay meals without suffering negative consequences, something that will accelerate the reduction of excess body fat. Out on the roads, you should be experiencing increased efficiency training at aerobic heart rates, something you can quantify by performing the MAF test regularly.

A great way to test your progress with fat adaptation is to delay your morning meal until you experience true sensations of hunger. Right now, hunger might occur as soon as you wake up, especially if you've been accustomed to a classic high-carbohydrate endurance athlete's power breakfast of a mixing-bowl-sized serving of cereal or a huge stack of pancakes. Over time, you will become so efficient at burning fat that you will be able to get up and go—not just off to work but for an actual workout—without an obligatory early-morning calorie fest before hand.

## HOW FAT-ADAPTED ARE YOU? TRY DELAYING YOUR MORNING MEAL UNTIL YOU GET HUNGRY AND TRACKING YOUR PROGRESS OVER TIME.

If you typically have gone around twelve hours between your evening meal and morning breakfast (e.g., 7 p.m. to 7 a.m.), occasionally or regularly extending your fasting period out to sixteen hours (11 a.m.) or even eighteen hours (1 p.m.) will deliver a host of metabolic benefits. This is what primal/paleo folks call "Intermittent Fasting (I. F.)," or a "compressed eating window." Training your body to function without ingested calories constantly circulating in the bloodstream will further optimize your ability to burn fat and ketones in place of glucose. It will deliver a potent anti-aging effect by slowing the rate of cell division and optimizing *autophagy*, which is a complex process of cellular degradation, repair, recycling, and regeneration. This downscaling of cell division and optimized autophagy is a hard-wired survival mechanism for the body to operate more cleanly and frugally when dietary calories are restricted, which has been the case for almost all of human history on the grand timeline.

In addition to the metabolic benefits of I.F., waiting until you are hungry to eat in the morning (and at any other time!), delivers a greater appreciation for the natural sensations of hunger and satiety that are often masked by the modern propensity for excessive carb intake, regimented eating patterns, and overfeeding in general. When you optimize your appetite hormones and eat according to your natural appetite, you will require fewer total calories in a day, and a lifetime, to not only survive, but thrive, and feel totally satisfied by one of life's greatest and most fundamental pleasures. Being able to thrive on fewer calories is known as metabolic efficiency, and it happens to be one of the most profound anti-aging strategies ever discovered. In fact, across all living species, the individuals who produce the least amount of insulin over a lifetime live the longest.

# THE DELICATE BALANCE BETWEEN FASTING AND RECOVERING

With my commitment to primal-style eating well into its second decade, my first meal of the day is never before noon. So with my eating window falling between noon and around 7 p.m., I effectively engage in a seventeen-hour fast every single day. This requires no special commitment or restraint; it's simply become a daily routine that brings me a maximum amount of pleasure along with the aforementioned anti-aging, cellular repair, and metabolic benefits. I'm never hungry in the morning, and I can easily conduct a high-intensity strength workout, a bicycle sprint session, or a two-hour hike in a

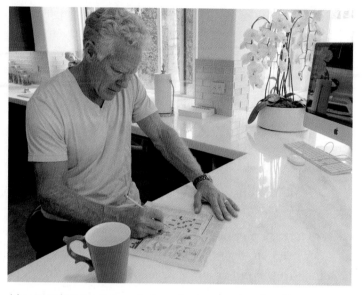

*My morning routine entails enjoying a cup of coffee (including a pinch of sugar, shhhh!), and killing the vaunted LA Times crossword puzzle in under twenty minutes. But no food—not until after noon on most days—even if I conduct an intense workout.*

twelve- to-fourteen-hour fasted state. I also make a point to fast for one to three hours after my intense workouts to maximize the impact of the anabolic hormones that flood my bloodstream. If I were to quickly consume a high-carbohydrate meal after this session, per conventional athletic training advice, the resultant insulin spike would clear the testosterone and human growth hormone out of my bloodstream.

Granted, after an intense, glycolytic (glucose-burning) workout, restocking muscle glycogen is essential for recovery, but I approach this issue from a different angle in the primal paradigm. First, I have trained my body to require less glucose, even at high intensity, through a sustained pattern of primal-style eating and sensible (not chronic) exercise patterns. My compressed eating window, low-insulin-producing diet, and training patterns that require fewer carbs help improve my *insulin sensitivity*—and this is a good thing. This means that whatever carbohydrates I consume are readily accepted into my liver and muscle glycogen storage depots without me having to produce a lot of insulin. The cells are highly sensitized to the signal of insulin knocking on their doors and asking to deliver precious cargo of carbohydrate, amino acids, or fat into the cells for storage. Second, my high-intensity workouts rarely last longer than thirty minutes, so I don't run my glycogen stores down to the "I-need-a-large-pizza-or-I'm-gonna-pass-out" level.

Hence, my abundant intake of vegetables, selective in-season fruits, moderate starchy tubers, and incidental other carbohydrates (like that pinch of sugar I like in my morning coffee) provide all I ever need to keep liver and muscle glycogen levels optimal. Even if I don't obsessively refill my glycogen tank to the very top every single day, I'm not out there the next day re-draining that tank. This gives my body plenty of time to recover completely before my next high-glycolytic session. One way this is achieved is through *gluconeo-genesis*—the conversion of ingested amino acids (protein) into glucose on a moderate, as-needed basis. This means that if I burn a bunch of carbs in a workout and don't wolf down the requisite amount right away, my body will adapt by making glucose internally, and prioritizing other fuel sources like fat and ketone bodies.

In contrast, the chronic exerciser/obsessive refueler might experience a different fate. First, it's likely that overfueling will occur occasionally, or even frequently, due to the severe disturbance in appetite hormones caused by excessive carb intake and chronic training patterns. This results in insidious lifelong weight gain for most people, as evidenced by the disturbing stat that the average American gains 1.5 pounds of fat (and loses a half-pound of lean mass) each year from ages twenty-five through fifty-five.

If you are a hard-training endurance machine, your carb overfeeding habits might not result in you packing on a pound of fat every year of your adult life, but you will quite likely experience difficulty removing unwanted fat—especially those final stubborn four to eight pounds of fat that represent the difference (in quantifiable performance terms on the fin-ish-line clock) between your age division placing and a spot on the podium.

If you wonder if you are overfeeding, simply monitor your body composition over time. If you aren't trending toward or arrived at where you want to be despite devoted efforts in training, you are consuming too many dietary carbohydrates, period. If you think it's nor-mal and customary to add seven to ten pounds of bodyweight when you reduce training load each winter, you might want to reconsider this belief. Endurance athletes packing on pounds in the winter might be commonplace, but it's an indication of overfueling and also perhaps hormonal irregularities caused by chronic training patterns.

As with the *Biggest Loser* contestants who drop massive amounts of weight during the televised competition only to gain it back and then some over time, our bodies react to overly stressful, depleting lifestyle patterns by forcing the pendulum to swing too far in the other direction. After a bout of starvation and extreme exercise for viewer entertainment and cash prizes, or after a season of chronic training, not enough sleep, and too much stress in general, your major appetite hormone, ghrelin, will run wild and your major fat storage/satiety hormone, leptin, will send your central nervous system powerful signals to eat and eat, and to store those calories as fat. There is a much better, easier, and healthier way to effortlessly maintain ideal body composition, moderate stress levels, and protect your health as you pursue ambitious fitness goals; it starts with slowing down workouts and cutting out refined carbohydrates.

— *Mark Sisson*

## STILL ON THE FENCE? GIVE IT A 21-DAY TRY!

For further validation that this primal stuff works, Chapter 7 features success stories from real live low-carb endurance athletes who are killing it on the race course and feeling healthier, stronger, and leaner with the primal approach. The ultimate validation will occur when you take twenty-one days to experiment with a primal-aligned diet and experience the immediate beneficial effects for yourself. The momentum you build in your first few weeks of ditching sugars, grains, and bad oils and eating primally—a reduction in body fat, more energy, fewer sugar cravings, faster recovery from workouts, and improvement in inflammation-related conditions—will allow you to effortlessly transition into a long-term primal-aligned eating style.

When it comes to performance, your improved body composition will be a big help, but the metabolic benefits of primal eating might provide an even bigger boost. When you become fat-adapted from primal eating and sensible training (aerobic emphasis, stress/rest balanced, and periodized) you require less glucose to perform at all intensity levels. To say this is huge is a serious understatement. This ability to depart from extreme carbohydrate dependency during training (not to mention during life in general) represents one of the greatest breakthroughs in the history of endurance training and performance. Dr. Tim Noakes tried to emphasize this—for the benefit of the *Cereal Killer* documentary-filming cameras in his office—when he theatrically tore out an entire chapter, page by page, from *Lore of Running* that pertained to the central role carbohydrate played in fueling sustained exercise. "The material isn't bad, it's actually quite good; there just wasn't enough written about the role of fat in endurance performance," Noakes explains.

Instead of training under the constant risk of bonking, having caloric absorption problems, or digestive distress from the gels, bars, and drinks endurance athletes live or die by (a study published in the journal *Medicine & Science in Sports & Exercise* reported that *31 percent* of Ironman distance triathletes experienced serious gastrointestinal distress during their event!), you will become expert at accessing and burning internal sources of fuel for long-duration workouts and races.

**DID YOU KNOW?** *The end-all endurance performance goal of sparing glycogen can be accomplished through both years of hard training and also by immediate dietary modification to ditch processed carbs and promote fat adaptation.*

Sure, you will still require and benefit from additional ingested calories during long efforts (especially as your speed increases, as seen at the elite level), but it will no longer be the most dicey, inconsistent, and frustrating X-factor for competitive success. We'll learn some specific tips from our group of athletes in Chapter 7, but it's interesting to note that Primal Endurance athletes are favoring high-fat, real-food fuel sources during workouts and races, stuff like avocados, coconut butter, almond butter, or homemade energy bar concoctions made with nuts, seeds, coconut, and perhaps some honey for a little sweetness.

# GOING PRIMAL LIBERATES YOU FROM THE CONSTANT RISK OF BONKING AND DIGESTIVE DISTRESS DURING PERFORMANCE; INSTEAD YOU WILL BECOME EXPERT AT BURNING INTERNAL SOURCES OF FUEL.

There are also some interesting cutting-edge products offered as an alternative to the usual sugary supplements taken during exercise, such as UCAN SuperStarch, a long-chain carbohydrate formula that doesn't spike insulin; Iskiate (IS-kee-ah-tay) Endurance, an all-natural superfood concoction modeled after the legendary Tarahumara runners' performance fuel (author Chris McDougall called it "10,000-year-old Red Bull"), and 3Fuel, a whey protein, coconut milk, and long-chain carbohydrate mixture promoted by CrossFit Endurance leader Brian MacKenzie, author of *Unbreakable Runner*.

## ADIOS, ARNOLD—GETTING BACK TO SENSIBLE EATING AND HEALTHY LIVING

As you ditch chronic cardio and gain more mastery balancing stress and rest, you break free from the sugar dependency cycle that is fatiguing, immune compromising, pro-inflammatory, and promotes excess body fat storage. With your chronic exercise patterns mitigated and dietary insulin production moderated, you can eat like a normal person again instead of a pig! Yep, I get to call you that because my nickname in college was actually "Arnold," after the pig in the television show *Green Acres*. I was called that because I was a bottomless pit of caloric consumption; I could put any football player at Williams College to shame with the volume of calories I inhaled each day to fuel hundred-mile training weeks and a still-growing body.

In fact, food was such a big part of my life that I started on my entrepreneurial track in college, renting out a local meeting hall every Tuesday for "Arnold's Beef & Brew" night. I'd order up a couple kegs, barbeque chuck steak that I purchased from the local distributor for sixty-two cents a pound, and charge five bucks to guests for all they could eat and drink. Turns out, I cleared a profit off the females and lost money on the hungry males that shaved and tapered for these Tuesday events.

Indeed, I bought into the philosophy that my diligent running efforts allowed me to eat whatever I wanted with impunity. Millions of other runners and endurance athletes touted this free pass to the all-you-can-eat buffet of life as one of the primary fringe benefits of being a runner. The tagline (attributed to assorted luminaries, including the late Jim Fixx, author of the 1977 bestseller *The Complete Book of Running*) "if the furnace is hot enough, anything will burn," came to describe the dietary selectivity standards of the typical endurance athlete.

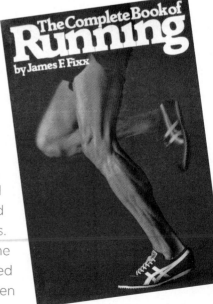

Everyone started to sober up a bit when Fixx, whose book was credited with turbo-charging the running boom, dropped dead of a heart attack during a routine training run at the age of fifty-two in 1984. Personally, my marathon career came to an abrupt and painful end when I was debilitated by an assortment of injuries and health problems while still in my prime competitive years. I was a lean, mean, eating machine—impressive on the outside in the brightly colored Dolfin shorts that defined the era. Inside, I was overstressed, inflamed, and broken down. I had chronic fatigue, osteoarthritis in both of my feet, severe tendonitis in my hip joints, strange and painful gastrointestinal maladies that today we call leaky gut syndrome, and suffered from six or more upper respiratory tract infections every single year.

During my career as an elite runner and triathlete, I was always open to trying new training or dietary strategies to gain a competitive edge, but by the end of my run I was searching for a way to simply feel healthy and pain-free. The first step is ditching chronic exercise patterns, and thus those chapters preceded our discussion here about diet. Once you have your exercise habits and your mindset in order, you can proceed with a dietary strategy that will not only improve your performance, but also make you healthier and more energetic, delay the aging process, and quite possibly save your life if you have elevated risk factors for heart disease.

If you have any trepidation about this controversial high-fat, low-carb primal/ paleo stuff, especially as an endurance athlete with high calorie demands and minimal concern about excess body fat, I ask that you hear me out and proceed with an open mind. Remember, this is Arnold speaking—a guy who has never had body fat concerns, who raced at the front of the pack for years, and who walked and felt like an eighty-year-old when he was forty...until he changed his diet.

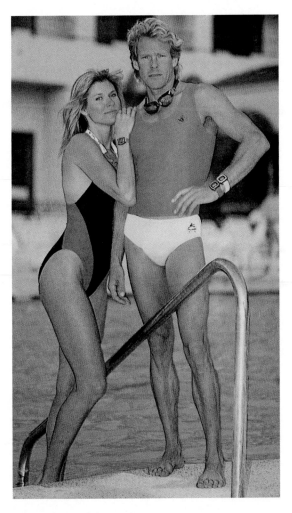

*Poolside in Palm Springs, late 1980s. Yep, Carrie and I have been together for neons...I mean eons.*

# CHAPTER SUMMARY

- Ditch grains and sugars
- Emphasize satisfying primal foods
- Moderate insulin = lose excess fat
- Sporadic meals, honor appetite

Transitioning away from carbohydrate dependency is not easy, particularly for endurance athletes who burn tons of calories and often drift into chronic training patterns that cause carbohydrate cravings. **The benefits of becoming fat- and keto-adapted are remarkable: excess body fat can be reduced easily, endurance performance improves due to more abundant and easily accessible fuel sources and less reliance on external calories, and inflammation, oxidative damage, and disease risk factors are minimized.**

Of particular interest to endurance athletes is the ability to easily reduce excess body fat when eating primally, because endurance athletes commonly struggle to remove those final few pounds despite careful attention to caloric intake and extensive training volume. Genetic predispositions to storing excess body fat become insignificant when insulin is moderated through primal eating.

**Going Primal Step 1** involves ditching the three most offensive foods in the modern diet: **sugars, grains, and highly refined polyunsaturated vegetable oils.** Sugar is pro-inflammatory and devoid of nutrition, and it locks you into a fat-storage pattern by stimulating excessive insulin production. Grains—"beige glop"—are commonly believed to form the foundation of a healthy diet—especially for endurance athletes. However, even whole grains offer minimal nutritional value compared to primal foods, and they promote carbohydrate dependency and excessive insulin production. **Sensitive individuals suffer from the negative effects of anti-nutrients like gluten, lectins, and phytates that are present in whole grains,** such as a destruction of delicate intestinal lining in the condition called *leaky gut syndrome*.

**Highly refined "industrial" vegetable/seed oils inflict oxidative damage directly upon our cells,** accelerating the aging process and increasing our risk for serious disease. Remember what Dr. Cate Shanahan says: That pleasant-looking bottle of organic canola oil offered at finer health food stores and grocers is "no different than eating radiation."

The flawed conventional wisdom that fat- and cholesterol-filled foods are unhealthy and promote heart disease and obesity is finally being countered by respected science showing that excess carbohydrate intake and overly stressful lifestyle patterns are the true catalysts for the oxidation and inflammation that promotes cardiovascular disease.

**Going Primal Step 2** involves emphasizing primal foods like meat, fish, fowl, eggs, vegetables, fruits, nuts and seeds, **highly nutritious supplemental carbs,** assorted other approved modern foods like high-fat dairy products, and an occasional sensible indulgence of dark chocolate. Far from a regimented diet, primal-style eating is driven by personal preference, flexibility, fractal eating patterns, and most of all maximum enjoyment of one of the greatest pleasures in life. Absent is the struggling, suffering, and deprivation that are so common in efforts to reduce excess body fat.

Dialing in carb intake as a Primal Endurance athlete starts with the question: **Are you carrying**

**excess body fat? If yes, carb restriction is advised until you attain your desired weight**. Otherwise, personal experimentation can help you dial in an optimal level of nutritious carbs to ensure you maintain ideal body composition and recover adequately, especially from high-intensity workouts. Carb intake can vary according to training periods and personal considerations like hormone optimization for females.

Even if you have low body fat, there is no justification for consuming significant amounts of pro-inflammatory, nutrient-devoid sugars and refined grains. Instead, Primal Endurance athletes can strive for the goal of becoming ever more fat-adapted—less reliant on external sources of carbohydrates during workouts, and during everyday life.

**The Primal Blueprint Carbohydrate Curve** predicts body composition results according to various levels of average daily carbohydrate intake. Primal-aligned eaters consume 150 grams per day or below, with some allowances for additional intake in conjunction with vigorous workouts. Ketogenic endurance athletes consume 50 grams per day or less, a practice which requires strict adherence, to remain in this delicate metabolic state.

**To become a fat-adapted endurance athlete, first slow down (minimizing the demand for glucose to fuel workouts), then ditch processed carbohydrates** so insulin production is moderated. A twenty-one-day commitment is necessary to up-regulate fat-burning genes and down-regulate glucose-burning genes. Don't worry about shedding body fat early in your primal transition; be sure you eat to satisfaction and minimize energy lulls that might occur when escaping carbohydrate dependency. Gene reprogramming requires a serious commitment, because both sugar and grains have addictive properties—triggering the same pleasure centers in the brain as hard drugs.

Test your level of fat adaptation by waiting until you get hungry to consume your first meal of the day. This enables a daily period of "**Intermittent Fasting**," which will further improve your ability to prefer fat for fuel, your insulin sensitivity (a good thing!), and your ability for cells to repair and regenerate (delivering an anti-aging effect). Just understand that a balance is necessary between fasting benefits and refueling to recover from intense glycolytic workouts.

# KETOGENIC ENDURANCE TRAINING

*– The Final Frontier?*

**4**

## IN THIS CHAPTER

After many months of successful primal eating and training, you can consider experimenting with ketogenic endurance training. Elite athletes have delivered some incredible performances to validate the effectiveness in prioritizing the use of ketones for brain fuel and fats for muscular fuel. In essence, becoming fat- and keto-adapted makes you "bonk proof."

Being in ketosis is a fragile metabolic state that requires a strict devotion to limiting dietary carbohydrate intake to around fifty grams per day. This equates with cutting out all carbs except vegetables, and perhaps tracking your carb intake with an online food calculator.

The potential of ultra-low-carb ketogenic endurance training is remarkable. A fat- and keto-adapted endurance athlete can perform for hours on end without worrying about bonking or trying to absorb ingested carbohydrate calories successfully. Even greater potential exists for ketogenic eating to address the global epidemics of obesity and type 2 diabetes.

Committing to ketogenic eating and endurance training can be daunting, but its perfectly acceptable to dip into and out of a ketogenic state and enjoy the performance and body composition benefits that come from low-carb, primal-style eating in general.

. . . . . . . . . . . .

BY ITSELF, AN ANCESTRAL-STYLE EATING pattern is considered so effective that some other low-carb books for athletes (including *The Art and Science of Low Carbohydrate Performance* by Volek and Phinney and *The Paleo Diet for Athletes* by Cordain and Friel) focus almost exclusively on the eating variable as it applies to endurance performance. As you will see in the discussions of breaking science in this chapter, and with the success stories in Chapter 7, an underground revolution is afoot. Elite and casual performers alike in ultrarunning, triathlon, and other endurance sports are experimenting with this novel low-carb training approach and performing amazing feats—completing all-day Ironman races in a fasted state with zero supplemental carbs, rowing from San Francisco to Hawaii in forty-five days eating 70 percent fat and only nine percent carbs, and winning the national 100K championship, *running sixes for six hours* with minimal supplemental calories.

At the cutting edge of this revolution is the *ketogenic endurance training strategy*. Here, dietary carb intake is greatly restricted to the extent that the athlete becomes adapted to burning almost entirely fat and ketones for fuel, and being almost completely liberated from needing any supplemental carbs. Ketones are an energy-rich byproduct of fat metabolism in the liver that provide around five calories per gram of energy. They are manufactured in the liver when glucose and insulin levels are low due to extreme carbohydrate restriction in the diet. The brain, cardiac, and skeletal muscles burn ketones in the same manner as glucose. Ketones have been a fabulous source of internally manufactured energy for over two million years of human evolution—a critical element of human survival when dietary calories were inconsistent.

Ketones are an excellent internally produced alternative fuel source to glucose, produced in the liver when dietary carbohydrate intake is restricted.

When you strictly limit dietary carbohydrates, you can enter a state of *ketosis*, which literally means you are accumulating ketones in the bloodstream faster than you are burning them. Contrary to common misunderstanding (or the surprisingly common confusion of the term *ketosis* with the life-threatening condition of *ketoacidosis*, even by medical professionals who should know their stuff), being in a state of ketosis is not unhealthy or dangerous, it's simply a state where you haven't consumed any carbs in a while and are consequently choosing other fuels over the easy-burning, low-octane glucose that's made from dietary carbohydrates. In fact, all metabolically healthy people start making and burning ketones pretty much every morning, because we haven't ingested any carbs during our overnight sleep. Unfortunately, as soon as we ingest even a small amount of carbohydrates, ketone production shuts down, knowing our bloodstream has an ample supply of quick-burning glucose.

Entering and remaining in a ketogenic state entails consuming in the neighborhood of fifty grams (two hundred calories) of carbs per day on average, with some variation based on your activity level, sex, and size. You can consume a decent amount of high-antioxidant veggies and still be ketogenic, but you are definitely eliminating all sugars, grains, sweetened beverages, starchy tubers like potatoes, and even restricting fruit intake to make sure you up-regulate those fat- and ketone-burning genes and down-regulate those sugar-burning genes.

While it takes a sincere commitment to transition from the Standard American Diet high-carbohydrate patterns and adhere to a ketogenic diet, the amazing news for endurance athletes is that you can literally become bonk-proof when you train ketogenically. Contrary to common misunderstanding, bonking occurs not when the muscles run out of energy per se, but when the brain runs out of the precious glucose that it relies on to function and direct the muscles to perform work. When insufficient glucose is available for the brain, it starts to shut down your physical and mental operations in short order. By training the body to operate mostly on fat, and training the brain to rely on ketones instead of, or in addition to, glucose, you can continue to perform endurance activities without living or dying by whether you ingest and successfully assimilate sufficient carbohydrate calories.

As long as you are burning fat, you are producing ketones. Remember that primal humans routinely lived, and performed great physical feats, with little to no dietary carbs for long stretches of time—as in winter! As in still having to forage for calories, build and maintain shelter, and evade predators, without the luxury of FuelBelts packed with gels, or even so much as a modest dinner after a long, hard, often unsuccessful day of hunting and gathering. Instead, because and only because they were magnificently fat- and keto-adapted, they fueled performance internally, until they were eventually able to succeed in securing some proper meals.

**KETOGENIC DIET**
- PROTEIN
- FAT
- CARBS

*(approximates)*

PROTEIN 20%
CARB 10%
FAT 70%

Becoming bonk-proof is great news for an endurance athlete, but it's interesting to note that the potential of ketones in medicine extends far beyond the racecourse. Certain biological compounds, including the neurotransmitter adenosine, increase in the brain when you're eating a ketogenic diet. This has a calming effect on neuron membranes, and is a reason why ketogenic diets have been used for a century to calm mental patients, and to lessen the incidence of epileptic and brain seizures.

Encouraging scientific studies and anecdotal success stories suggest that operating in a ketone-burning state significantly improves conditions like autism and ADHD. Ketogenic diets deliver a potent anti-inflammatory effect (the opposite of a high-carbohydrate diet), which helps moderate autism symptoms in particular. Ketones simply burn cleaner than carbs, leaving less mitochondrial trash and fewer free radicals behind when they are metabolized as fuel. That keeps the membranes in the mitochondria of the brain and the muscles healthier. Consequently, people eating ketogenic diets report improved mental clarity, and ketogenic endurance athletes report faster recovery from exercise stress.

Burning ketones makes you bonk-proof during long workouts, and improves your health by reducing inflammation and free radical damage in comparison to burning glucose, and also by stimulating mitochondrial biogenesis.

We discussed the performance and health benefits of mitochondrial biogenesis through aerobic and anaerobic exercise in a Chapter 1 sidebar. Science also supports the idea that mitochondrial biogenesis can be spurred by caloric restriction and ketogenic eating patterns. Remember, the stress adaptation for mitochondrial biogenesis is the depletion of cellular energy. This occurs when you exercise for long duration or vigorously, and it also occurs in the course of fasting or eating ketogenically. Interesting animal research spawns speculation that caloric restriction stimulates a "spontaneous uncoupling" of mitochondria (no connection to Gwyneth Paltrow's relationship status updates), resulting in greater protection against free-radical damage. When you are a fat-burning beast with primal-aligned exercise and dietary habits, mitochondria do cleaner work. Fat and ketone burning produce fewer free radicals and generate less inflammation.

# WHEN YOU BECOME KETO- AND FAT-ADAPTED, YOU ARE VIRTUALLY BONK-PROOF.

The recent breakthroughs in keto- and fat-adapted endurance performance, in both the lab and the competitive arena, suggest that this concept may one day revolutionize our entire approach to endurance training. For the past fifty-plus years, we've been obsessed with the challenge of sparing glycogen and improving fat oxidation during exercise, but have failed to look outside the carbohydrate dependency paradigm. The pendulum is now shifting at a faster rate each day, thanks to the great science delivered by Volek, Phinney, and others on the topic of keto-adapted endurance performance, and legit performances by elite-level ketogenic endurance athletes, several of whom you will meet in Chapter 7.

Dr. Noakes, for decades one of the leaders in studying and shaping this carbohydrate dependency/glycogen-loading paradigm as it relates to endurance performance, has done a magnificent job in recent years publicly rethinking the basic assumptions of endurance exercise physiology to embrace a new paradigm with all-new assumptions. Let's call it the *fat-burning beast paradigm* (maybe it will catch on!), where fat can become the preferred fuel source of both the exercising athlete and the healthy eater. On a 2015 *Endurance Planet* podcast, Dr. Volek spoke enthusiastically about the great potential for fat-adapted endurance performance, but reminded listeners that the worldwide pandemic of obesity, universally agreed to be caused by high-carbohydrate, high-insulin-producing diets across the globe, could be an even bigger target for this revolution!

The ketogenic endurance strategy is definitely an advanced strategy that might not be appealing to a casual enthusiast. Although ten years from now it may very likely be de rigueur to be a fat- and keto-adapted endurance athlete, today it requires a serious commitment and a willingness to break free from the conventional approach with perhaps minimal support or alliance in your athletic community, general community, and even your own family. For one thing, being in a ketone-burning state is very fragile. Ingestion of even a moderate amount of carbohydrates—grabbing a banana or an energy bar as you pass by the break room—will immediately bump you out of ketosis and back to a glucose-preferred state. Carbs are easy to obtain, easy to burn, and easy to become dependent upon. They are today's low-octane fuels for our DumbCars!

Interestingly, scientists have known for decades that trained athletes can switch over to a low-carb eating plan without hurting their performance, as any body (athletic or not) will train itself to run mainly on fat, break down and deliver fat quicker to the muscles, store more intracellular fat within the muscles, and turn glycogen into more of a supplementary fuel.

# BENEFITS OF FAT-FUELED ENDURANCE PROVEN SCIENTIFICALLY...OVER THIRTY YEARS AGO!

Way back in 1983, Dr. Steve Phinney conducted a study at Chico (CA) State University (Phinney et al, "Human metabolic response to chronic ketosis without calorie restriction; preservation of submaximal exercise capability with reduced carbohydrate oxidation," published in *Metabolism*) that produced mind-blowing results attesting to the benefits of dietary keto- and fat-adaptation on endurance performance. He took a group of lean, mean, highly trained cyclists (VO$_2$ max above 65 mL/kg—serious racer dudes!) and had them pedal to exhaustion. These guys were burning nine hundred calories per hour, so they were really hammering. Lots of exercise performance studies use untrained volunteers, and this potentially compromises the relevance of the study to real athletes. On their typical high-carbohydrate diet, these fit cyclists went for an average of 147 minutes before cracking. Four weeks later, after consuming a diet of 80 percent fat and almost zero carbohydrate (fewer than *10 grams per day*), they pedaled 151 minutes to exhaustion.

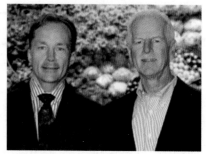

*Dr. Jeff Volek, PhD, RD (L) and Dr. Stephen Phinney, MD, PhD (R), the world's scientific leaders in low carb endurance training*

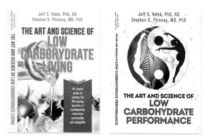

*Phinney and Volek detail the science of how the body performs exceptional endurance feats on a low carbohydrate diet.*

The study was covered prominently in cycling magazines and there was widespread disbelief and even disdain from seasoned endurance athletes. Those in the know basically scoffed at the concept of performing better to exhaustion on greasy sausage and pork rinds instead of pasta and oatmeal. Even Dr. Noakes admitted recently that the scientific community basically ignored the provocative results generated by Phinney's early work studying fat-adapted endurance exercise. Consequently, the study was quickly forgotten and we carried on with our sugar-burning ways. In the years that followed, the energy bar, sports drink, sports gel scene became a billion dollar industry, as endurance athletes became summarily brainwashed that ingesting carbs was the key to preserving glycogen during sustained efforts.

What we have disastrously failed to recognize in our quest for endurance success is the role diet can play in improving your ability to metabolize fat and preserve glycogen during exercise. We know how difficult it is to get fitter through hard work on the roads, so now you can take comfort and inspiration knowing that every meal you eat can also contribute to your success on the race course. I appreciate the value and satisfaction of making gains through hard work, but I certainly don't mind trying an easy way to get an edge on the race course!

## THE SCIENCE BEHIND KETOGENIC ENDURANCE TRAINING

Recent science in this burgeoning topic of low-carb and ketogenic endurance training has been nothing short of astonishing. As Noakes has so boldly proclaimed, endurance exercise physiologists the world over are being forced to completely rethink the major carbohydrate paradigm assumptions and parameters they have operated in for decades.

One 2015 study by Dr. Jeff Volek and his graduate students at the University of Connecticut is really moving the needle away from the status quo with some shocking results. The FASTER study (Fat Adapted Substrate Oxidation in Trained Elite Runners) recruited a group of carefully screened elite-level ultrarunners from two distinct dietary camps. One group, the Low Carb Fat-Adapted, consumed 10–12 percent of daily calories from carbs and 70 percent from fat. These folks were handpicked for having followed a sustained pattern of low-carb eating prior to the study. Individuals from this group were paired with runners of equal ability and body compositions in a High Carb Conventional group. These athletes ate a more typical endurance athlete diet comprised of 60 percent carbs and only 25 percent fat.

Prior to this study, exercise science suggested that well-trained humans can burn a maximum of one gram of fat per minute, with most athletes burning at a rate of .45–.75 grams per minute. The FASTER study shattered accepted limits by showing a *mean* fat oxidation rate among Low Carb Fat Adapted athletes of 1.1 grams of fat per minute and a maximum rate in one athlete of 1.8 grams per minute—nearly twice the rate of what was believed to be the absolute human limit!

At comfortable heart rates in a three-hour sub-maximal (65 percent of $VO_2$ max—in the neighborhood of the aforementioned maximum aerobic heart rate) treadmill run performed by each athlete in the study, fat-adapted elite runners burned over 90 percent fat for hours on end, while the High Carb Conventional athletes burned between 40 and 55 percent fat, obtaining the rest of their energy from that scarce and rapidly depleting commodity known as carbohydrates (they weren't allowed any supplemental calories during the three-hour treadmill test).

*In the FASTER study, fat-adapted elite ultrarunners burned over 90 percent fat for hours on end. Zach Bitter, pictured here, burned 98 percent fat at a seven-minute mile pace!*

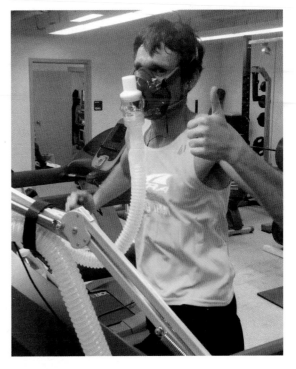

Zach Bitter, who is profiled in Chapter 7, reached a maximum of *98 percent fat burning* at a comfortable intensity of 75 percent $VO_2$ max during a separate $VO_2$ max test that escalated him from a comfortable pace up to maximum effort. Bitter was not dawdling at 75 percent of $VO_2$ max—he was clicking off seven-minute miles and still burning almost entirely fat. At his Mad City 100K national championship victory that happened near the time of the study, Bitter ran faster than 6m:30 miles for nearly *seven hours*, while only ingesting 156 calories per hour!

On his popular blog, zachbitter.com, Bitter shared an important take-away from the study: "I strongly believe that the less you have to fuel during a race, the better. Heat, for example, can greatly affect how the body accepts (or on super hot days, rejects) the calories you give it. This is why you see so many more stomachs turn at hot weather races. Less eating means your body can use its precious blood stores for cooling and muscle function, rather than for digestion."

Dr. Peter Attia, the San Diego physician and deep experimenter we introduced in Chapter 1, conducted a methodical before and after test of the ketogenic endurance training hypothesis, which you can read all about at eatingacademy.com. Before Attia transitioned to a ketogenic eating pattern, he performed a sustained sub-max effort (he described it as "all-day pace" of 60 percent of $VO_2$ max) and tested the ratio of glycogen to fat he used for fuel. He then repeated the same test while immersed in a sustained period of ketogenic eating. The ratio of fuel usage can be measured using a value called Respiratory Quotient (RQ). You wear a tight mask over your nose and mouth, and a machine measures the ratio of carbon dioxide produced to oxygen consumed. On a scale of 0.70 to 1.0, 0.70 equates with 100 percent fat usage, while 1.0 (expelling carbon dioxide at a rate equal to oxygen consumed) means 100 percent glucose usage.

On the test he performed before going ketogenic, Attia burned 95 percent carbs and only 5 percent fat at that comfortable all-day pace. At a heart rate of 104 beats per minute (very slow pace), he hit a point of burning half carbs and half fat. After a strict twelve-week period of eating ketogenically, his repeat test results were nothing short of astounding. At the all-day pace, Attia burned 22 percent glycogen and nearly 80 percent fat! The heart rate where he hit the 50/50 ratio increased to 162 beats per minute—hammering pace! Also, when he bumped his pace up to the red-line anaerobic threshold (AT), he burned 100 percent glycogen before, but 70 percent glycogen and 30 percent fat at AT during ketogenic eating.

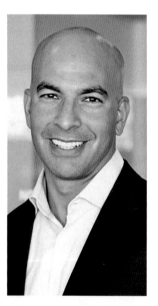

*Dr. Peter Attia is one of the leaders in the science of low-carb endurance performance, and walks his talk with tons of heavy-duty personal experimentation.*

Furthermore, Attia reached AT at a higher wattage as a ketogenic athlete. This caused him to speculate that ketones may blunt the effects of acidosis on the bloodstream, enabling improved performance not only at comfortable fat-burning intensity, but also at red-line pace. Interestingly, when Attia completed his test by revving up to all-out $VO_2$ max pace, he experienced a slight decline in performance while ketogenic. His carefully recorded data suggests that ketogenic eating and endurance performance offers a substantial benefit at virtually all intensity levels short of absolute maximum effort. While there is a sentiment on the street that ketogenic endurance performance can mainly benefit extreme ultra athletes going very slowly but is difficult for athletes competing at shorter events, the research disproves this notion.

World champion amateur 70.3 triathlete Sami Inkinen has also shown with precise laboratory data that ultra low carb (less than 10 percent of total calories) eating patterns can dramatically improve endurance performance. In only three months of a high-fat, low-carb eating pattern, Sami went from an extreme sugar burner (around 95 percent of total fuel usage while pedaling at a relatively high intensity 300 watts) to a remarkably fat-adapted endurance machine. At that same 300 watts of

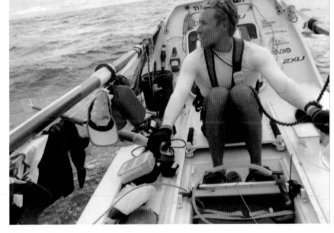

*Sami Inkinen pushes the limits of human endurance and fat adaptation with his elite amateur triathlon exploits, and other superhuman feats you'll learn about in Chapter 7.*

energy output after his dietary modification, Sami transformed his substrate utilization from 95 percent glucose to around a 50/50 split between glucose and fat, and doubled his fat oxidation to 400 calories per hour. Mind you, this is at a super legit 300 watts energy output rate equating to pedaling around 25 mph on flat ground!

Even more amazing was Sami's "time to bonk" calculations at lower intensity, extrapolated from substrate utilization percentages at his three performance tests. The calculation predicts when the subject would run out of energy, assuming no additional ingested calories. At his first test as a sugar burner, he calculated a bonk time for 5.6 hours at the low intensity of 200 watts output. At his 2014 test, after five years of fat-adapted eating and training, the time to bonk at 200 watts increased to *87 hours!* Chapter 7 details Sami's carefully recorded fat-adaptation experiments, and the superhuman feat he and his wife, Meredith, accomplished in 2014—rowing from Northern California to Hawaii in forty-five days!

Phinney and Volek also relate in *The Art and Science of Low Carbohydrate Performance* that ketogenic eating helps athletes preserve lean muscle tissue, because they always have easy access to fats and ketones for energy. Conversely, a carbohydrate-dependent athlete will kick into fight-or-flight mode and trigger gluconeogenesis whenever glucose levels run low. This means that hard-earned lean muscle tissue is stripped away to prioritize a steady fuel supply for the brain. Unfortunately, this is a catabolic process that significantly delays recovery and overstimulates the delicate stress response.

In summary, being carb dependent pretty much sucks on an assortment of levels. You live and die by the fickle ability to assimilate enough ingested glucose during long workouts and races; you put your hard-earned lean muscle at risk of catabolic gluconeogenesis whenever you run a little short on glucose (this is true even at rest, when you are carb-dependent and miss a meal); and you flat-out compromise your health by burning a dirty, inflammatory, oxidative fuel—at a much greater severity than the average Joe or Jane who is minimally active.

Being carb dependent pretty much sucks on an assortment of levels; you flat-out compromise your health by burning a dirty, inflammatory, oxidative fuel.

Before you get too excited—or intimidated—about taking the big leap to a ketogenic approach, let's back up and prepare for a gradual transition into primal-aligned eating. This entails a much more liberal intake of well-chosen carbohydrates, without worrying about the extreme and carefully regulated patterns necessary to enter and remain in ketosis.

We will apply a triage strategy and make the first step to going primal an elimination of the most offensive foods from your diet—the stuff that can quite possibly kill you no matter how many hours a week you burn these crappy, highly oxidized and inflammatory fuels: sugars, grains, and highly refined industrial oils. In their place, you'll start to emphasize the nutrient-rich primal-aligned foods of meat, fish, fowl, eggs, vegetables, fruits, nuts, and seeds. You will be pleased to discover that primal eating offers an incredibly broad selection, is extremely flexible and customizable by personal preference, and emphasizes the enjoyment of delicious, satisfying meals. You will not have to suffer or struggle or get overly regimented or restrictive in your approach.

You'll make a total commitment to primal eating for the first twenty-one days to kick-start the process of gene reprogramming and eventually progress to the level of fat-burning beast. As you build momentum with sensible, aerobic-emphasis training and primal-aligned eating for around six months, you can then explore the world of ketogenic endurance training. The following sections will take you step by step through this sequence.

## LEVERAGING EXERCISE TO REWIRE YOUR BRAIN

Engaging in that traditional post-workout carb feeding frenzy can make you especially vulnerable to carbohydrate dependency, because your appetite hormones are highly sensitive when you are in this depleted state. Dr. Cate Shanahan explains:

> Exercise is one of the most powerful ways to influence appetite hormones, especially ghrelin (pronounced "grell-in"; *ghrelin* gets your stomach *growlin'*), an extremely fast-acting hormone that causes sensations of hunger in both the brain and the stomach. When you get depleted during a workout, ghrelin will spike big time. When you slam carbs after a workout, your body releases dopamine and endogenous opioids to deliver that strong sensation of pleasure. So the ghrelin spike (in response to depletion), and the dopamine and opioid spike (in response to eating) all act on the nucleus accumbens in the hypothalamus to control neural mediation of food reward.
>
> In that post-exercise depleted state, your appetite hormones are very sensitive and primed for rewiring. Hypothetically, if you were to fast for a spell that you could endure, or satisfy your ravenous hunger with a high-fat meal, you could moderate your neural mediation of food reward—the nature of your cravings. This could up-regulate your fat- and ketone-burning genes, since you are teaching your body to rely on something besides carbs when your energy needs are high. Similarly, if you get yourself into a hunger frenzy and then serve up nutrient-dense foods that you know are good for you but you dislike—sardines and liver anyone?—your body will learn how to use those raw materials for high-octane cellular fuel and repair. Consequently, because you feel good after eating them, you may come to look forward to them in the future.
>
> On the other hand, if you reward yourself with sweet treats of minimal nutritional value, you lose that potential opportunity to recalibrate appetite and reduce your sugar cravings in the future. Instead you literally become wired for sugar, like a lab rat. This is true not only after workouts but all the time, because workouts at 10, 20, or 30 MET have such a profound influence on your metabolism. Furthermore, as anyone who's ever had a sweet binge can relate, replenishing with low-nutrient-value foods triggers cravings for more and more, because your desire for actual nutrition to promote recovery is not being met. Similarly, the old adage about not going to the grocery store when you are hungry has some validity, because the influence of appetite hormones can indeed affect your purchasing decisions.

While Dr. Cate says "hypothetically" in the second paragraph of her explanation, real-world anecdotes support the claim that fasting after workouts can be beneficial. Tour de France cyclists looking to shed those last few pounds of body fat before the Tour like to fast after long rides to stimulate accelerated fat burning. When you are already super lean, homeostatic forces refute ordinary efforts to drop even more pounds, so cyclists have to take extreme measures. Of course they are mindful of that fine line between dropping more fat and inhibiting muscle recovery by fasting for too long, but the advantages of being as light as humanly possible for that brief period of time coinciding with the Tour are phenomenal.

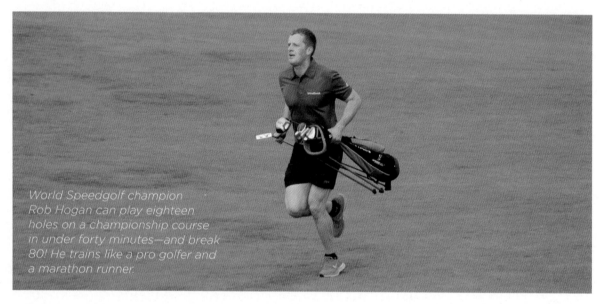

World Speedgolf champion Rob Hogan can play eighteen holes on a championship course in under forty minutes—and break 80! He trains like a pro golfer and a marathon runner.

On the Primal Blueprint Podcast Episode 49 (available at iTunes, Stitcher, or blog.primal-blueprint.com), Dr. Cate comments about a remarkable story from World Speedgolf champion Rob Hogan (shared on Primal Blueprint Podcast Episode 48), whom Dr. Cate believes rewired the appetite center in his brain by completing a series of seventeen-mile runs on successive weekends, all with no added calories or fluids. This story is presented in detail in Chapter 7. In short, Hogan claims that after pushing through a bonking episode—where powerful visions of Fanta soda (his typical post-run treat) consumed his thoughts in the latter stages of his fourth consecutive weekend seventeen-miler—he finished the run and noticed that the Fanta vision was gone and that he had no craving for sugar.

Furthermore, Hogan's sugar cravings in daily life vanished after the run, never to return. Dr. Cate says, "These intense, novel, and unique experiences are powerful signal generators that message the body that it needs to change, and the body responds accordingly." Hogan essentially hacked the typical transition from sugar burner to fat-adapted that might take weeks of gradual dietary transitions and aerobic training, by pushing his body to the limit while starving it of calories.

# EXPERIMENTING WITH KETOGENIC ENDURANCE TRAINING

When you have a periodized, stress-balanced, aerobic-emphasis training strategy coupled with a primal-style, low-insulin-producing eating pattern, you will start performing amazing athletic and metabolic feats that you previously thought impossible. You'll discover that you can complete long aerobic workouts in a fasted state, eat in a compressed eating window, shed excess body fat and keep it off indefinitely with no trouble (even if you train less!), and generally enjoy a much more stable daily appetite and energy level. As a finely tuned fat-burning machine, you can now aspire to testing out the advanced and quite possibly revolutionary strategy of ketogenic endurance training.

As this fringe idea has gained some serious momentum and real-life credibility from top-performing athletes (you'll meet several in Chapter 7), it's easy to envision with great excitement a potential complete transformation in the conventional approach to endurance training and performance. While the word "revolution" is used in a cavalier manner in every other magazine ad ("Try our *revolutionary* new gel flavor: Cookies 'N Crème with extra caffeine!"), this could be a true revolution—from carbohydrate dependency to carbohydrate aversion—in both dietary habits and inside the metabolic machinery of the athlete.

Ketogenic endurance training could revolutionize endurance sports; fat and ketones are more abundant, more efficient, and vastly cleaner burning than carbs.

The revolution will occur because fat and ketones are more abundant, more efficient, and vastly cleaner burning than the beloved carbohydrates we live and die by today. Aside from the potential performance benefits of being fat- and keto-adapted, athletes can greatly reduce the accelerated aging and oxidative damage that's an inevitable byproduct of doing things the conventional way. If you are ready to see for yourself and join the elite group of pioneers experiencing performance breakthroughs with the ketogenic approach, here are the steps you can take.

**Become Fat-Adapted:** Complete your twenty-one-day transition and stick with it! Strive to accumulate at least six months of primal-aligned eating and training to achieve successful gene reprogramming before trying the ketogenic approach. You can probably get 80 percent of the way there after twenty-one days, but you want to eventually land at 100 percent.

**Do *Another* Twenty-One-Day Transition—Go Keto:** This time, you are going to go full ketogenic by strictly limiting carb intake to around fifty grams per day. You can still enjoy generous servings of vegetables, and perhaps a handful of seasonal berries, but that's really about it. Hold off on the extra fruit and sweet potatoes that are ordinarily okay. Completely restrict grains and sugars. Use fitday.com to log your food intake and make sure you are eating in the ketogenic range, since it's obviously easy to leak out of this ultra-low-carb intake pattern. Remember, a single diversion into a bit of carbs will throw you out of ketosis and potentially compromise your progress with the experiment. Again, eat to total satisfaction by enjoying rich, nutrient-dense, high-satiety primal foods.

How do you know you are in a ketogenic state? It's difficult to quantify, but being able to do workouts fasted or skip meals effortlessly are telltale signs that your fat- and ketone-burning genes are up-regulated. You may have heard about people using measuring devices like Ketostix (strips that change color when activated by urine) or even expensive blood meters to measure ketone levels, since a reading of 2.0 mmol/L indicates a state of nutritional ketosis. You don't need to bother with this approach, because any readings you obtain may be misleading for a couple of reasons that are particularly relevant to endurance athletes. First, a high score for urinary ketone levels might mean that you are excreting a lot of ketones instead of them being taken up by muscle tissue, heart, and brain for an energy source.

Furthermore, studies from Phinney and Volek, authors of *The Art and Science of Low Carbohydrate Performance* and distinct leaders in this field, suggest that you can go through some interesting metabolic phases in the process of keto-adaptation. When you first radically cut carbs, your muscles burn ketones and fat for fuel. As adaptation improves, it seems that your muscles express a preference for fat, in order to preserve ketones for use by the brain. This might deliver a confusing result of low blood ketones, because your brain is burning them!

The process of keto-adaptation is a fascinating phenomenon with major evolutionary repercussions. In times of famine, perhaps combined with extreme physical demands (i.e., looking desperately for some food!), we couldn't accomplish much without sharp brain function. The brain is an organ that relies almost exclusively on glucose, or the excellent glucose substitute of ketones, for fuel. And for such a small organ, the brain has massive caloric demands—consuming around 20 percent of our total daily energy! For millions of years, ketones have been an essential and precious commodity to promote our survival during tough times. They have always been put to the highest-priority task of keeping the brain well fueled and functioning optimally.

Ketones are a magnificent energy source…unless your body receives a lifelong onslaught of sugar. In this scenario, which essentially characterizes the advent of civilization and the caloric abundance that enabled civilized life, ketones aren't even produced. Or if they are produced, such as after an overnight fast, they are largely excreted due to poor adaptation—lack of experience—with ketone burning.

KETONES ARE A MAGNIFICENT ENERGY SOURCE… UNLESS YOUR BODY RECEIVES A LIFELONG ONSLAUGHT OF SUGAR.

So when we envision the ultimate fat- and keto-adapted endurance athlete, we have a specimen who is burning ketones in the brain to remain sharp for hours on end, without being dependent upon the next gel coming down the hatch. Meanwhile, the muscles are burning mostly fat, while sparing precious muscle glycogen to help stoke the fat fire a bit, and perhaps be utilized for a final finishing sprint. Remember, our ancestors needed that glycogen to be ready at a moment's notice for a life-or-death supreme physical effort. The fat-adapted muscles, which could burn ketones if they wanted, instead generously and wisely give the brain first crack at this precious fuel.

## YOUR PRIMAL ENDURANCE DIETARY/ FUELING OPTIONS

Now that you understand the distinctions between being carbohydrate dependent, becoming fat-adapted, and going into full ketogenic endurance training, you might wonder exactly what your best long-term fueling options are. A great thing about the primal approach is that it offers tremendous versatility. When you have programmed your genes to prefer fat as the primary fuel source around the clock, you can consume a varied level of carbs depending on your current body composition, or your training goals of the day or training period. Following are three broad categories of fueling/metabolic function that you can transition into and out of at your leisure.

**Full Ketogenic:** When you diligently restrict carbs to around fifty grams per day or less, you experience best results with rapid removal of excess body fat, ultra-sharp, bonk-proof brain function, moderated inflammation, and enhanced mitochondrial biogenesis (making new and improved mitochondria to enhance energy production and protect your entire system against the oxidative stress of training, and life). Because this is a delicate state to arrive at and stay in, it's best to try full ketogenic when training and life stress are moderated, such as during an aerobic period or rest period. It's not advised to try during a high-intensity period, due to the extreme glycolytic demands of strength and speed workouts.

**Cyclic Ketogenic:** Remember that a single moderate-to-high-carbohydrate meal will spit you right out of the sweet zone of full ketogenic, and that's actually okay. Your forays into full ketogenic training can last as long as you feel comfortable and experience great results. Some athletes remain ketogenic for months on end without a second thought. Some might go ketogenic for a defined period of a couple weeks or a month in alignment with a particular training micro-period, or a focused fat-reduction goal. Mark's strategy of eating in a compressed time window spits him into and out of ketosis every single day. He doesn't notice any discernable effects of this, particularly since his meals are invariably low enough in carbohydrate to not stimulate an extreme insulin response—even as they may bump him out of a full ketogenic state. Remember, all of us operate in a cyclic ketogenic state when we go to sleep every night and go without food for eight hours or more. The problem is that most people get violently spit out of that mild to significant ketogenic state each morning when they slam their power breakfast.

**Classic Primal:** While the science and the performance potential of ketogenic endurance training are fascinating, you may not be inclined to dive in that deep right away, or anytime soon, for that matter. Making the transition from carbohydrate dependency into a generally fat-adapted state, and a diet of vastly superior nutritional value and less inflammation and oxidative stress, will transform your health and your body. This is true even if you prefer to consume more carbs than are required to enter the ketogenic club. Your macronutrient intake levels, as with the rest of the guidelines in this book, are subject to modification and final approval based on your personal experience.

Furthermore, a fundamental principle of the Primal Blueprint is the 80 Percent Rule (detailed in the *Primal Blueprint* book and in numerous MarksDailyApple.com articles). Here, Mark suggests that you strive to do the best you can with your primal lifestyle goals, but accept that the realities of modern life might create a few detours here and there. If you strive for 100 percent compliance and end up being 80 percent compliant, you can consider that a success. Just make sure you don't misconstrue this message to mean that going for 80 percent out of the gate is okay, or that "cheat" days and other such self-destructive gamesmanship is part of the primal philosophy. Since you are an athlete and a healthy-living enthusiast, it's critical to make a sincere commitment to eliminating unhealthy foods from your diet, regardless of how hot your furnace burns. Instead, enjoy the performance, recovery, health, and pleasure benefits of eating—and training—primally!

# CHAPTER SUMMARY

- Ketogenic endurance could become future norm
- Becoming fat- and keto-adapted = bonk-proof
- Okay to dip in and out of ketosis
- Rewire brain to escape sugar dependency

**Ketogenic endurance training** represents the cutting edge of endurance exercise science, and offers a potential for remarkable performance breakthroughs. **Ketones are an energy-rich byproduct of fat metabolism in the liver when blood glucose levels are low**. The brain, heart, and skeletal muscle can burn ketones very efficiently. Our ability to manufacture ketones internally is a hard-wired evolutionary adaptation that was critical to human survival when calories were scarce, which was often! Ingesting even a moderate amount of carbs kicks you quickly out of ketosis, so this is an advanced strategy requiring a sustained period of primal-style eating and training before attempting.

Elite ultrarunners in Dr. Volek's FASTER study **burned fat at nearly twice the rate that was previously believed to be the human limit!** In Dr. Peter Attia's well-chronicled ketogenic eating and performance experiment, he transitioned from burning mostly carbs to burning mostly fat at a comfortable pace, and improved his wattage output at anaerobic threshold while eating ketogenically. Triathlete Sami Inkinen extended his laboratory verified "time to bonking" from 5.6 hours to 87 hours after becoming fat-adapted.

After many months of successful primal eating and training, you can consider experimenting with ketogenic endurance training. Taking the next step entails cutting back on all carbs except vegetables, and perhaps tracking your carb intake with an online food calculator to stay below fifty grams per day. Once you are a fat-burning beast, you can choose to train full ketogenic, cyclic ketogenic, or classic primal in accordance with personal preference, training periods, and peak performance goals.

# STRENGTH TRAINING

*Become more powerful, resist fatigue, and preserve form and mobility with Primal Essential Movements (PEM) and Maximum Sustained Power (MSP) workouts*

# CHAPTER 5

## IN THIS CHAPTER

You will learn the rationale for endurance athletes conducting brief, high-intensity strength workouts of the proper format and timing in the annual periodization cycle. The focus will be on improving raw strength and explosive speed, and preserving proper technique while fatigued. The Primal Endurance approach to strength training differs from the typical endurance athlete strategy of conducting "blended" workouts that stimulate both cardio and strength energy systems. These exhaustive sessions can compromise improvements in raw power and also lead to overtraining.

Properly conducted strength workouts complement your hard work on the roads, allowing you to preserve form and power output while fatigued. Strength training also delivers a potent anti-aging effect by stimulating the release of adaptive hormones like testosterone and growth hormone.

Two approaches to strength training are covered. First is the simple **Primal Essential Movements**, where you perform pushups, pullups, squats, and planks on a regular basis to improve functional, full-body strength and mobility. For devoted athletes looking to improve explosive power and the ability to sustain a better percentage of that power over long duration, the **Maximum Sustained Power** training strategy is presented. You lift heavy weights for fewer reps and take more rest. The focus is on increasing maximum raw power and sustaining maximum power throughout the workout. Favored exercises are full-body, functional movements like deadlifts, squats, presses, and vertical jumps.

• • • • • • • • • • • •

**IF YOU'VE READ THIS FAR** and bought into the fundamentals of the program, congratulations are in order for building an exceptional aerobic base. As an endurance machine fitter than 99.9 percent of the humans on Earth, you are delaying the aging process, improving your cognitive function, managing stress effectively, and priming your body for peak performance in endurance competition. Of course, all this glowing praise assumes you're doing everything right—right?! If your endurance efforts drift into a chronic pattern, you are literally accelerating the aging process, causing a decline in cognitive function, adding more physical stress to an already stressful modern life, inflicting damage and scarring upon your heart and arteries, and falling far short of your competitive potential.

If you are feeling strong and healthy, and have progressed steadily with your aerobic function over at least two months of strictly aerobic workouts, never exceeding your aerobic maximum heart rate, you are ready to add some strength workouts to your schedule (and sprint workouts, which we'll cover in the next chapter). Because you are already an aerobic machine, you needn't worry about generating a cardiovascular training effect during your strength-training sessions. By contrast, the stated goal of CrossFit is to "forge broad, general and inclusive fitness" through "constantly varied functional movements performed at relatively high intensity." The desired result is an all-around athlete in the model of an Olympic decathlete or, hey, a CrossFit Games competitor. There is nothing objectionable about this approach, and CrossFit has experienced an incredible growth in popularity since its birth in 2000.

Here's a great light-resistance, high-rep workout for a runner: go run six miles!

With the assumption that you have distinct endurance goals as your top priority, Primal Endurance takes a different approach to strength training than the "broad, general" CrossFit model, or the typical regimen recommended to endurance athletes from a book, magazine, or personal trainer at your local gym. Rather than striving for a well-balanced strength session that involves a cardio endurance component, try to zero in on the most critical weaknesses revealed by the typical endurance athlete: raw strength, explosive speed, and general physical mobility and motor control.

The truth is, you already have plenty of endurance and do plenty of training to build and preserve it. We might also assume that you are mainly interested in endurance performance rather than broadening your skills to knock off Ashton Eaton in the decathlon at the next Olympics. Hence, we are going to address getting strong and explosive (*relatively* strong and explosive that is, at a level appropriate to your endurance goals), improving your mobility and motor control under load, and thereby being able to preserve good technique and power generation even as you fatigue.

PRIMAL ENDURANCE EMPHASIZES RAW STRENGTH, EXPLOSIVE POWER, AND GENERAL PHYSICAL MOBILITY AND MOTOR CONTROL.

This approach counters the common misconception among endurance athletes that the paltry strength and speed sessions they might throw into the mix have to include, and even emphasize, an endurance component. It's like they need repeated confirmation that yes indeed, they are relatively weak and frail, but are capable of suffering long after explosive athletes have finished their workout. You hear skinny endurance folks all the time say, "My gym circuit features light resistance and high reps." Unfortunately, these types of sessions aren't difficult enough (and last too long) to truly get you strong and explosive, nor do they markedly improve your mobility or motor control. Here's a great suggestion for a light-resistance, high-rep workout for a runner: *go run six miles!*

We are going to get you truly strong, fast, explosive, mobile, and well aligned with workouts that are ridiculously short and ridiculously intense. It's gonna be fun, and a refreshing break from the drudgery of a narrow approach focused on miles and more miles. Remember, just a handful of very brief workouts can stimulate breakthroughs in endurance performance that you couldn't obtain through your routine aerobic efforts lasting ten or twenty times longer.

Don't believe us? Pause your reading here and drop for a set of twenty air squats. Don't worry about laying a barbell across your back, just lower your butt all the way down (as close as you can to the ground) and raise back up, making sure to track your knees on the same plane as your feet (not caving inward, knock-kneed). So, how did your twenty reps go? It's surprisingly difficult for even a supremely fit endurance athlete to do a basic warmup set of squats or a handful of pullups. And if you think these skills aren't relevant to your marathon or triathlon time, your awakening comes right now—read on!

## BUT...DO I REALLY NEED STRENGTH TRAINING?

This heading poses an important question. Honestly, strength training requires lots of energy and recovery time, and is an entirely different athletic endeavor from sustained endurance performance. It's also been unequivocally confirmed by science that *specificity* is the most effective way to improve in any competitive endeavor. To swim faster, best results come from swimming. To run faster, it really helps to run. To master the violin, you have to practice the instrument often.

However, because endurance training is so physically stressful and technique-dependent, you have to follow best practices for technique and recovery to get maximum return on investment for every lap that you swim or mile that you run or pedal. This is an obvious statement, but unfortunately one that is widely disregarded out on the roads. As we discussed earlier, there is no direct correlation between more hours or miles and improved performance. Even a violin player can practice in an ineffective manner or get fried from excessive practice to the extent that additional practice hours can actually compromise skill development.

When you get fatigued during endurance workouts, technique falters, bad habits become ingrained, and recovery time is delayed.

In order to generate maximum return on investment with your training, you have to execute proper technique at all times. When you get fatigued during endurance workouts, technique falters, bad habits become ingrained, and recovery time is delayed. And endurance athletes spend an awful lot of time getting themselves tired and broken down!

Dr. Kelly Starrett, the larger-than-life CrossFit/Mobility/physical therapy industry leader who started the viral MobilityWOD.com (Mobility Workout Of the Day), and wrote the bestseller *Becoming a Supple Leopard: The Ultimate Guide to Resolving Pain, Preventing Injury, and Optimizing Athletic Performance* and *Ready to Run* (where he applies his revolutionary movement and mobility philosophy to the injury-plagued world of running), has a lot to say on the subject of how endurance athletes can benefit from strength training and other complementary movement practices.

In his inimitable brash style, K-Star hits endurance athletes with a sobering message: "Endurance athletes seem to care only about time. But imagine if we ran our lives with this mentality: 'Hey, I got to work faster today! Uh, I hit three parked cars and ran seventeen red lights, but I got there faster.' We need to value our endurance performances with a bigger-picture perspective."

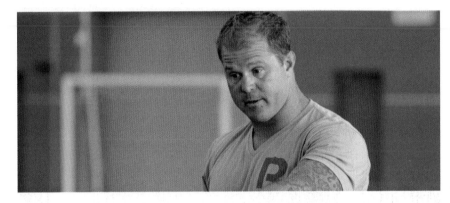

*Dr. Kelly Starrett, perhaps the world's leading mobility expert and a one-man quote machine. Some pearls: "Squatting regenerates defunct mechanics," and, on the subject of how diet influences peak performance and recovery, "You can't eat like an asshole, you just can't."*

Starrett advocates resistance and mobility training to improve proprioception (awareness of your body moving through space) and motor control (ability to exhibit proper technique, even when you are under load or fatigued). Starrett asserts that poor technique results in muscle tension and poor biomechanics during your workout, things that have a disastrous effect on power output. When you are misaligned, you down-regulate your ability to produce force (such as wattage on the bike) in an attempt to protect your body from damage (due to being misaligned).

## MOBILITY AND RESISTANCE TRAINING IMPROVES PROPRIOCEPTION AND MOTOR CONTROL, ALLOWING YOU TO PRESERVE MAXIMUM POWER OUTPUT WHILE FATIGUED.

Starrett explains, "We've seen up to a 30 percent decline in $VO_2$ max due to compromised breathing and a misaligned load anywhere along the spine during assorted endurance efforts. For example, cyclists, especially in the aero position, have radically hinged neck and shoulders, and that curved back position places a huge load on the lumbar spine.

They look like a dog taking a poo on the bike. When runners fatigue, they too become destabilized. The pelvis gets overextended and their man-bellies hang out. Mechanically, the nervous system becomes compromised and unable to generate maximum force or transfer energy into the ground, the pedals, or the water efficiently. Furthermore, when the eleven-pound head is destabilized and the neck is destabilized, the athlete defaults into a shallow, 'stress breathing' pattern. This over activates the sympathetic nervous system—the fight-or-flight response —and makes workouts more stressful than they should be, and more difficult to recover from."

*"Endurance athletes seem to care only about time, disregarding the important subtleties of spinal alignment, musculoskeletal mobility, breathing patterns, recovery techniques, and sleeping habits."*
— Dr. Kelly Starrett

Recovery is compromised because your body is still reeling from the tension caused by spending hours training in a misaligned position during the time it should be getting relaxation and restoration. The overstimulation of the sympathetic nervous system results in prolonged elevation of cortisol and excessive stress on the adrenal glands—fatal flaws for endurance athletes trying to manage their training amidst hectic daily schedules. Starrett mentions that many athletes grind their teeth at night, a sign of an over-stimulated sympathetic nervous system that can't calm down and enable sleep to happen smoothly.

After a busy day of life and training, the parasympathetic system— often called the "rest-and-digest" system, in contrast to the "fight-or-flight" sympathetic—should kick into gear and help you relax, unwind, digest and assimilate nutrients, and eventually transition comfortably into a good night's sleep. If you can relate to having more difficulty unwinding after a particularly stressful day at work, the same is true for unwinding after an unnecessarily stressful, misaligned workout.

Even if your session was enjoyable and comfortably paced, misalignment during the session overactivates and prolongs the fight-or-flight impact of the session. For this reason, Starrett recommends devoting fifteen minutes of each endurance workout to working on correct positioning and alignment. This might include those often overlooked running drills (such as hopping, high knees, or kickouts) that help your nervous system integrate and preserve correct form in the midst of fatigue. Similarly, exceeding aerobic maximum heart rate too often and training in a chronic pattern also promotes sympathetic dominance and eventual burnout. Meanwhile, the parasympathetic system can be stimulated by stretching, foam rolling, and massage therapy, all important big-picture elements of the endurance athlete's training program.

"This is why it's time to look beyond the straightforward training parameters and look at the subtleties of spinal alignment, musculoskeletal mobility, breathing patterns, recovery techniques, and sleeping habits to pursue performance breakthroughs," Starrett argues. "Whatever activity we are doing, we need to put our body in a position where it can generate the most force, and the most *mechanical ventilation efficiency*. Unfortunately, this stuff is subtle. You might not notice how your breathing is impinged or how you have super tight calves, because the immediate sensations of pain are not there. Instead, you just go home from races wondering why you keep getting beaten by your training partner!"

Starrett continues, "Resistance training and also complementary movement and mobility practices such as yoga, Pilates, CrossFit, kettlebells, and so forth, are essential for an endurance athlete. As you fatigue, you want to fatigue into safe mechanical positions and have your efficiency increase, not decrease. But unfortunately, when you fatigue, your proprioception gets blown out, so you don't even realize your technique is falling apart. I'll observe people in the gym, even world-class athletes, and say, 'Hey, your back is starting to round, better stop.' They don't even believe me—they have to see it on video!"

This is a compelling argument for a broader training regimen that develops motor control and proprioception over a narrow obsession with time and mileage. Going back to Starrett's driving example, hitting parked cars and blowing through red lights as a commuting strategy will eventually slow you down when your car breaks down or you have to answer to the police—injuries or burnout being the athletic corollaries here. Indeed, the current stats suggest lots of hit-and-run crimes are going on. Starrett says there are an estimated thirty million runners in America, and that 80 percent of them get injured in a given year. According to a *Runners World* magazine survey, 13 percent of runners experience knee injuries, 8 percent get Achilles tendinitis, 7 percent suffer hamstring pulls, 10 percent deal with plantar fasciitis, 10 percent have shin splints, 14 percent report iliotibial band syndrome, and 6 percent get stress fractures.

# "STRENGTH TRAINING ALLOWS YOU TO CONNECT THE DOTS AND IDENTIFY WEAKNESSES THAT CAN CAUSE YOUR FORM TO BREAK DOWN DURING AN ENDURANCE WORKOUT."

## —DR. KELLY STARRETT

When you do resistance training, you improve overall motor control and your ability to sense and make corrections when you break down under fatigue. As Starrett explains, "Strength training allows you to connect the dots and identify weaknesses that can cause your form to break down during an endurance workout. Loading positions makes the invisible, visible. Even doing basic assessments in the gym like a ten-minute squat test (yep, holding a squat pose for ten minutes) can identify shortcomings in your indigenous range of motion that can lead to injuries and compromised performance. If we can identify and improve these shortcomings and restore full range of motion, we can eliminate 99 percent of the reason for injuries and inefficiencies that compromise power. This is like free money for your endurance performance!"

## STRENGTH TRAINING DELAYS AGING

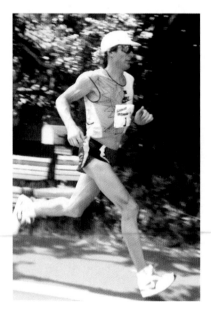

*Astute observers noticed Grip looking ever more jacked in the latter years of his career. Here he runs to the annual Gun Show at the Kailua-Kona Convention Center.*

While the improved technique, motor control, and proprioception benefits of strength training are relevant to the youngest bucks on the starting line, strength training is especially critical for endurance athletes over thirty-five years of age. It's widely accepted that sharp declines in explosive strength occur with chronological aging to a greater extent than declines in endurance. Endurance athletes seem to be able to build on years of base and continue to excel at the elite level all the way up to the big 4-0 and beyond, while sprinters and power athletes seem to peak in their twenties. While outliers occasionally prove this generalization wrong (swimmer Dara Torres, a 50- and 100-meter sprint specialist, won three silver medals in the 2008 Beijing Games at age forty-one—the oldest US Olympic swimmer ever), there are more cases of aging endurance athletes extending their careers.

Consider some legends of the Hawaii Ironman: Mark Allen winning six times in succession until he finally retired on top with his last victory at age thirty-seven; Australian Craig Alexander culminating a long career in the sport by winning his third

Hawaii title at age thirty-eight, breaking the oldest-winner record; and six-time Ironman champ Dave Scott coming out of a five-year retirement in the mid-90s to place second at age forty and then fifth at age forty-two. Ethiopian distance-running legend Haile Gebrselassie, after a long career on the track setting twenty-seven world records and winning six world championship and Olympic gold medals, set the marathon world record at 2h:03:59 at a reported age of thirty-five (but was possibly as old as forty!).

On the power end of the spectrum, science suggests that age-related muscle mass deterioration begins in most people around age thirty-five. The chronic and catabolic (muscle-wasting) nature of high-level endurance training exacerbates this decline in power. While an endurance athlete can get away with power declines more than an NFL football player or Olympic 100-meter sprinter, losing explosive power absolutely slows you down even when you go long. This is true for an elite as well as a five-hour marathoner whose hip flexors blow out at mile twenty, forcing him to waddle through the final ten kilometers.

Consequently, an aging endurance athlete who still wants to be competitive can benefit greatly from doing carefully structured high-intensity strength and sprint workouts to delay that inevitable decline in power. Especially if you are over thirty-five years old, you might seriously reconsider your longtime devotion to aerobic volume and instead transition into a program with more explosive strength and sprint workouts, fewer total hours, and more rest in general. After a decade or two or three of hard slog on the road, it's pretty easy to max out on your aerobic benefits, and preserve most of the functionality of your Tesla engine for more years than you think.

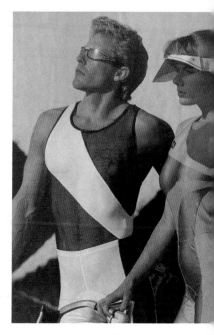

*Activewear modeling—a tough job but someone's gotta do it. And hopefully they spend enough time in the gym to fill out the lycra suit!*

As you age, you lose power more quickly than you lose aerobic capacity, so strength and sprint workouts are particularly beneficial for athletes over age thirty-five.

With performance declines associated with chronology becoming more and more relevant as you pass those decade milestones, you can fight back against slower times and increased injury risk by paying more attention to power and intensity—within the careful guidelines of periodization and stress/rest balance previously discussed. Mark Allen has mentioned frequently that he experienced great benefits from spending more time and energy strength training in the latter years of his career than when he was younger.

Here's how the hormonal benefits occur when you strength train: When you perform an intense strength session, micro-tears occur in the proteins that control the muscles' contraction. The damaged muscle sends a message to the brain that it needs some extra protein to heal the tears and rebuild itself even stronger in order to withstand a similar future assault.

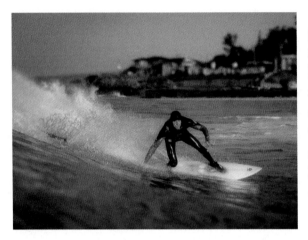

*Yes, that's Grip under the hood, "carving" a niche in his current favorite sport. He spent fifteen years pushing his body to the limits of human endurance on the lava fields of Kona, Hawaii, the mountains above Nice, France, and the trails of Boulder, CO, but preserved his strength and vitality from a stress-balanced approach.*

To supervise the rebuilding, the body dispatches an army of hormones, including the fountain-of-youth dynamic duo, human growth hormone and testosterone. Growth hormone, responsible for growing young bodies to adult size, helps glue adults' torn muscles back together and promotes youthful vitality at any age by regenerating muscle mass, bone, cartilage, hair, nails, and skin, stimulating deeper sleep, and even reducing body fat. Testosterone influences energy, motivation, mental focus, and libido, and also plays a critical role in recovery and the maintenance of an athletic body composition (promoting lean muscle mass and turbo-charging fat burning).

These so-called "adaptive" hormones are released in large doses during all forms of intense exercise. These hormones also decline with age—steadily in a best-case scenario, or precipitously if you engage in adverse lifestyle practices such as prolonged sedentary periods, chronic exercise, poor stress management, insufficient sleep, or a high-carbohydrate, high-insulin-producing diet. Hence, particularly for athletes over thirty-five, stimulating pulses of these important hormones through intense exercise can deliver a potent anti-aging, performance-enhancing effect.

Again, the sustained low-to-medium-intensity cardiovascular workouts that are your bread and butter provide an assortment of health benefits and disease protection, but they simply do not deliver a similar hormonal fountain-of-youth effect that brief, intense sessions do. In fact, they quite often deliver the opposite effect—a suppression of adaptive hormones when you drift into a chronic pattern. This is why even the emaciated Tour de France riders favor the same anabolic steroids (literally, a term for assorted artificial testosterone agents) that hulking bodybuilders and homerun hitters use.

# WHY STRENGTH TRAINING IS EFFECTIVE FOR ENDURANCE PERFORMANCE

**Resist Fatigue/Preserve Technique:** Like it or not, slowing down is a fundamental element of every endurance competition. In fact, many pundits like to clarify that the winner of an endurance contest is not the "fastest" athlete, but the one who *slows down the least.* Fatigue that causes you to slow down in the latter stages of workouts and races is always muscular rather than an exhausted cardiovascular system or a lack of mental focus. Your muscles weaken, your technique falters, and your power output diminishes. Then you get passed by the pack and start to lose focus!

With your proprioception "blown out," as Starrett says, when you're fatigued, you hardly realize that your technique is breaking down, or how to correct it. You just plod along, making noisier footsteps on the ground, bigger splashes in the water, or more herky-jerky pedal or oar strokes—an epic waste of whatever precious energy you have left in the latter stages of your performance.

High-intensity strength training will make your muscles more resilient against breakdown during endurance efforts. You can preserve good technique even as you fatigue, generate as much power as possible, and stay focused. Furthermore, with the improved proprioception you gain under load in the gym, you will also be able to better notice your form breakdowns and take corrective action to fatigue into the most efficient mechanical positions.

**Anti-Aging/Hormonal Benefits**: Endurance training is a high-risk endeavor for your hormones, due to the constant danger of drifting into a chronic pattern. Cortisol, the primary stress hormone that is elevated for too long in overtraining patterns, is the antagonist of testosterone, the primary vitality and anti-aging hormone. When cortisol is elevated, testosterone is suppressed. This delays recovery, accelerates the aging process, promotes the catabolization of lean muscle tissue, and even causes declines in cognitive function.

In contrast, brief, intense workouts stimulate a spike in testosterone and human growth hormone. Because they are over with quickly, they carry little risk of the catabolic effects of chronic endurance training. These brief spikes of adaptive hormones that happen in response to high-intensity exercise deliver an anti-aging, muscle-building, accelerated-fat-burning effect. Strength training gets you pumped up instead of worn out!

**Ventilatory Efficiency:** Being able to preserve a strong, stable spine position for the duration of your endurance efforts will enable maximum oxygen exchange from deep, diaphragmatic breaths, moderate the fight-or-flight response caused by being in inefficient spinal positions, and help you ease into recovery mode soon after workouts.

## WHAT KIND OF STRENGTH TRAINING WORKOUTS SHOULD I DO?

Hopefully you're convinced about the necessity of and the incredible benefits to be obtained from strength training. You also might be a bit confused, annoyed, or even intimidated by the prospect of picking up an entirely new fitness endeavor, especially when you get hit with all the questionable "bro-science" that pervades the muscle world. Don't worry, we are going to keep things simple and do-able for any endurance athlete who wants to make an honest effort to get stronger and more functional.

This chapter details two disparate approaches that will have excellent direct application to endurance performance and be easy to adopt and become expert in, even for a novice. The first one, the **Primal Essential Movements**, is a simple concept that entails lifting heavy things (Primal Blueprint law number four), even for just a couple of minutes at a time, on a regular basis in daily life. You can really ramp things up with formal thirty-minute workouts during your intensity-training phases, but you can still put in a baseline level of general everyday strength efforts when you are base building or even during your off season.

The second one is a more sophisticated strategy called **Maximum Sustained Power (MSP)** training. MSP training involves lifting heavy weights in the gym during carefully structured workouts designed to improve your maximum power and your ability to sustain maximum power even as you fatigue. If you are a novice to strength training, professional guidance is advised, but even MSP is scalable to all levels of ability. It's all about heavy weight, low reps, and a patient progression in degree of difficulty over time to build true explosive power, and power sustainability, with minimal risk of overtraining or injury.

## GROK'S STRATEGY—JUST LIFT HEAVY THINGS

Law number four of the Primal Blueprint lifestyle is "Lift Heavy Things." We need to lift heavy things regularly to optimize gene expression, delay the aging process, and also set ourselves up for success with endurance endeavors. Unfortunately, high-tech modern life has largely negated the necessity of putting our muscles under any form of significant load during the day. Unless we are in a unique job requiring an assortment of physical exertions, we can skate through our days without lifting anything heavier than a backpack, briefcase, or grocery bag.

YOUR CARDIOVASCULAR FITNESS CONFERS MANY HEALTH AND PERFORMANCE BENEFITS, BUT IT'S ONLY A SMALL SLIVER OF TOTAL FITNESS. IT'S TIME TO GO LOOKING FOR WAYS TO LIFT HEAVY THINGS!

It's great that we don't have to build our own huts anymore, but it's disastrous to your health to proceed through your decades without challenging your muscles under load. Your cardiovascular fitness confers many health and performance benefits, but it's only a small sliver of total fitness. It's time to go looking for ways to Lift Heavy Things—not necessarily weights in a gym or a home gym machine. You can become exceptionally strong using only your own bodyweight for resistance. Consequently, we present the Primal Essential Movements—four of the most simple and effective exercises ever known to humankind: **pushups, pullups, squats, and planks**.

Collectively, these exercises work all the muscles in your body and promote functional fitness for a broad application of athletic and daily life activities. These are movements our bodies have executed (in some semblance or another) on a daily, near-constant basis to promote survival for over two million years. They can be done virtually anywhere with no equipment (save a bar for pullups), with no expert guidance or knowledge required, and with little injury risk when done properly.

They can be done in an intermittent, fluctuating, and intuitive manner, where you always balance the effort expended with your energy level at the time. So on a busy day of work, travel, or a serious endurance session, you might drop for a set or two of pushups while watching TV and that's it. You know that tree branch along the side of your house, by the garbage barrel? How about establishing a rule that every time you pass by, you do at least one set of max effort pullups? How about agreeing to do a couple sets of planks to failure time for every twenty-two-minute show that you binge watch from your Netflix queue? Just make it part of your daily routine around the house and think nothing of it!

Endurance athletes deserve to do more of this kind of stuff, because it really, really adds up over time to something significant. Furthermore, it's easy to pat yourself on the back as you fill that logbook with big numbers and totally negate the importance of not only strength training, but regular everyday movement (detailed in Chapter 8).

Here are some suggested guidelines to implement the Primal Essential Movements: Lift something heavy most every day, even if it's just your weary body up to the pullup bar a few times. During the intensity phases of your training, where aerobic volume is reduced significantly, you can pay more attention to this edict and conduct a proper full-length strength session lasting twenty or thirty minutes (but no need to ever go longer than that, really!). If you are doing PEMs, this might entail two or three sets of maximum reps in each of the four exercises. Two full-length PEM (or other) strength sessions per week is plenty, even when you are focused on this type of training during the intensity phase.

Meanwhile, change your mentality that you have a stack of free passes to escape all other forms of exercise and movement besides your precious miles or hours of cardio, and start looking for small and large ways to challenge your muscles in daily life. This can include doing a set of twenty or fifty air squats or holding the plank pose for a couple of minutes at the end of a comfortably paced run or bike ride—just to improve motor control and stimulate the preservation or development of lean muscle tissue.

Realize that you can become strong without doing the prolonged, exhaustive workouts that most people associate with strength training. The muscle hypertrophy favored by bodybuilders indeed comes in response to prolonged exhaustive workouts, but hypertrophy (building more muscle fibers) is not synonymous with strength and power. Increasing your strength involves your brain and nervous system stimulating more of your existing muscle fibers to perform the work. Consequently, if you do a single set of pullups each day, you most likely won't get any bigger, but such a habit will definitely contribute to getting you stronger.

> Slight mobility or strength inefficiencies can add minutes to your finish time, at the *exact same energy expenditure*.

While you might question the relevance of your paltry time-to-failure in the plank position to improving your time in a 10K or a 70.3 triathlon, any shortcomings you exhibit in strength will compromise your proprioception, motor control, and ability to exhibit and preserve good technique, especially as you fatigue. For example, if you have weak core muscles as a runner, you might have a tendency to collapse your hips into the ground a bit with each footstrike, instead of preserving an elongated spine with a balanced center of gravity and an optimal footstrike that generates maximum propulsive force with each landing. A slight overstride pattern with an inefficient distribution of your center of gravity can literally add minutes to your time in a 10K or triathlon, at the exact same energy expenditure. Even a cyclist who doesn't have to worry about fighting gravity nevertheless requires a resilient and stable platform—the core musculature—from which the hips and thighs can power the pedals.

# PRIMAL ESSENTIAL MOVEMENTS: BASELINE STANDARDS AND PROGRESSION EXERCISES

In consultation with expert trainers, the Primal Blueprint has established a baseline mastery level for males and females for each Primal Essential Movement. Reaching baseline mastery indicates that you have a respectable level of total body strength, and are likely making a decent effort to lift heavy things in your everyday life. If you can't achieve each of the four baseline standards, you can conduct the PEM Progression Exercises. These are easier variations of the baseline Essential Movements. For example, doing pushups with arms resting on a bench or chair enables you to stimulate the identical muscle groups as a regular pushup while completing a substantial number of reps to get a good training effect.

Your first Primal Essential Movement workout will be an assessment session, where you see where you rank with each movement and determine the correct progression or baseline exercise to start with. When you reach a 20 percent improvement from your starting point with a particular progression exercise, you can attempt the next more difficult progression exercise, and continue to work toward the goal of eventually reaching the mastery level for each of the baseline PEMs. If you have reached mastery level in one or more essential movements, you can pursue more creative and challenging advanced level exercises, such as doing the PEMs with a weighted vest, or elevating the legs for decline pushups or planks.

Here are the baseline mastery standards for the Primal Essential Movements:

## Males
- 50 pushups
- 12 pullups (overhand grip)
- 50 squats
- 2-minute hold of forearm/feet plank

## Females
- 20 pushups
- 5 pullups (overhand grip)
- 50 squats
- 2-minute hold of forearm/feet plank

Here, briefly, are the progression exercises for each PEM, along with a performance standard that suggests it's time to move up to the next progression exercise. To see how to do each progression and baseline exercise with correct form, please go to YouTube and search "Pushup Progression – Primal Blueprint Fitness", "Pullup Progression – Primal Blueprint Fitness", and so on to see an assortment of instructional videos published on the MarksDailyApple channel. Even though these are simple movements, proper technique is essential to prevent injury and get maximum muscular benefits.

## PUSHUPS

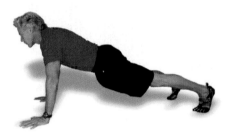

Easy: Wall pushup (standing, arms pushing off against wall—males 50, females 30). Medium: Incline pushup (hands pushing off chair or raised object—males 50, females 25). Advanced: Decline pushups or weighted vest pushups.

**Baseline pushup (on ground, arms extended and body in plank position).**

## PULLUPS

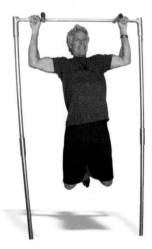

Easy: Chair-assisted pullup (one or two legs on chair, raise to bar using legs just enough to clear bar with emphasis on arm effort—males 20, females 15). Medium: Chin-up (inverted grip, raise to bar—males 7, females 4). Advanced: Weighted vest pullups.

**Baseline pullup (overhand grip, raise to bar).**

## SQUATS

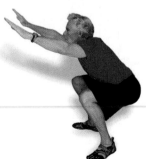

Easy: Assisted squat (hold pole or other support object, lower buttocks as far as possible to ground with spine straight and knees tracking in alignment with toes—males and females 50). Advanced: Weighted vest or barbell squats.

**Baseline squat (arms extended in front, lower buttocks as far as possible to ground with spine straight and knees tracking in alignment with toes).**

## PLANKS

Easy: Forearm/knee plank (Forearms and knees contact ground, body in plank position, hold till failure—males and females 2 minutes). Medium: Hand/feet plank (Arms extended, hands and feet contact ground, body in plank position *à la* pushup—males and females 2 minutes). Advanced: Spiderman planks (drive knee to touch elbow, then return to plank position—repeat till failure).

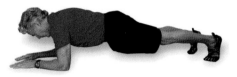

**Baseline elbow/feet plank (forearms on ground, aligned with shoulders, and feet contacting ground).**

While a suggested complete strength session is two or three sets of maximum reps in each of the four exercises, keep in mind that you can do any variation or abbreviation of a complete workout in the interest of lifting heavy things in daily life. Have some fun and take a morning to focus on a single PEM and try to do, say, one hundred pushups in the span of thirty minutes. Perform as many reps as you can until failure and then take brief or prolonged breaks (depending on what other stuff you're doing, like making morning phone calls) until you finally hit your number. Don't feel constrained by any rules about exactly how a strength-training session should look, and don't be afraid to just haul off and do a single set of a single PEM if you happen to pass a pullup bar or feel like hitting some squats while waiting for your teakettle to boil.

Hopefully this description of the Primal Essential Movements will lower that intimidating entry barrier to the world of strength training and allow you to get going and have some fun. Of course, you can explore assorted other strength-training options, such as home gym machines, health club stations, free weights, CrossFit workouts, or guided sessions with a personal trainer. Even a simple set of Stretch Cordz (a length of quality surgical tubing with handles on either end and a center that hooks onto a fixed object, like a doorknob) can deliver a fantastic full-body workout—and it fits into your carry-on luggage! If you have sufficient momentum and interest in breaking through to the next level of raw power and explosive strength, check out a revolutionary new strategy called Maximum Sustained Power Training.

## MAXIMUM SUSTAINED POWER TRAINING

Maximum Sustained Power (MSP) training is a program developed by Jacques DeVore, an innovative strength and conditioning and cycling coach with private gyms in Los Angeles and Santa Barbara called Sirens and Titans Fitness. It's a revolutionary approach that leverages decades of the best strength-training science and takes a logical, intuitive leap to deliver a beautiful complement to the aerobic sessions that form the foundation of endurance training.

Embracing MSP and other explosive, high-intensity strength work is an enlightened new way to view the endurance training paradigm. You are now attacking your performance goals from a new dimension—training for not just endurance but also for the development of more raw, explosive power, and the delivery of a higher percentage of maximum power for the greatest length of time, and the preservation of optimal technique while fatigued.

> YOU ARE NOW ATTACKING YOUR PERFORMANCE GOALS FROM A NEW DIMENSION: INCREASING MAXIMUM POWER, AND PRESERVING THE HIGHEST PERCENTAGE OF THAT POWER FOR AS LONG AS POSSIBLE.

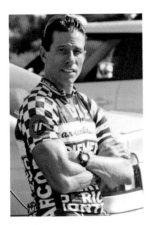

Southern California trainer and competitive cyclist Jacques DeVore, the innovator behind MSP training

The essence of Maximum Sustained Power training is to first improve your absolute power (e.g., your highest vertical jump in a single rep, or maximum weight you can deadlift for five reps), then conduct MSP workouts that help you *sustain the highest possible percentage of your absolute power for as long as possible, relative to your competitive event*. For example, an extreme power athlete like an Olympic shot putter gets six throws in competition. He or she summons 100 percent maximum power for only a split second, and repeats six times with plenty of rest between throws. And that's it—Olympics are over. On the other end of the spectrum is an ultra-distance runner or triathlete, who wants to sustain a lower percentage of a much lower maximum power level, but for a much longer duration, and with no break.

MSP workouts are appropriate for all types of athletes, but the nature of your MSP workouts should sync with the average power output and duration of your goal event. DeVore calls this the workout's *correlation coefficient*. An MSP session for a shot putter involves vastly heavier weights, fewer reps, and more rest than an endurance athlete's MSP workout. However, even an endurance athlete will deliver a highly explosive, short-duration workout lasting no longer than twenty minutes—even for an Ironman athlete!

To understand the MSP concept, let's discuss a sample workout consisting of deadlifts—lifting a weighted barbell from the ground to your hips. This simple movement is considered by many strength-training aficionados to be the ultimate full-body, compound exercise. If you are a novice, you'll start by learning correct form using nothing heavier than a PVC pipe, or perhaps an unweighted Olympic bar (typically forty-five pounds). Then, as you gain some practice in the gym with this strange new activity, you can work to improve your absolute power, best represented—for endurance athletes—by how much weight you can lift five times. This is safer than messing with one-rep max measurements, since these have little application to endurance performance and obviously carry a higher risk of injury. If you spend some time off the roads and in the gym, ideally under the supervision of a skilled trainer ensuring you exhibit excellent form, you will soon improve your best five-rep set deadlift from an embarrassing 80 pounds to a more respectable 180 pounds.

To conduct an MSP workout, you'll lift your new five-rep max weight 180 pounds three or four times, then rest for ten to twenty seconds. Then you'll do three more reps at 180, rest a bit, do two more at 180, rest a bit, do two more at 180, rest a bit, do two more at 180, rest a bit, then perhaps only muster up one rep on your final "mini-set." That, friends, is a beautiful Maximum Sustained Power workout! In contrast, consider the typical approach of trying to execute your five-rep max deadlift weight consecutively, with no rest break. You might hit five reps the first set, another five reps on the second set, and then be crapped out like a Vegas high roller.

By conducting mini-sets (where you stop before total failure) separated by rest breaks, you can lift significantly more total weight in the workout. It's kind of like doing four-hundred-meter intervals or mile repeats to get acclimated to fast pace running, instead of always running an exhaustive five-kilometer time trial for your speed workout.

In the MSP example described, the athlete lifts his 180-pound bar a total of fourteen times, in mini-sets of 4-3-2-2-2-1 reps (total 2,520 pounds). In the contrasting example, the athlete lifts the bar only ten times in full sets of 5-5 (total 1,800 pounds).

# IN MSP WORKOUTS, YOU "GO MAX OR GO HOME," BY DOING MINI-SETS WITH FREQUENT REST BREAKS.

That's a stunning 40 percent increase in what DeVore calls the "total overload" of the workout. Remember you are not lifting any more than your max of 180 pounds, but you are conditioning your body to lift this weight more times—to produce force at maximum for a much greater length of time.

It might be hard to imagine how such a brief workout can help drop your Ironman time from 13h:00 to 12h:21, but consider this: has your endurance performance ever suffered on account of cardiovascular fatigue? You know, running short of breath during your thirteen-hour Ironman or four-hour marathon? Of course not! From an ultra all the way down to a 5K, we have plenty of wind and plenty of blood supply to working muscles. The performance limiter is always muscular fatigue, or—if you prefer—central nervous system fatigue that results from repeatedly firing muscles that become overwhelmed trying to sustain the desired power output and duration.

So how does improving your deadlift (or other great MSP contributing exercises like squats, vertical jumps, or one-legged leg presses) translate to a faster marathon or Ironman? For endurance athletes, twenty-minute MSP workouts put your body under a similar load as you face when you've ridden for several hours and need to power up that final climb, or when you hit mile twenty on the marathon and need to hold it together on the final six miles. By training to deliver that brief explosive effort required to hoist 180 pounds again and again in that short MSP session, you will be able to plug along on your twenty-six-mile route, preserving correct form and generating the natural explosive propulsion that your Achilles tendon and other muscles and tendons can supply on each footstrike when they are not completely fried.

Theoretically, you could save massive amounts of time over a marathon—a minute per mile or even more—over a strictly endurance-trained athlete whose hip flexors start shutting down and calves start cramping up at mile twenty. Even for the top elite performers, it's difficult to replicate the state of your muscles at mile twenty or at hour eleven of Ironman. You just can't take yourself to that dark place very often in training! Similarly, MSP workouts might help you climb the third tall mountain of a Tour de France stage at a similar wattage output to what you generated on the first climb of the stage. First, with more baseline force production and subsequently more absolute power (e.g., going from lifting 80 pounds to 180 pounds), the early climbs (or early miles of a marathon) are less taxing, and second, thanks to MSP workouts, you can deliver a respectable percentage of that absolute power even as you fatigue.

Don't misunderstand: you absolutely, positively have to go long to stimulate adaptations in your central nervous system, cardiovascular system, and metabolic system in order to succeed in endurance sports. It's exasperating to read articles or listen to blowhards talk about how you can excel in endurance events with an assortment of hacks like intense plyometric sessions, low mileage, all-interval workout patterns, amazing nutritional supplements, visualization exercises, and other follies. There always seems to be an undercurrent of hype in the endurance world, of people trying to "hack" the reality that success is a product of smart hard work and adequate rest.

YOU ABSOLUTELY HAVE TO GO LONG TO STIMULATE TRAINING ADAPTATIONS, BUT MSP WORKOUTS HELP LIMIT DEGRADATION OF FORM AND POWER AS YOU FATIGUE.

Every elite performer in every endurance sport for the past fifty years has put in the major hours required to win, period. However, as Dr. Starrett alluded to earlier in the chapter, challenging the muscles you use during endurance efforts with short-duration, explosive efforts in the gym will limit the degradation of form and power output that occurs in everyone—even elites—over the course of sustained workouts and races.

## WHY MSP BEATS TRADITIONAL "BLENDED" STRENGTH WORKOUTS

Endurance athletes, as well as many recreational fitness enthusiasts at the gym, seem to favor what might be described as "blended" workouts—sessions that stimulate both endurance and strength energy systems. They take a moderate weight or resistance and perform around twelve reps to failure. With heart rate elevated into the anaerobic zone, they move quickly to the next workout station or exercise, carry on for a total of forty-five or sixty minutes (remaining anaerobic for long periods, due to only minimal recovery breaks between work efforts), and leave the gym feeling tired and depleted. Blended strength workouts are strategically and metabolically similar to doing a challenging tempo or interval workout. Tiring yourself out on the roads one day, and then doing so in the gym on a different day, can be risky for endurance athletes in particular. Can you say *overtraining*?

In contrast, Maximum Sustained Power workouts are much less taxing on the cardio endurance component and instead focus on going for max power or going home. Literally, you end your mini-sets when you can't lift the heavy bar again due to accumulated fatigue. Or, in the case of vertical jumps or calibrated exercise equipment, you stop the set when you fall materially short of your baseline absolute power performance standard that you started the workout with. Hence, mini-sets rarely last longer than a minute or two.

For example, if your vertical jump maximum is seventeen inches and you perform a bunch of mini-sets where you get up to seventeen inches a dozen times total (absolute max power), but then only get to fourteen inches on your next attempt due to accumulated fatigue, you shut it down. This is a key point. If you are jumping less than seventeen inches, or lifting less than 180 pounds in the previous deadlift example, then you are training at a submaximal level. This will not help you maintain maximum power longer and will turn your session into a blended workout. In MSP workouts, you don't fool around with diminishing power outputs where you get progressively more tired and generate less power or hoist lighter weights as the sets accumulate. You don't feel exhausted and depleted at the end, and you don't add unwanted muscle bulk as a consequence of these depletion workouts.

In essence, there are several major reasons why the traditional blended "multiple failures till exhaustion" sessions are less effective and more risky for serious endurance athletes:

**Overtraining**: Blended workouts are too similar to anaerobic time trial and interval work, thus bringing high risk of overtraining and burnout.

**Less Explosive:** Blended workouts limit improvement in pure strength and power, since you go to failure with lighter weights and are never truly explosive during these grueling sessions.

**Promote Bulk**: Blended workouts leave you in a depleted state, and the body responds during the recovery period by inducing muscle hypertrophy—the classic bodybuilding scenario of breaking muscle down to gain size. Endurance athletes don't need more mass, they simply need to improve the efficiency and explosiveness of their existing fibers, which is what MSP workouts accomplish. Rather than stimulating the addition of more fiber, the neuromuscular response of MSP workouts is to recruit more of the existing fiber that is dormant without this type of training stimulus.

**Injury Risk**: Technique errors and accidents causing injury are more common in fast-paced, exhaustive sessions. Reducing the weight or degree of difficulty and doing more reps till failure reduces the injury risk a bit, but makes the workout even more aerobic and less explosive.

**Stressful**: In isolation, long-duration, fast-paced, short-rest blended workouts deliver an excellent full-body fitness benefit for the typical exerciser. However, for those with sophisticated fitness goals, blended workouts interfere with aerobic development during base-building periods, challenge your immune and hormonal systems to the edge of burnout, and ultimately—for a serious athlete—promote mediocrity in both endurance and power.

*"Do you need a spotter?"*

*76, 77, 78... 87, 88??*

*"No, I need a counter..."*

# THE ORIGIN OF MAXIMUM SUSTAINED POWER TRAINING

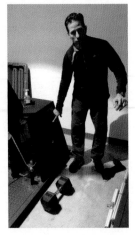

*Jacques at his Sirens and Titans Fitness center in Los Angeles, CA, patiently explaining MSP training to a skinny endurance geek*

Jacques DeVore came up with the idea of Maximum Sustained Power in the early 2000s when he realized that he couldn't match the weight of younger guys anymore. So he wondered, "What's the logic of three sets of ten reps to failure, anyway? Who said that's the right way to train?" He couldn't do ten straight 200-pound deadlifts in a row, but found that he could do five deadlifts of 225 pounds, rest a few seconds, then do five more—in the process racking up 250 additional pounds lifted, cumulatively, over the old seven or eight lifts of 200 pounds.

What about results? Well, DeVore noticed significant strength gains while doing squats, deadlifts, one-leg presses, and isokinetic jumps in this heavy, "maximum sustained power" style, which aligns with the traditional strength-building strategy of doing fewer reps with heavier weight. He also liked that it was a fun, logical, and engaging way to track his progress.

> "For strength development, harder isn't always better; *heavier* is better."          —Jacques DeVore

But when the longtime cyclist discovered he was also getting faster on his bike, he knew he was onto something that could be a game changer for endurance athletes. (Today, by the way, DeVore's deadlifts are up to over three hundred pounds.) DeVore explains, "It's simple: If you want better performance, you have to train in the gym at maximum output—not at sub-maximum output. That means to push very heavy weight, repeat-

edly, and to constantly strive to elevate both your baseline numbers and the total weight lifted at the workout—until you start to reach a natural limit relative to your competitive goals. This will deliver improvements in strength and subsequent improvements in endurance performance, and also maximize the hormonal, anti-aging benefits of the workout."

DeVore explains the practical application of MSP for endurance athletes. "Since endurance athletes are not competitive weightlifters, you don't need to worry about constantly increasing your baseline weight—once you get to a respectable level, that is. If you are a marathoner or triathlete playing around with 180-pound deadlifts, that's great. Going heavier offers diminishing return on investment (and more risk of injury) because of the long duration of your competitive event. Stick with a respectable but not crazy baseline weight, and focus your efforts on the MSP protocol. The mathematical application of MSP to endurance peak performance is simple: If you can increase your ability to sustain power by 10 percent, then times drop quickly. We see improvements between 5 and 15 percent in all of our endurance athletes who spend four to eight weeks training in this fashion."

# CASE STUDY: ROAD TESTING MSP WITH CYCLING GREAT DAVE ZABRISKIE

Dave Zabriskie, retired American professional cyclist and former Tour de France yellow jersey wearer, was one of the only elite professional athletes in the world to give MSP training an honest go, with excellent, but extremely underpublicized, results. He kept meticulous records of his improved climbing time trial performances while integrating MSP training for the first time, in the final season of his career.

Dave raced at the highest level of professional cycling from 1999 to 2013. A skilled time trialist and climber, he is one of only four Americans to wear yellow during the Tour, and the only American ever to win stages at all three of cycling's grand tours (Tour de France, Giro d'Italia, and the Vuelta a España). Since Dave's career coincided with the doping era in professional cycling, he took his lumps and served a six-month suspension in 2012–2013 for admitting to past doping practices. Coming off his suspension, Dave realized his days in the peloton were numbered, and that the doping-influenced training methods of the past would have to be replaced with an approach that was legal and effective.

Being an adventurous type of athlete with little to lose during his comeback, Dave decided to take a radical departure from the training methods favored in the highly traditional world of cycling, and decided to introduce MSP training to complement his requisite hours pedaling on the road. The results were astounding, but unfortunately have not become widely recognized because Dave's story—and career—ended with a crash that broke his collarbone and sent him into retirement.

Dave started working with Jacques DeVore in late 2012, while serving his suspension from pro racing. When he arrived at the gym, he had never lifted weights before (save for some occasional core work) and couldn't do a single pullup! "He was skeptical, but open to it since he had nothing to lose," DeVore remembers.

Along with his voluminous road work, Dave started strength training twice a week under DeVore's supervision. He kept at it all winter and made huge gains from his modest starting point. His maximum hex-bar deadlift weight went from 150 pounds to 245 pounds. His max single-leg press went from 210 pounds to 470 pounds. Without dieting, his weight dropped to 152 and stabilized in-season at 154–156, compared to his normal racing weight of 158.

This effortless default into peak body composition is notable for a professional cyclist because of the extreme effect that weight has on hill-climbing performance. These guys are obsessed with every gram that goes onto their machines and into their mouths, because it translates directly into a slower time up the mountain. It takes months and months of riding literally all day long and counting calories to carefully carve away those last few pounds of extra body fat in time for the start of the three-week grand tour stage race, yet here was Dave dropping effortlessly into the sweet spot during the off-season.

It's possible that the extremely high-intensity Maximum Overload workouts triggered an acceleration in metabolism without a corresponding increase in appetite. In contrast, long endurance sessions burn tons of calories and also stimulate a massive increase in appetite, because you are depleting your glycogen stores after pedaling for hours and hours.

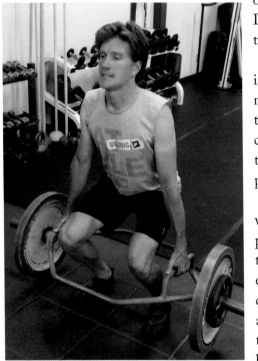

*DZ doing a bread-and-butter exercise of MSP: deadlifts (using a hex-bar)*

Dave's massive increases in raw strength combined with a lower bodyweight naturally improved his cycling performance, especially for climbing. His benchmark time trial was climbing a five-mile hill four times, with each ascent taking about twenty-five minutes. Um, don't try this "Tour workout" at home! Dave improved an amazing 18 percent after a devoted period of MSP training. He also produced over six watts per kilogram of bodyweight while riding at anaerobic threshold on the climbs. This value is simply power generated divided by body weight.

As detailed in Daniel Coyle's excellent book *Lance Armstrong's War*, watts per kilo at threshold is the single most critical metric that Tour de France cyclists use to determine with great accuracy whether they are fit enough to contend for the overall title when the going gets tough in the mountains. If you don't hit your numbers in training, you will not be able to hang with the big boys on the long climbs of the tour, period. In the doping era, the magic number for riders hoping to contend for the yellow jersey was 6.7: get that strong and that light or go home. For a clean rider to achieve a 6.0 value is exceptional.

Dave was primed for a huge 2013 season. The early-season Tour of Catalonia, a seven-day stage race in Spain, confirmed Zabriskie's improved fitness. The historically average climber held his own on the climbs and returned to the States psyched up for the Tour of California in May, where he'd finished second on four occasions. Sadly, a broken clavicle early in the Tour ended Dave's hopes for a win in his favorite race, and ushered in his retirement from the cutthroat world of professional cycling. However, to astute observers he proved something that has the potential to revolutionize cycling and other endurance sports: You can get into world-class form with the help of innovative strategies like MSP training.

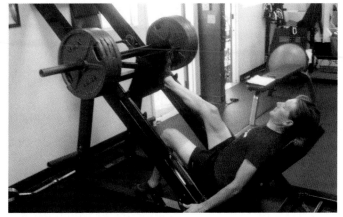

*DZ doing single-leg presses to promote balanced power output while pedaling*

What exactly did Dave do in the gym? Besides the deadlifts and single-leg presses (specifically single, in order to independently equalize each leg to optimize pedaling efficiency), he also did an assortment of upper-body exercises that involved pushing, pulling, and rotational core work, in all cases holding maximum output and power for as long as possible via mini-sets and frequent rest breaks.

Dave also worked with DeVore's unique isokinetic machines. These machines allow you to do vertical and horizontal squat jumps against resistance, and have a distinct application to cycling. Dave would do isometric jumps at a pace of two all-out jumps per ten seconds (two jumps, then eight seconds of rest until the next ten-second round), and ultimately progressed to six all-out jumps per ten seconds, continuing for six minutes straight.

The logic should be familiar by now: Dave was able to extend the time he could do maximum-output jumps because his early jumps got easier as he got stronger, saving more of his energy for the later jumps. That directly translated to his improved hill climbing on the long rides, as evidenced by his time trial performances on the repeated long climbs. DeVore's Sirens and Titans gym in Los Angeles definitely has some cool stuff, but obviously a good old barbell and plates for squats and dead lifts will work just fine too.

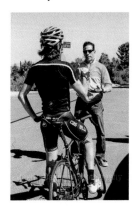

*Hard work in the gym translates directly to improved endurance on the road. DeVore consults with Zabriskie before he attacks some big climbs in Southern California.*

# HOW TO CONDUCT AN MSP WORKOUT

If you are new to strength training, enlist the services of a qualified trainer and start conservatively by lifting moderate weights and focusing intently on executing each lift with perfect form—even if it's just a PVC pipe. For power development, Jacques (and most other trainers) recommends the major full-body, functional strength exercises like deadlifts (his favorite for endurance athletes), squats, and single-leg presses. "These are your primary lower body strength exercises. Power exercises would be standing jumps, stairs (sprints or jumps), plyometric box jumps, single-leg explosive jumps, and Olympic lifts," explains Jacques.

"Strength exercises are easier to measure because you just add weight to the bar. Power exercises are ballistic and are measured in distance or height. This can be trickier but is still doable. You do not have to be exact. If the box you are using for your jumps is twenty-four inches and you can jump what seems like twenty-seven inches, that's okay. You just want to feel comfortable that you are delivering something close to maximum effort. These full-body, 'primal' movements recruit maximum amounts of muscle fiber and have a great application to complex real-life movements like swimming, paddling, running, or pedaling a bicycle. MSP is not about doing tons of mini-sets of bicep curls (not enough muscle fiber recruitment) or even bench presses (which have a relatively low functional component because you are lying down). Stick with the more functional moves that develop maximum explosive power throughout your kinetic chain," he concludes.

Once you gain basic competency, you will use weights heavy enough that you max out at five reps when fresh—where completing a sixth rep would seriously compromise your form or be difficult to impossible due to temporary muscular exhaustion. You can focus on a single exercise such as deadlifts for the whole workout, or do two or three exercises to compose a workout. Don't worry if you have limited equipment and can only do one exercise. DeVore reassures you that it's just about getting weight onto a bar and eliciting the hormonal and neuromuscular benefits of maximum sustained power training.

Take your time and enjoy gradual progression to some respectable baselines—increasing one-rep max deadlift from 80 to 180, or improving your vertical jump from eleven inches (dunking: ain't gonna happen) to a more respectable fourteen inches  (still no dunking, but an impressive 27 percent increase in maximum power). With respectable five-rep max baselines, you can proceed to proper MSP workouts.

**Rest Equals More Explosive Power:** Taking short rest breaks between each mini-set and taking long breaks between full sets gives you a sense of comfort that breaks are okay and always looming around the corner. The "permission to rest" concept is nothing to scoff at—this is a seriously important component of rest that goes beyond the obvious physical elements of allowing your heart rate, respiration, and muscle fibers to somewhat normalize before the next hoist. Whether it's delivering maximum explosive effort or prolonged endurance efforts, the central nervous system plays a big role in governing your performance. The mini rest breaks give you a chance to refresh your psychological and spiritual energy so you rekindle the desire to perform another set. Check out the Central Governor Theory sidebar to get a little deeper into the fascinating concept of how your brain governs your physical performance.

"MSP WORKOUTS EMPHASIZE FUNCTIONAL, FULL-BODY MOVEMENTS THAT DEVELOP MAXIMUM EXPLOSIVE POWER THROUGHOUT YOUR KINETIC CHAIN."

—JACQUES DEVORE

# THE CENTRAL GOVERNOR THEORY

Dr. Noakes's *Central Governor Theory* refutes the long-held notion that sensations of physical discomfort (e.g., lack of oxygen or burning muscles) are the main limiters of physical performance. He suggests that symptoms of fatigue are "utterly and completely illusory," that they are generated by your brain and "have nothing to do with the state of your body." In Noakes's model, your brain processes feedback from your body and generates symptoms of fatigue. This response helps protect your body against potential damage. For example, you slow down when exercising in oppressive heat, or stop lifting heavy weight after five reps, because your brain senses that you will, under the current conditions without rest, collapse from exhaustion or tear muscles to shreds. However, with fatigue, it only feels like we're going to die. "The actual physiological risks that fatigue represents are essentially trivial," says Noakes.

What's more, Noakes asserts that fatigue often worsens as you approach the finish line (or pre-designated finish point of a workout or a set of reps), not because the muscles are out of energy, but because your brain knows the finish or final rep is imminent. You feel like you cannot continue much longer, primarily because *you know* you are almost done and won't have to continue much longer! If you were still a mile from the finish line or had a drill sergeant screaming at you to complete twelve more reps or run a five-mile penalty loop in combat boots, your brain would delay the transmission of fatigue messages, and you would discover a magical second wind.

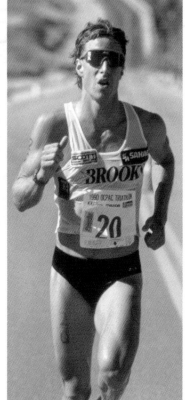

*Brad off the front in Mission Viejo, 1990. His central governor enjoys winning, and skillfully coerced his screaming legs to continue for one more mile to the finish. Later that summer, running along in 17th place in Cleveland, Brad's central governor directed him to a nearby taxicab for a ride back to the finish line...*

Along these lines, Noakes contends that the physiological capabilities of leading athletes are so similar that brain function is what separates the champion from the other contenders. He suggests that even a localized muscle tear is a brain-based phenomenon. Here's Noakes: "It's not the muscle tearing because it's weak, it's because the nervous system causes excessive activation of muscle fibers [because you are extending beyond your physical capabilities]. The fibers eventually go into spasm and as a consequence, the whole muscle goes into spasm to try to protect the area of damage."

Noakes believes that the outcome of a race (or any other activity) is what you believe it will be, and that you will use these illusory symptoms of fatigue as an excuse or explanation for the end result. For example, "Gee, my leg muscles were sluggish during this race. No wonder I ran so poorly." But the reality is your mind generated the symptoms, and more severely than they really needed to be, which gives you a ready excuse to justify your less-than-stellar performance. Saying something like "Oh, gee! I really tried my hardest, but I was exhausted," is not a statement of fact but a justification. Once you understand that most symptoms are generated by inner conflict instead of actual circumstances, you begin to realize how you can influence the outcome of an event.

Obviously, applying this "mind over matter" concept to your workouts has some nuances, as you might want to govern your central governor judiciously to avoid the overstress/burnout scenarios we have discussed at length. For example, if during a workout you start getting messages (from your muscles or your brain—maybe it doesn't matter who's knocking on your pain door!) that you are getting tired, it's wise to respect this feedback and put the weight down or not do any more intervals. Acknowledge that if your life depended upon it, you could go further by willing yourself to.

If you are at the magnificent peak performance race that you have trained months and months for and start to experience negative thoughts in the latter stages ("My quads are aching; I don't think I can stay with this guy much longer; Where the heck is the finish line?; Man it's hot today!; Why didn't I just sign up for the half?"), this might be a great time to get some inner dialog going that honors Noakes's assertion that "the outcome will be what you believe it to be."

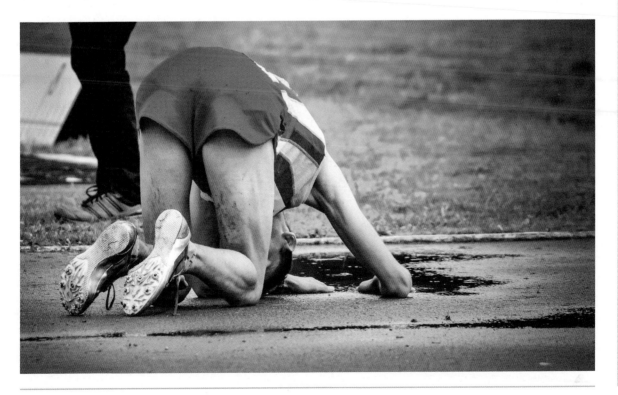

Mini-sets with frequent rest breaks keep you fresh and enthusiastic to continue performing at a high level and improving your maximum sustained power. Consider that carefully worded statement and see if it gets your endurance juices going a bit: "…*keeps you fresh and enthusiastic to continue performing at a high level.*" Sounds a lot like a magic formula for success in a marathon, half-Ironman triathlon, or long-distance paddle, doesn't it?

## FREQUENT REST BREAKS KEEP YOU FRESH AND ENTHUSIASTIC TO CONTINUE PERFORMING AT A HIGH LEVEL AND IMPROVING YOUR MAXIMUM SUSTAINED POWER.

If you can train yourself to generate explosive power again and again during an MSP workout, you will minimize the breakdown of technique and the decline in power that happen during the latter stages of an endurance event, and you will be more fresh and enthusiastic to continue performing at a high level for miles longer. While less easily quantified than increasing your maximum deadlift or your total workout weight lifted, there is a profound psychological benefit to the endurance athlete in going to that dark and mysterious place when you have to once again lift two hundred pounds after several such explosive efforts.

So, take the rest you need between mini sets, which will usually be ten to twenty seconds. If you go much longer than this then you can begin to lose the increased muscle recruitment that comes from being in a partially fatigued state. You might feel the urge to return to the bar after a quick pace around the mat—a ten-second break and you're re-focused and ready to roll. On your final segment, it might take thirty seconds to get pumped to go for it one more time. The idea is to come back to the bar or the apparatus feeling psyched and explosive. Go ahead and grunt, or chalk up your hands and clap up a cloud of dust if you need to.

It's not recommended to rest longer than twenty seconds between mini sets because you might lose some of the peak performance benefits of your elevated heart and respiration rate and the high volume of blood in the muscles you are challenging. The rest between sets can extend to at least 90 seconds and up to a few minutes if necessary. Bodybuilders believe that ATP regeneration takes 90 to 120 seconds, while creatine replacement in the muscle can take up to six minutes of rest. You want to feel as fresh as possible before going for another set of explosive efforts (don't worry, you'll get the blood pumping again after one mini-set!).

**Increasing Your Baseline and MSP Values:** Along with appropriate rest, another key MSP rule is to *never lessen the baseline weight* during a workout. The common strength-training strategy of doing a descending pyramid of weights (one hundred pounds, ninety pounds, eighty pounds, etc.) is worthless, according to DeVore. After all, he says, to make strength gains you need to *raise* the weight, not lower it. You want to train in your peak performance zone as long as possible, and avoid performing in sub-optimal performance zones.

That naturally raises the question: *When do you increase your baseline weight?* After a few good sessions, you might be able to go to eight or nine reps before temporary exhaustion in a baseline test. Alternatively, you might notice that the second and third segments of mini-sets don't decline much or at all from your initial effort (i.e., you can do five reps on your first, second, and third segments). In our example of a 180-pound deadlift, it's time to raise your baseline weight up to 200 or 220 pounds. Under this load, it's likely that you will be back at six-rep max and can proceed with an MSP workout accordingly, expecting a decline in reps as your mini-sets accumulate.

While DeVore points out that continually adding weight is unnecessary once you get strong, you might really get into this MSP stuff and make such great improvements over time that your typical workouts become too easy again and again. If this happens, strive first to increase weight instead of adding a bunch more reps or adding sets to extend the duration of the workout. Remember, you're already getting an A+ in endurance! If you continue to add weight over time and again hit a point where your typical workout feels too easy, you are either still progressing to an optimal baseline weight or you are spending too much time in the gym and not enough on the road!

At some point you should arrive at baseline weights or performance standards in the various exercises where you can perform highly effective, highly challenging short duration workouts. These MSP sessions will wonderfully complement your bread-and-butter endurance workouts, but not overwhelm your program in terms of energy expenditure and recovery time required.

GO MAX OR GO HOME! NEVER LESSEN THE BASELINE WEIGHT DURING AN MSP WORKOUT.

# CHAPTER SUMMARY

- Delay aging, optimize hormones
- Improve mobility and technique efficiency
- Beware wimpy "blended" workouts
- Go max or go home (MSP!)

The Primal Endurance approach to strength training focuses on developing **explosive power with brief, high-intensity, maximum-effort workouts.** This differs from the endurance athlete's typical strength-training strategy of engaging in "blended" workouts that develop both cardiovascular endurance and strength. Blended workouts are great for novice enthusiasts looking for a general fitness adaptation, but sophisticated athletes with specific performance goals can benefit from focusing on high-intensity workouts that develop explosive power, and are conducted with respect to the broader periodization principles of building an aerobic base, introducing short-duration intensity phases, and always balancing stress and rest.

Endurance athletes need strength training to improve proprioception and motor control, which happens when you place the body under more load than occurs during a typical endurance session. **Strength training allows you to identify and directly address technique and mobility shortcomings,** subtleties that might only be revealed during endurance exercise by form degradation and diminished performance. With improved strength and mobility, you can better notice technique breakdowns, **and fatigue into safe and functional mechanical positions.**

**Strength training also helps to delay the aging process by preserving muscle mass and explosive power,** both of which are believed to decline more quickly than endurance as you age. Strength training delivers profound hormonal benefits by stimulating brief pulses of "adaptive" hormones, like human growth hormone and testosterone, which deliver a potent anti-aging effect. In contrast, the prolonged stimulation of the fight-or-flight response that is common in **chronic endurance exercise can accelerate the aging process via the excessive production of the catabolic stress hormone cortisol.**

The Primal Essential Movements offer a simple, entry-level way to include strength training in your lifestyle. They entail conducting **pushups, pullups, squats, and planks** on a regular basis, with more attention to paid to formal workouts during the intensity training phases. Each Primal Essential Movement is scalable to all ability levels through a series of progression exercises (modifications to the baseline movement that make it easier to achieve the desired number of reps), that help you progress toward a level of baseline mastery.

Maximum Sustained Power (MSP) training is a novel approach that improves absolute power, and your ability to sustain the highest possible percentage of your absolute power for as long as possible, relative to your competitive event. **MSP workouts involve full-body functional movements like deadlifts, squats, leg presses, and vertical jumps.** MSP workouts feature **heavy weights, few reps, and more rest.** By doing a succession of mini-sets, you **"go max or go home."** Once you fall significantly short of delivering maximum power, the set or the workout is over. MSP is appropriate for all athletes, from highly explosive to ultra endurance, but workouts are designed to have a strong *correlation coefficient* to your competitive goals. Even for ultra athletes, workouts need not last more than twenty minutes.

The **typical endurance athlete's "blended" sessions featuring light weights, high reps, and performing multiple failures till exhaustion, carry a high risk of overtraining**. Blended workouts can interfere with aerobic development, fail to improve explosive power, promote unwanted muscle bulk, and carry a high risk of injury. Endurance athletes with already impressive cardiovascular development can benefit from focusing on short-duration explosive workouts and build endurance through sport-specific activity.

# SPRINTING

*The ultimate primal workout to optimize gene expression and deliver massive performance breakthroughs in minimal time*

## IN THIS CHAPTER

For endurance athletes, a little bit of sprinting goes a long way. The occasional short-duration workout, performed only during high-intensity training periods, can generate exceptional improvements in endurance performance. Sprinting improves cardiovascular function, helps muscles buffer lactic acid, and extends "time to fatigue" markers at all intensity levels. Sprinting elicits a spike of adaptive hormones into the bloodstream, delivering a potent anti-aging effect. Sprinting improves resilience to physical (muscle contractions) as well as psychological fatigue, allowing you to go longer and faster during endurance efforts. Sprinting, especially high-impact sprints (running), strengthens muscles, joints, and connective tissue. Finally, sprinting can get you over the hump with difficult body composition goals by turbo-charging fat metabolism around the clock.

Deliberate and focused warmups are essential to ensuring a safe and effective sprint workout. Endurance athletes might have to adjust their mindsets to minimize the importance of suffering and enduring and instead focus on delivering high-quality explosive performances, only when they are 100 percent rested and motivated for peak performance.

Each sprint you perform should be of *consistent quality*—a similar measured performance and perceived exertion level. If you slow down significantly, or have to work significantly harder to maintain the same performance standard, it's time to end the workout. A good general recommendation for endurance athletes is a sprint workout consisting of five repetitions of fifteen-second sprints. Rest intervals vary, probably from thirty seconds to one minute, with the main goal of ensuring you are rested and psyched for the next rep!

Stacking an MSP strength training with a sprint session can deliver performance benefits via the concept of *postactivation potentiation*. You literally "pump up" your muscles and central nervous system by challenging muscles under load prior to sprinting.

Conducting an effective sprint session entails picking the right day (rested?), the right exercise (high impact, unless injury risk or sport goals dictate otherwise), a deliberate, focused warmup, the appropriate number of work efforts, reps, and rest intervals, a deliberate cooldown, and finally recovering completely before the next sprint workout.

. . . . . . . . . . . . .

**BELIEVE IT OR NOT, SPRINTING** does have a place in the picture for endurance athletes and even ultradistance endurance athletes. By sprinting, we're talking about all-out efforts, short in duration and performed only occasionally. When you properly integrate sprinting into your program, you enjoy an assortment of health and fitness benefits as follows:

**1. Fitness Boost:** Improving your all-out explosive performance stimulates profound physical changes that have a direct application to performance at lower intensities. Modern research confirms that the health and fitness benefits of sprinting in many ways surpass the benefits of cardiovascular workouts that last several times as long. Sprinting improves capillary profusion and mitochondrial biogenesis—building a bigger engine for use at all intensities. Sprinting turbocharges the oxidative enzymes that burn fat and glucose, enhances oxygen utilization and maximal oxygen uptake in the lungs, improves the ability to store and preserve glycogen, improves muscle buffering capacity (the ability to process and eliminate lactic acid and other waste products from the bloodstream), and extends the "time to fatigue" marker at all levels of intensity. After only a few sprint sessions, you'll be lighter, faster, more explosive, and more comfortable at whatever pace you perform at.

**2. Anti-Aging Effect:** Occasional short bursts of maximum-effort sprints trigger a cascade of positive neuroendocrine, hormonal, and gene expression events that deliver a potent anti-aging effect. The spike of adaptive hormones like testosterone and human growth hormone that occur in response to sprinting stimulates lean muscle development or preservation, accelerated reduction of excess body fat, increased energy and alertness, enhanced insulin sensitivity, improved lipid profiles, and increased mitochondrial biogenesis. Sprinting also improves cognition and elevates mood by decreasing inflammation in, and improving oxygen delivery to, the brain. High-impact sprinting (running) helps to increase bone density and strengthen bones and connective tissue.

Sprinting stimulates an immediate and significant spike in cortisol, but this is an example of a genetically optimal activation of the fight-or-flight response to support an extreme effort of brief duration. Scientists call the positive effects of a brief natural stressor like sprinting *hormesis*. Our genes expect occasional short-term shocks, which we can adapt to and become stronger from. Cold-water plunges, relaxing in a sauna or hot tub, or getting some exposure to direct sunlight all deliver a hormetic effect at the proper dosage, but—like chronic exercise—can be unhealthy when excessive.

## A SINGLE THIRTY-SECOND BIKE SPRINT BOOSTS GROWTH HORMONE LEVELS BY 530 PERCENT OVER NON-EXERCISERS' BASE LEVELS.

Once a brief sprint workout concludes, cortisol levels moderate, while the so-called "adaptive" hormones (testosterone, human growth hormone) circulate in the bloodstream and target specific organs to promote enhanced health and vitality and deliver assorted anti-aging effects. Adaptive hormones help preserve or increase lean muscle mass, reduce excess body fat, enhance cellular repair and regeneration, and increase bone density and libido. Testosterone is elevated for fifteen minutes to an hour after intense exercise, while growth hormone, produced in the pituitary gland, sticks around for twenty-four hours. That's plenty of time for both agents to effect a host of positive changes.

A 2003 study in *Sports Medicine* lauded the hormonal benefits of intense exercise in general, while taking an indirect dig at chronic exercise: "...the impact of some of the deleterious effects of aging could be reduced if exercise focused on promoting exercise-induced growth hormone response." A 2003 study in the *Journal of Clinical Endocrinol-*

*ogy and Metabolism* said, "…the beneficial effects of intense exercise can mimic the effects of (artificial) HGH treatment." Indeed, a study in the 2002 *Journal of Sports Sciences* showed that a single thirty-second cycling sprint increased growth hormone levels by 530 percent over non-exercisers' base levels. "The harder you work the more you produce," is the message of a 2002 University of North Carolina-Greensboro study in the journal *Sports Medicine*, which found that greater intensity of both aerobic and strength training stimulates greater release of HGH.

Testosterone, produced in the testes of males, is considered the quintessential male hormone. However, it is also produced in the ovaries of females and has a similar vitality effect, even though females have only about one-seventh the amount circulating as do men. As you probably know, these vitality hormones decline with chronological aging—the effects of this decline pretty much represent the essence of aging—so you might be particularly interested in nurturing healthy circulating levels of these hormones through exercise and other lifestyle behaviors once you hit the big 3-0 and beyond.

Females might be a little taken aback reading about the importance of their testosterone (and might consider a new quip to yell out the window when victimized by aggressive drivers). Interesting research cited by authors Ashley Merryman and Po Bronson, in their outstanding book *Top Dog: The Science of Winning and Losing*, indicate that testosterone's beneficial effects extend far beyond the narrow layperson view that it increases aggression. Merryman elaborates on this concept: "Testosterone is primarily a social hormone, providing the motivation for behaviors that are most valuable—under whatever particular circumstances you are facing—to bring you social status and approval. Sure, sometimes that's aggression—especially when your social status is being threatened. Other times a testosterone spike can fuel focus, or cohesion within a team.

Testosterone is about more than just aggression; it provides motivation for behaviors that are most valuable to your particular circumstances; it can fuel focus or team cohesion, too.

"For example, when paramedics and firefighters work in an emergency situation, testosterone motivates the firefighter to rush into the building, save the people, and then go back and try to save the goldfish too. For the paramedic, testosterone enables him or her to stay conscientious while treating a victim, taking meticulous notes to assist the doctors when the patient arrives in the emergency room."

**3. Resilience to Physical and Psychological Fatigue:** Sprinting trains your brain to become more resilient to fatigue, lowering the rate of perceived exertion at all intensities. It's like jumping up for the rim ten times while wearing ankle weights, then taking them off and jumping again. You feel like you can fly! This is not superficial commentary; the psychological resilience you develop while sprinting literally makes your competitive pace of five-minute, six-minute, or eight-minute miles seem easier. We've mentioned Dr. Noakes's Central Governor Theory a few times, and it applies here as well. When you train to become competent at maximum output, even for a very short time, you are firing not just your hamstrings but the neurons in your brain—making them more adept at sending signals to generate explosive force and more resilient to fatigue.

But let's not discount the hamstrings! Over a decade ago, Jens Bangsbo of the University of Copenhagen published research popularizing the idea that muscle fatigue during exercise is primarily caused by a depletion of the minerals sodium and potassium in the muscle cells. Muscles need an electrical charge across the cell membrane to contract effectively, and this requires sodium outside the cell and potassium inside the cell. Sodium-potassium pumps in the cell membranes ensure high concentrations of each mineral and efficient recycling of potassium back inside the cell after each contraction. The sodium-potassium pumps are fueled by ATP, the familiar energy source for muscles during activity.

When you challenge muscles with maximum-intensity contractions, such as when sprinting or strength training, pumps become more effective, leading to improved endurance. Triggering the fight-or-flight response will also turbocharge the sodium-potassium pumps, bringing literal significance to the term "pumped up." By the way, it's believed that muscles can contract at maximum force for only around thirty seconds before fatiguing, so your sprint efforts should never exceed thirty seconds—otherwise they are not really considered sprints. This characterization is similar to the commentary about MSP workouts, where you want to "go maximum or go home."

**4. Stronger muscles, joints, and connective tissue:** When you put your body under the intense load of sprinting—demands of up to 30 MET, and in the case of running fast, generating five to six hundred pounds of impact force per stride (a thousand pounds if you're Usain Bolt!)—your body responds during the recovery period by strengthening those moving parts. If you can sprint safely, your injury risk when running at low intensity drops substantially. Obviously, this benefit is maximized when you are doing weight-bearing activity like running. However, even if you're doing low- or no-impact sprinting (rowing, cycling, swimming, cardio machines), you are still generating much greater forces than during a typical endurance workout, and building more resilient muscles, joints, and connective tissue.

**5. "Nothing cuts you up like sprinting":** This is Mark's favorite spicy, but dead serious, reply at Q&A seminars when people ask how to overcome stalls in weight-loss progress. Even if you are fully fat-adapted through diligent primal-aligned eating, honoring your natural appetite to eat only the calories you need to feel satisfied, and putting in substantial training hours, genetic predispositions and homeostatic drives make it difficult to lose those final few or dozen stubborn pounds. Enter sprinting. Performing at 30 MET sends a strong adaptive signal to your genes to pare away any unnecessary weight—again, to prepare for future (perceived as life-or-death) maximum physical efforts.

While carrying excess pounds through a 70.3-mile triathlon or a 26.2-mile marathon is no fun, extra non-functional weight presents an exponentially greater hindrance to sprinting performance. Watch sprinters perform at a meet or on TV or YouTube and you will quickly realize there is no such thing as excess body fat in their world. It's simply impossible to train and perform at an elite level (or even a moderate level, like quality college or high school athletes) with excess body fat jiggling along at over twenty miles per hour. Conversely, it is commonplace to see excess body fat crossing the finish line of a triathlon, marathon, or ultramarathon. In a landmark 1994 study published in the journal *Metabolism*, researchers found that short, intense bursts of exercise zap considerably more fat than sustained aerobic activity. The explanation, according to Dr. Mark Hyman, the author of *Ultrametabolism: The Simple Plan for Automatic Weight Loss*, is that your mitochondria, the little engines in your cells that burn calories and create energy, run hotter all day after intervals. You metabolize fat at an accelerated rate for up to twenty-four hours after a sprint workout, according to a 1985 study in the *American Journal of Clinical Nutrition*.

We're not talking about totally revamping your program and your competitive goals and running out to buy spikes and a form-fitting body suit. The idea here is to integrate just a bit of sprinting into your game and enjoy huge fitness benefits. You conduct sprint sessions only during intensity phases, and only when you feel 100 percent rested and energized to deliver a maximum effort. The total duration of your sprint workouts, including warmup and cooldown, will be no more than twenty minutes, with the work efforts totaling up to only a handful of minutes.

## SPRINTING ACCELERATES FAT METABOLISM FOR UP TO TWENTY-FOUR HOURS AFTER A WORKOUT.

Believe it or not, going out and doing four to six hundred-meter sprints is a perfectly respectable workout for an endurance athlete. That's only a couple minutes total of hard work, and the entire session might take only fifteen to twenty minutes. A workout like this will elicit the aforementioned spike of adaptive hormones, turbo-charge fat metabolism, and condition the brain to become more comfortable with lower-intensity endurance efforts, but it won't blow out your stress hormones for three weeks like a block of excessive volume or black hole intensity zone training will. It also won't ruin your work productivity that afternoon like a grueling 5:30 a.m. Master's swim session of 4,500 meters might.

Despite the extreme physical effort, you should feel pleasantly pumped after a sprint workout. You probably won't feel like going out for a fifty-seven-mile bike ride in the hills right afterward, but you can definitely go about your daily business. You'll likely feel some moderate to significant next-day muscle soreness, especially early into your sprinting practice, and should consequently take a day or two of recovery, where you either don't exercise beyond walking, or are certain to keep your heart rate in the recovery zone of 65 percent of maximum heart rate or lower.

It's important that your Type-A, endurance-oriented brain approaches sprint sessions with the proper perspective. More is not better when it comes to sprinting—and that goes for workout frequency as well as number of repeats. The goal is to signal optimal gene expression and the profound physical and psychological adaptations that come from 30 MET efforts.

## CHILL LIKE USAIN—SPRINTING MINDSET AND WORKOUT GUIDELINES

Sprinting comes with a high risk of injury, especially if you are a novice and even if you are highly experienced. The first and foremost rule is to only attempt these sessions when you feel 100 percent rested and energized to deliver a maximum effort. If you have low energy at rest, elevated stress factors in daily life, lingering soreness, or injury hot spots, don't even consider sprinting until you are champing at the bit with a green light on all systems checks.

Besides the injury risk, central nervous system fatigue is a major factor in sprinting, as well as high-intensity strength training. It's a major effort for the brain and the nervous system to fire those muscles at maximum capacity and produce maximum force, even for only a short time. You can definitely burn out on high-intensity training, just as you can with chronic cardio, if you aren't extremely vigilant about not only muscular fatigue (soreness, weakness), but also central nervous system fatigue.

CENTRAL NERVOUS SYSTEM FATIGUE IS A MAJOR FACTOR IN SPRINTING; BE SURE YOU ARE MENTALLY REFRESHED AND FOCUSED FOR EACH WORK EFFORT.

Sprinting in a pre-fatigued state not only risks poor performance and muscle damage, but literally slows down your central nervous system's messaging process, according to a study by periodization guru Tudor O. Bompa, PhD, in his book *Periodization Training for Sports*. That means that even if you run the same speed as usual, your fatigued body can't accurately process that effort fully, so you don't get as much benefit from the session as you should. It's like studying your tail off to score 100 percent on a test, but only getting credit for 90.

Technically, here's how sprints improve you: When you sprint, you force the billions of neurons of your central nervous system (CNS) to process messages and motor responses faster and more accurately. Information signals are transferred from muscle to brain to muscle by moving from "receptor" cells to "effector" cells through the CNS. To move the body as fast as possible when sprinting, the speed of this signal itself also needs to be super-fast in order to recruit the optimal amount of fast-twitch muscle fibers for the job. Therefore, an athlete's receptors and effectors need to be primed for action—"optimally excited and uninhibited," explains Bompa.

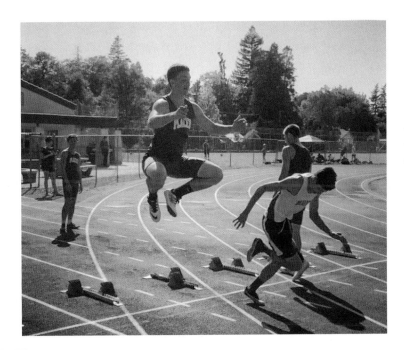

Owen "O-train" Scott, an elite California high school sprinter and running back, primes his central nervous system for maximum effort with explosive hops. Thanks to his efficient warmup, he threw down an 11-flat 100 meters after the photo was snapped.

The trouble is that fatigue will slow down the ability of the receptors and effectors to get excited and uninhibited, particularly those within fast-twitch fibers, which fatigue much more rapidly than the oxidative slow-twitch fibers that power aerobic workouts. Bompa says you can identify central nervous system fatigue by the subjective sensation of "quickness." If you feel quick and springy, this indicates you're rested and ready. Check out sprinters as they assemble in their lanes before receiving the command to enter the blocks. Nearly all of them perform the same preparatory exercise of a series of explosive jumps in the air, where they bring their knees up high as if trying to land on a plyo box. If your feet feel too slow in leaving the ground as you run, your speed in lifts is lagging, or your ability to hit a tennis ball or other sports skill is off, you probably are fatigued.

When you feel rested and ready to go, it's imperative to create a carefully structured, high-quality workout, featuring an optimal warmup period, preparation drills that reinforce good technique and get the central nervous system excited and uninhibited, a main set of all-out efforts with plenty of rest to ensure *consistent quality* of the efforts (details shortly), and finally a deliberate cooldown to smoothly transition back to a resting state. This will minimize the stress of the session and promote a speedy recovery.

# THE IMPORTANCE OF ADEQUATE WARMUP BEFORE HIGH-INTENSITY WORKOUTS, ESPECIALLY SWIM STARTS!

The endurance athlete mindset is more calibrated to going long instead of going fast and explosive. Warming up properly is of minimal concern when you are heading out for a twenty-miler, but unfortunately many endurance athletes warm up insufficiently before hard workouts and races. While it's true our primal ancestors didn't warm up before those chance life-or-death encounters with saber-tooths, they also didn't sit at a computer screen for hours prior to their physical efforts. Preparing for an intense workout requires a serious warmup, especially if you are coming out of a prolonged inactive state, as with morning workouts.

The term "warmup" has a literal connotation, as the most important element of preparing for activity is elevating body temperature and shunting more blood from the torso area (where it is concentrated in the vital organs at rest) and into the extremities, where it is needed for exercise. If you just do a few minutes of light cardio exercise of any kind, you will get the heart rate and body temperature up, and direct blood into the extremities. Then you want to commence further warmup activities that are directly related to your upcoming max efforts. For strength training, you can do some specific movements to engage the muscles in question, such as arm circles, air squats, or gentle trunk rotations, then transition into doing the exact activity with really light weight—such as squatting or deadlifts with an unweighted bar, or vertical jumps onto a lower platform.

Warming up properly for a high-impact sprint session requires that brief cardiovascular exercise to start, followed by extensive dynamic stretches and drills that prepare joints and muscles for sprinting. These sequences, which all elite sprinters engage in without fail prior to maximum-effort sprinting, serve to further elevate body temperature and increase bloodflow to the extremities. They also optimize joint mobility, reinforce proper sprinting technique (e.g., a "high knees" running drill), and focus the mind for the hard work ahead. These mental aspects of proper warmup before

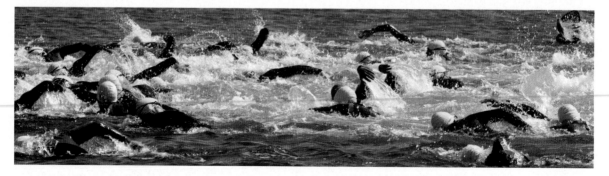

*Proper warmup before intense exercise will improve performance, lessen the stress impact of the workout, and reduce injury risk. Before a swim race, it could save your life!*

a peak performance effort are relevant for enthusiasts of all levels, as a deliberate sequence of mindful drills and stretches ensures optimal focus, boosts confidence, and heightens motivation and arousal in anticipation of the peak efforts.

"Warmup" has a literal connotation: you want to elevate body temperature and move blood from the organs to the extremities.

Here is a checklist of sensations associated with a proper warmup:

*Temperature elevated*: Your skin feels warm and a bit moist, and your respiration is increased. When your muscles heat up, they receive blood and nutrients more efficiently, enabling them to contract faster and more powerfully.

*Fluid:* Creaky joints become lubricated and stiffness subsides as your warmup gains momentum. Make sure that your warmup movements are precise and do not unduly stress joints. Particularly with rotations of the spine, you should never compress discs during a stretch or drill, nor add extra force or resistance beyond the natural pull of gravity.

*Focused:* The psychological components of a proper warmup are critical, especially for high-intensity sessions. Going through the deliberate motions of drills or light resistance activities primes your central nervous system to respond optimally to the forthcoming more difficult efforts.

*Dynamic:* All your pre-workout preparations should be movement oriented. If you feel the need to perform a static stretch, find another way to engage the joints or muscle groups with movement. For example, foam rollers (stiff foam cylinders that provide resistance for muscles to roll against) have become popular tools for warmup, recovery, and injury prevention. Static stretching is most appropriate for after workouts, or in the course of a prevention or rehab prescription from a physical therapy professional.

Insufficient warmup is especially disturbing before swims, and is a likely contributor to the alarming number of triathlon swim deaths in recent years. Over forty swim deaths have occurred in triathlon events in the United States since 2006. All of these fatalities had a mysterious cause. The victims had adequate swimming ability, and ranged from novice triathletes to highly experienced and competitive.

According to Rudy Dressendorfer, PhD, a longtime exercise physiology professor and world-level age group triathlon competitor, the combination of insufficient warmup and immediate demand for high-intensity performance in the swim start shocks both the body and brain. The sudden exertion along with physiological changes due to immersion, often in cold water requiring a restrictive wetsuit, promote shortness of breath that can lead to swim failure and unconsciousness. In contrast, a swimmer who is warmed up adequately acclimates their body and brain to the cold water, the tight wetsuit, and the physiological changes to become race ready. Warming up can help you perform better in a sprint workout, but it can save your life if done before a triathlon swim start.

WITH SPRINTING, THE FOCUS SHOULD BE ON
PERFORMING INSTEAD OF SUFFERING. TAKE YOUR
TIME TO ENSURE A PROPER WARMUP, SUFFICIENT
REST BETWEEN EFFORTS, AND A GOOD COOLDOWN.

Sprinting effectively requires that you switch hats and lay aside many of the principles that frame your endurance workouts. Intervals, tempo sessions, and time trials are distinct workouts with different objectives from a true sprint session. These anaerobic endurance sessions, with work efforts ranging from one to ten minutes on minimal rest intervals, are designed to get you comfortable with performing at or near your anaerobic threshold—as you would when racing for an hour or longer. You are training your brain and body to keep pace despite lactate accumulating in the bloodstream. You have to bear down, stay focused, and stay with the group despite your legs and lungs begging for respite.

With sprinting, it's time to don your Usain Bolt cap and think about *performing* instead of *suffering*. Here's a guy who will travel across the globe and pack a stadium full for a single glorious effort lasting less than ten seconds. Not a bad way to earn a few hundred grand, eh? With your sprint workouts, take your time with careful warmup and drill preparations, and adequate rest between work efforts—just like MSP sessions in the gym. Have some fun stretching in the sun, chatting with your workout mates, and generally operating at a relaxed pace instead of worrying about workout duration on the stopwatch, mileage on the GPS, heart rate zones, and how much raw work you can squeeze into whatever time you have allocated for a workout. Leave the toys and the OCD noise at home and go to the track or chosen venue focused on opening up the throttle and having some fun!

*Brad hanging out with—okay, photobombing—some Olympic gold medal sprinters during their track workout at UCLA. These elite athletes spend two or more hours at the track most every day. They'll deliver only a handful of total minutes of serious hard work, while the rest of the time is devoted to jogging, stretching, mobility exercises, preparatory drills, chatting with Brad, and generally moving at a leisurely pace, except when the coach blows the whistle for another repeat!*

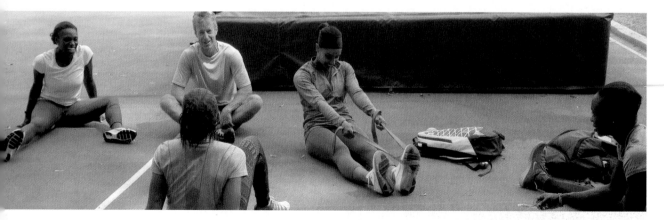

Along those lines, if you feel a twinge in your hamstring or other signs of suboptimal function, pull the plug on the session like a true Olympian. Yep, sprinters pull out of their races all the time, even as late as when they settle in the blocks, take a couple practice starts, and feel a small disturbance in their motor patterns. Just like a jet airplane or a rocket ship, these finely tuned explosive performance machines will not operate unless every single check light comes up green.

## DELIVERING A *CONSISTENT QUALITY* WORKOUT

Since the focus with sprinting is on developing explosive power, the duration of the recovery interval (how long you wait to start your next effort) should be sufficient enough for respiration to return to near normal, and for you to feel mentally refreshed enough to tackle another effort. It is common for athletes even at the elite level to experience mental fatigue along with physical fatigue during a difficult all-out sprint session, due to the incredible demand that all-out efforts place on the central nervous system. Consequently, in addition to physical markers such as respiration rate and muscle fatigue, you should be vigilant about mental fatigue. If you have difficulty focusing, concentrating, or even keeping your balance during a walk recovery interval, this is an indication that the nervous system is fried and that further sprint efforts are unwarranted.

*Consistent quality* means your sprints should be similar in both measured performance and perceived effort level. If you slow down or struggle, it's time to end the workout.

Each sprint should be similar in both measured performance (e.g., time over a certain distance) and perceived effort level. Consider the example of a sprinter deciding to conduct a workout of five times hundred-meter sprints at consistent quality of performance and effort. On her first effort, she covers the length of a football field in twenty seconds. Full recovery should be taken by walking and light jogging (perhaps back to the original starting point at the opposite end of the field) until respiration returns to near normal. Each subsequent effort should be delivered at a similar effort and also be around twenty seconds.

As the workout proceeds, a *slight* attrition in performance (slower time) is allowable and expected. In this example, the measured performance is the time it takes to run the length of the field; perhaps this athlete will clock twenty-one seconds on her third and fourth efforts. Measured performance can also include running or cycling uphill for twenty seconds and trying to make it to the blue house on the right each time, or performing on calibrated fitness equipment in the gym (e.g., cycling for twenty seconds at 25 mph or at a certain wattage output).

As physical and mental fatigue accumulate, it will be difficult to deliver a consistent quality effort on subsequent sprints. In the runner's example, a couple of scenarios might unfold after working hard on four efforts: First, delivering another twenty-one-second clocking will require significantly more effort—blowing out their engine with an "eleven" effort on a scale of one to ten, just to try and hit twenty-one again. This is not advised because it can result in exhaustion, extended recovery time, overstimulation of stress hormones, and increased risk of injury.

The ideal sprinting strategy is to deliver a *controlled* maximum effort—preserving your form, rhythm, and focus for the duration of each effort—not face-planting at the finish line. The second scenario is that another run at consistent effort will result in a substantially slower time than twenty-one seconds. When effort level is maintained but performance drops off markedly, it's a sure sign that it's time to end the workout and thereby preserve its quality and intended training effect.

Sprint workouts are not meant to be a steady march to exhaustion. The romanticized image of an athlete puking trackside after pushing through an extreme sprint workout is not aligned with optimal gene expression or sensible fitness progress. *Consistent quality* should be the foremost goal of your sprint sessions. Even if you don't measure your time or performance carefully, it can be very effective to regulate your perceived exertion on each effort so that your last effort isn't vastly more strenuous than your first, and to be aware of any attrition in performance (slowing down from fatigue).

As you get fitter, aspire to increase speed rather than add more repetitions

Remember, sprint workouts are always supposed to be challenging, high-quality efforts—there is no such thing as a "moderate" or "light" sprint workout! If you notice on your first couple of sprint efforts that your body isn't responding in the expected manner due to fatigue, you should end the session and attempt another sprint session when your energy and motivation levels are optimal. If you learn from experience that times drop off after the fourth or fifth repetition as in the aforementioned example, you can design future workouts with appropriate target times and number of reps.

As your fitness progresses, you should aspire to *increase speed* rather than add more repetitions. The sprinter doing five times a hundred yards in twenty seconds may one day improve to seventeen seconds for five efforts, but there is no need to ever escalate to ten repetitions. Going for quantity instead of quality will increase the risk of entering a chronic pattern and compromise the intended purpose of these types of workouts. As mentioned in the MSP discussion, you don't want to get into a "blended" workout situation where elements of endurance start entering the equation—too many reps, not enough rest, and so forth.

## BLENDING MSP WITH SPRINTS? TRY IT OUT!

If you currently have a high fitness level and some good sprinting experience under your belt, you can try an advanced strategy of stacking a sprint workout immediately after an MSP workout in the gym—a practice called *postactivation potentiation (PAP)*. PAP suggests that loading your muscles with heavy weights before a sprint workout primes the central nervous system to deliver a superior effort, so you get greater motor unit recruitment and force production during your sprinting. You become "optimally excited and uninhibited" before you even step onto the track, and we're not talking about getting up the courage to chat up the cutie running the stadium stairs that day! The turbocharging effect of PAP can last for up to thirty minutes in a well-trained athlete. For novice athletes, the effect might only last for five minutes before the body becomes debilitated by fatigue. Hence, it's obviously not worth experimenting with PAP until you are quite fit.

Research suggests that PAP works in two ways: First, after doing maximum voluntary muscle contractions (MVC) in the gym, the proteins in your muscles become more responsive to calcium ions released in the sarcoplasm (muscle cell environment) when muscles contract. This enables greater force production for longer duration, since the calcium ions hang around after these MVC efforts. Secondly, PAP helps to increase the efficiency and rate of nerve impulses delivered to the muscles via the spinal column, something known as the H-Reflex.

As you might surmise, this PAP stuff is really more the domain of explosive power athletes like sprinters and high jumpers. However, studies using triathletes and distance runners suggest that PAP workouts can help improve resistance to fatigue in the muscle groups they train with these workouts.

Experiencing a successful stacking of workouts confirms the important role the central nervous system plays in athletic performance. We tend to think in the narrow dimension of the muscles or the lungs doing all the work and then getting tired, but it's actually a complex interplay between the central nervous system and the peripheral elements (e.g., muscles, lungs, heart) that it directs like a symphony conductor.

Another fun example comes to mind here with ankle weights. Remember decades back when these Velcro cuffs first appeared on the scene and became all the rage? Runners or jumpers would strap on a set of five- or ten-pounders and then perform several jumps to the rim or sprints down the track. Then, when the artificial burden was removed, you experienced not only a psychological boost, but an actual performance boost. Indeed, guys who could never dunk would finally throw down, thanks to postactivation potentiation. The athlete can actually jump higher or run faster thanks to the increased efficiency and rate of nerve impulses delivered from the brain to the muscles in response to the extra resistance of the ankle weights.

## POSTACTIVATION POTENTIATION DELIVERS A "TURBOCHARGE" EFFECT TO YOUR MUSCLES AND CENTRAL NERVOUS SYSTEM FOR UP TO THIRTY MINUTES, ENABLING AN EFFECTIVE "STACKING" OF WORKOUTS.

Again, an adjustment in mindset is necessary to convince yourself that vigorous preparatory efforts won't make you tired, but rather prime the pump for maximum efforts. This is why the aforementioned world-class sprinters spend two hours at the track to deliver only minutes of maximum effort. They have the patience to do a leisurely warmup jog, engage in extensive stretching and mobility work, do a set of technique drills, recover, do a moderate sprint set such as practice starts (running for only fifteen to twenty meters), recover, and then and only then get into some meaty stuff. This is followed by more jogging, stretching, mobility work, and deliberate cooldown efforts. Yes, it helps to get the blood flowing and muscles warm before going hard, but there is much more to it than that. Elite power athletes also understand the importance of preparing the brain for maximum efforts.

Stacking strength and speed workouts has the additional benefit of allowing for more recovery time, since your high-intensity efforts are performed in a compressed window of time. Recall the example of Brad stacking his two most difficult endurance workouts of the week on consecutive days, then taking it easy for the next four days. This type of stress and rest balance might be more difficult if you adopted the conventional approach of, say, an MSP workout on Tuesday and a sprint workout on Thursday. Now, if you are intuitive and disciplined, both approaches can work just fine. My main point here is that stacking hard workouts is not taboo, and in fact might deliver some performance and recovery benefits.

# CONDUCTING AN EFFECTIVE SPRINT WORKOUT

Recall that an anaerobic period must never last more than four weeks, and that Dr. Phil Maffetone suggests that best results come from anaerobic blocks of only two to three weeks. Inside that anaerobic period you may aspire to deliver some killer gym sessions as well as race-preparatory anaerobic endurance sessions like tempo sessions, intervals, and time trials. Recall that the Primal Blueprint recommends sprinting only once every seven to ten days, and only when feeling 100 percent rested and motivated. That means you are not going to be doing a whole ton of sprinting over the course of a year, which is fine. A little sprinting goes a very long way, while a little too much can be dangerous and destructive.

If you are like most endurance athletes and have paid little mind to sprinting to date, let's start with a simple protocol to complete a safe, fun, and highly effective workout:

**Pick the Right Day:** Like the rocket or jet airplane analogy, make sure all systems are go before you even head out the door. First, this means high scores on the energy, motivation, and health tracker mentioned in Chapter 2. Second, this means you are respecting the periodization approach, have successfully built an aerobic base, and are in a brief high-intensity training period—a period characterized by significantly reduced training volume and with a focus on peak performance and extensive recovery.

**Pick the Right Exercise:** Running is the most beneficial type of sprinting because its weight-bearing nature enhances the cutting up effect and the bone density effect. If you have an insufficient general fitness base or significant injury concerns that preclude you from fast running, or have sport-specific competitive goals (e.g., cyclist, winter sport, or water sport athlete), you can certainly benefit from low- or no-impact sprinting. If you fall in the middle of the descriptions listed, you can choose uphill running sprints or sprinting in sand to lessen impact trauma but still develop your fast running abilities.

Here's an important caveat to mention if your sport is indeed low or no impact: you can sprint much more frequently than mentioned previously throughout the book, as these comments and guidelines are framed from the perspective of sprint running, with the high-impact trauma and consequent extended recovery time. All competitive swimmers sprint at virtually every workout. Competitive cyclists—even lower-level amateurs—include sprinting in their workouts several days a week, and obviously can race day after day in the grand Tours. Whatever your sport, it's critical to respect the periodization principles, but when you have an intensity period, you can proceed in accordance with the best practices in your sport.

**Warmup**: As described previously, get your mind and body ready for the main event with a deliberate, focused warmup. For running, this includes an assortment of technique drills that help ingrain good form and further prepare your muscles, joints, and connective tissue for the forthcoming maximum efforts. Following are some images of good dynamic stretch warmup drills for sprinting.

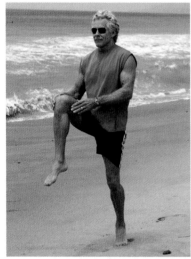

*Knee-to-chest:* Gently pull knees up to chest and release.

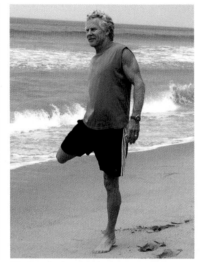

*Pull quads:* Grab foot and pull gently to butt, release with forward step.

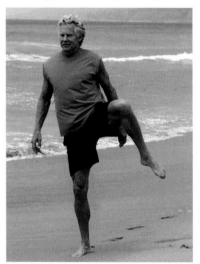

*Open hips:* Face forward, rotate knee up and along body line. Great for hip flexors.

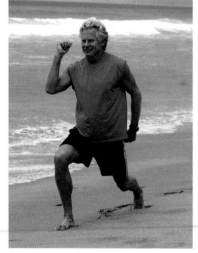

*Mini-lunge:* Take exaggerated-length steps, front thigh nearing parallel. Don't overdo this one; it's just a warmup!

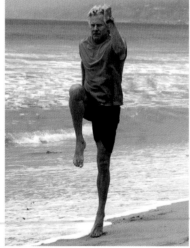

*Hopping drill:* Get the heart going now! Drive knee to chest while jumping up and forward, arms pumping. Land on same foot, repeat hop with other knee.

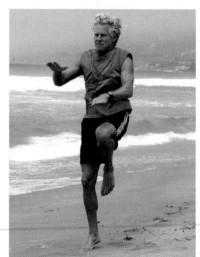

*High knees:* Toughest one last, almost ready to open the throttle and sprint! Exaggerate knee lift by slapping hands. Preserve tall, straight body, drive knees high, quick stride turnover. Remember these identical tips for actual sprinting!

**Choose Appropriate Work Efforts:** Sprints can last anywhere from ten to thirty seconds. This is little rationale for endurance athletes to attack sprints of less than ten seconds. Metabolically, these efforts burn pure ATP and are more applicable to athletes training for explosive sports like football, or the jumps, weight throws, and sprints in track and field. Max efforts from around eight seconds up to thirty seconds burn lactate for fuel, while going over thirty seconds kicks you into glucose burning. As stated previously, "sprinting" for over thirty seconds is not really sprinting; workouts with longer work efforts are categorized as intervals, tempo runs, time trials, or whatever. Here, we're gonna go max or go home. Consequently, try starting with efforts lasting around fifteen seconds. Perhaps this equates with a fixed distance, like a half, two-thirds, or full length of a football field. Having a finish line to reach every time will help with your efforts to deliver consistent quality sprints—same duration, same distance covered, same effort scale.

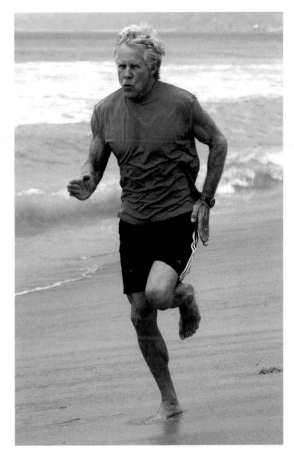

*Mark likes to perform a novel session on the packed sand as follows: 10 strides cruising, 10 strides fast, 10 strides all out. Each sequence takes around 30 seconds— repeated six times. If you are concerned about impact, hard or soft sand is a great option!*

**Choose Appropriate Rest Intervals:** With the aforementioned goal of delivering a consistent quality of sprint efforts, the main variable for your rest intervals is to ensure you are sufficiently refreshed and energized to deliver a consistent quality effort with each successive sprint. Your rest period should be sufficient enough for respiration to return to near normal, and for you to feel mentally refreshed enough to tackle another effort. Forget about stimulating any training effect from shortening your rest period and jumping into another sprint—save this type of training stimulus for interval workouts.

Besides getting your respiration under control and muscles refreshed, you should also be vigilant about recovering from mental fatigue during your rest periods. Sprinting places an incredible demand on the central nervous system; you might benefit from just walking around and staring off into space before even thinking about your next sprint.

If you have difficulty focusing, concentrating, or even keeping your balance during a walk recovery interval, this is an indication that the nervous system is fried and that further sprint efforts are not neces-

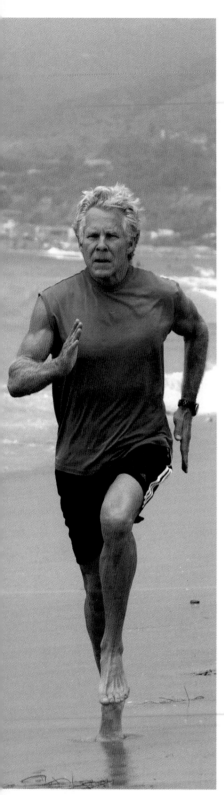

sary. All told, you will likely find yourself resting between thirty seconds to one minute between sprints fifteen seconds long.

**Choose Appropriate Number of Reps:** How many sprints to do? How about starting with five and seeing what happens? If you can only deliver a consistent quality effort for three, then that's where you are right now. You can deliver a couple or a few quality sprint sessions and add additional reps over time. No matter who you are, all you ever need to do is six sprints of fifteen seconds, or perhaps four sprints of twenty seconds, or some similar combination of the two different sprinting times. The rest of your workout progression and application of increased fitness will be directed at going faster, not doing more, and not resting less.

**Conduct Appropriate Cooldown:** Pretty simple instructions here. You simply want to gradually transition from an active, pumped up, highly stimulated state to a resting, calm, relaxed state. Abrupt transitions in either direction—jumping right into a tough workout or jumping right into your car after a tough workout—overstress the delicate fight-or-flight response. Make the workout easier on your body and speed recovery by winding things down gradually.

When you complete your final sprint, keep moving slowly for at least five minutes, jogging if you were running or otherwise doing the same activity—easy pedaling, stroking, or swimming. When you feel your body temperature and your sweat rate start to regulate a bit, you can stop moving. Of course, your heart rate and other metabolic markers are not going to regulate for many hours (and that's a good thing, as discussed with sprinting's impact on fat metabolism), but you want to pull back from pedal to the metal at least to the 55 mph highway speed limit.

**Recover Completely:** The Primal Blueprint recommends sprinting only once every seven to ten days, and only when your mind and body are fully rested and energized for peak performance. A good sprint workout takes at least forty-eight hours to recover from, so structure your strength workouts accordingly so that you can have a couple of easy aerobic recovery days after your sprint sessions. Again, these timeframes relate to running sprints. If you do low- or no-impact sprinting, you can recover much faster—probably in a single day—and perform more sprints during your high-intensity training periods.

# CHAPTER SUMMARY

- **"Nothing cuts you up like sprinting!"**
- **30 MET event = genetic adaptations**
- **Lower perceived exertion, delay aging**
- **Deliver consistent *quality* efforts**

Sprinting offers an assortment of benefits for endurance athletes. First, you get a fitness boost: more mitochondria, enhanced fat burning, increased lung function, improved lactic acid buffering, improved glycogen storage, and extended "time to fatigue" at all intensity levels. **Sprinting delivers a potent anti-aging effect, actualizing the "use it or lose it" maxim. The desirable short-term fight-or-flight stimulation elicits a flood of adaptive hormones (testosterone, human growth hormone) into the bloodstream**; you have more energy, improved body composition, improved blood profiles, improved oxygenation of the brain, and generally improved focus and vitality for a variety of peak performance goals.

The extreme difficulty of **sprinting builds improved resilience to physical and psychological fatigue when performing for longer duration at lower intensity levels.** Sprinting enhances the efficiency of the sodium-potassium pumps in the muscles. Consequently, your muscles can fire longer and stronger during endurance performances, and you have lowered perceived exertion so your pace feels easier too. Sprinting strengthens muscles, joints, and connective tissue by teaching your body to absorb much heavier loads than during endurance exercise. Even low- or no-impact sprinting builds more musculoskeletal resiliency. Finally, sprinting can help you break through plateaus with body composition goals. **The extreme shock of performing at 30 MET (Metabolic Equivalent of Task) sends a strong adaptive signal to your genes to shed excess body fat,** because excess weight is an extreme hindrance to sprinting performance.

For athletes with endurance priorities, **sprinting is best done only occasionally, only during high-intensity training periods**, and always balanced with extensive rest. Sprinting in a pre-fatigued state will destroy the intended benefits of the workout and increase overtraining risk. Beyond the familiar muscular fatigue, endurance athletes must be mindful of central nervous system fatigue associated with sprinting.

**Proper warmup is critical to optimize sprinting performance, reduce injury risk, and minimize the stress impact of the workout**. An optimal warmup elevates body temperature and respiration rate, lubricates joints, and gets the brain focused for the hard work ahead.

Endurance athletes might have to adjust their "suffer and endure" mindsets when it comes to sprint workouts. Instead, **strive to deliver a *consistent quality* sprint workout, which means that each effort is of similar measured performance and perceived exertion**. If you slow down significantly on a successive rep (a little slowdown is okay, but not a big drop), or during a successive rep it seems significantly harder to maintain a similar measured performance (e.g., running the straightaway in fifteen seconds), it's time to stop the workout.

Pursuing the goal of consistent quality will inform the optimal number of reps and the optimal amount of rest to take between reps. A general recommendation for endurance athletes is to **do**

**five sprints of fifteen seconds and rest for thirty to sixty seconds between reps.** Duration of rest intervals is intuitive, with the emphasis on feeling refreshed and energized for the next sprint effort.

An advanced strategy of *postactivation potentiation* entails performing high-intensity strength training prior to sprinting to promote greater force production and resistance to fatigue during the sprints. PAP primes the muscles to contract more forcefully, and gets the central nervous system "optimally excited and uninhibited" for sprinting (or any other explosive effort). In well-trained athletes, the PAP effect only lasts for up to thirty minutes. Novice athletes attempting PAP may become exhausted quickly, so PAP is best for those well adapted to explosive workouts. Be careful getting too tired during PAP workouts or you could fall on your face while sprinting and suffer a PAP smear...

The steps to conducting an effective sprint workout are as follows: Pick the **right day** (100 percent rested and energized); pick the **right exercise** (high-impact sprinting delivers the best weight loss and musculoskeletal benefits, but low- or no-impact sprints might be more appropriate, and still beneficial); complete a deliberate and focused **warmup**; choose the appropriate **work efforts** (ten to thirty seconds); choose appropriate **rest intervals** (intuitive, thirty to sixty seconds to ensure you're refreshed for the next effort); choose appropriate **reps** (five is a good start, and may be good forever—just get faster!); conduct appropriate **cooldown** (gradual transition from peak state to resting state lessens stress impact); and finally, **recover** completely before your next sprint workout.

# PRIMAL ENDURANCE
# SUCCESS STORIES

*Real-life primal endurance athletes*
*are killing it—here's how you can join them!*

**7**

We know that primal eating helps anyone lose excess body fat, increase energy, delay aging, and improve disease risk factors. We have literally hundreds of success stories, replete with stunning before/after photos, archived at MarksDailyApple.com. We have tens of thousands of user experiences reporting dramatic fat loss, often after lifelong struggles following conventional messages. Slowly but surely, mainstream authorities are admitting that carbs are the main problem of our fat society—not fats, as long believed.

Hopefully the previous chapters have given you a sense of the proper strategic approach to lose excess body fat, improve performance, speed recovery, and protect your health following the primal approach. Nevertheless, I can appreciate if you and your training partners have a little resistance to trying a low carb strategy, since it's so opposed to endurance tradition. And I can understand your hesitancy to hear "trust me" on this matter, especially if you've already plunked down your $85 entry fee for that season-culminating Ironman event (well, Hawaii cost $85 the last time I did it—has the price gone up?). Instead, we will strengthen the impact of the Primal Endurance message by meeting the following real-life athletes who have succeeded with a primal-aligned approach.

**Rich Airey:** A runner, triathlete, and CrossFit coach who went primal and became faster and leaner than ever, even as he pushes forty!

**Zach Bitter:** A fat-burning freak, with the highest rate of fat oxidation ever seen in the lab. Broke the American record for the hundred-mile run as a fat-adapted ultrarunner.

**Larisa Dannis:** Improved assorted injury and inflammation problems by going primal, and ran a 2h:44 Boston Marathon!

**Johnny G:** The fitness icon who invented Spinning indoor cycling was one of the first athletes to experiment with fat-fueled endurance performance when he completed the 1989 solo Race Across America (RAAM)—the old-school solo, non-stop format—in ten days.

**Matt Hart:** A fitness coach and ultrarunner who overcame lifelong asthma and allergies through dietary modification to win the Tahoe Rim 100 at the age of thirty-seven.

**Rob Hogan:** World champion professional Speedgolfer rewired his appetite hormones to eliminate sugar cravings not only during long runs but in daily life. Behold the unforgettable "Fanta story."

**Sami Inkinen:** Won the Hawaii Ironman world championship in 2011, rowed from California to Hawaii in 2014—an absolute cutting edge performer in fat fueled endurance and unique, time-efficient training methods.

**Ted McDonald:** Yoga teacher went from pre-diabetic to multifaceted ultra athlete, achieving performance breakthroughs with a total mind/body approach and a primal-aligned eating style.

**Timothy Olson:** Won the prestigious Western States 100-Mile Endurance Run two years in a row while eating a low-carb, primal-style diet. He cured lifelong digestive problems while his wife cured her juvenile rheumatoid arthritis through dietary modification.

**Dr. Klemen Rojnik:** A Slovenian Ironman triathlete who improved his Hawaii Ironman time by thirty-eight minutes in one year by going low carb.

These athletes succeeded because they stayed committed to a novel new way of eating and training long enough to reprogram their genes to transition away from inefficient sugar burning to highly efficient fat burning—even when they perform at the impressive speeds seen at the elite level. Reprogramming your genes to prefer fat for fuel will give you a boost during a friendly community mini-triathlon, but when you imagine how the body is tested during an extreme event like a hundred-mile endurance run, the difference in metabolic stress and performance potential is astronomical. Guys like Sami Inkinen, Timothy Olson, and Zach Bitter are racing their Teslas against a field of DumbCars.

The training and lifestyle habits of the elite endurance performers are always the major catalyst for a paradigm shift in the community as a whole. It's a completely sensible prediction to say that within five years, the best endurance athletes—pros and amateurs alike—will be fat-adapted and even ketogenic performers. As the level of competition escalates, marginal improvements in performance matter exponentially more than they do in the middle of the pack. For example, dropping from a four-hour marathon to a three-hour marathon requires a whole new level of commitment and hard work, but it's within reach of most four-hour marathoners. Even if they still have a bunch of training and lifestyle flaws, they can put in some extra miles or implement some focused aerobic base building and chop off huge chunks of time. To drop from a 2h:10 marathon to 2h:07 is a whole different story. Here, the tiniest improvements in workouts, sleeping habits, and dietary patterns must be scrutinized in the quest for an extremely minimal (by comparison to four hours versus three) improvement in finishing time.

If you aren't terribly interested in making the Olympic team, or even the podium, in the near future, it's important to remember the primary benefit of fat-adapted endurance training: *it's healthier!* Transitioning from carbs to fat will minimize the inflammation and oxidative damage caused by carbohydrate dependency and high volume endurance training. However speedily, or patiently, you complete your workouts and races, you'll have a longer, healthier, more enjoyable, more successful career using the wonderfully clean burning and highly efficient solar power plant we saw in the Chapter 1 illustration.

## PRIMAL PIONEERS: WINNING ON LOW-CARB

Let's meet the first wave of stars to fuel world-class wins on low-carb diets.

**RICH AIREY:** A lifelong athlete and bi-coastal running, triathlon, and CrossFit coach from New Jersey and San Diego, Rich keeps improving even as he pushes forty. Rich was a champion distance runner in college and continued to compete at a variety of distances from track races to ultras after graduation. Meanwhile, he was building a unique coaching business that integrates traditional running coaching with sophisticated strength training through a program called RunningWOD (workout of the day). Over the past seventeen years, Rich has coached over thirty high school

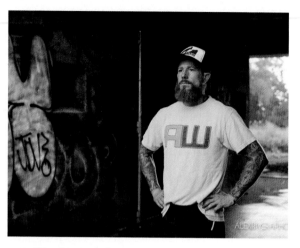

All-American runners, NCAA qualifiers, and Olympic Trials qualifiers.

Rich was thirty-six when he first transitioned to a primal-style eating pattern. Within a year, he delivered his best results ever—a second place 50K finish in 2012 and third place at two trail marathons in 2013. Best of all, when he replaced gluten, dairy, pretzels, Gatorade, and "other garbage" with almond butter, coconut oil, and fruit, he slimmed down to his high school waist size (28 inches) and weight (135 pounds).

Rich explains that the benefits of his primal-style eating extend beyond the race course. "As my diet and my mood improve, I have a greater appreciation for healthy living, and a deeper appreciation for the idea that time is fleeting. You want to maximize your time on Earth, and stay as happy and healthy as possible. My improved dietary habits are a huge part of that. When people resist experimenting with dietary changes, I ask them, 'What's 30 or 60 or 90 days in the scope of your life?' Experimenting with a potentially healthier approach can't hurt, and it might just change your life!"

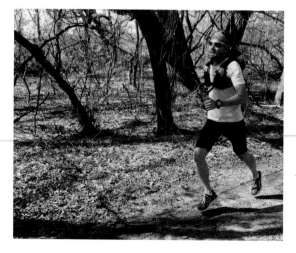

**ZACH BITTER:** Zach was a virtual unknown in the ultrarunning world on the morning of December 13th, 2013, just before the start of the Desert Solstice 24 Hour race in Phoenix. The twenty-seven-year-old Wisconsin schoolteacher was a self-described "former mediocre college 10K runner" who possessed a good-but-not-great 2h:31 marathon PR. So eyes popped and jaws dropped when Bitter had the sweetest (or perhaps we should say, "fattest"? Okay, how about "phattest"?) day of his running career, setting a new American hundred-mile record of 11h:47:21. That's right, a hundred miles in under twelve hours, or 8.3 miles per hour, or running at a 7m:04-per-mile pace *all day*!

Bitter gave the credit for his explosion onto the world elite ultrarunning scene to his primal-style, high nutrient value, and comparatively low-carb diet that he adopted for two years prior to his record run. "It made me really efficient at metabolizing fat," explained Bitter. A few months after Bitter's big win, with the ultra scene still buzzing about a low-carb runner busting out seven-minute miles on minimal ingested carbs (recall Bitter won than national 100K title in 2014, running 6m:30-pace for *seven hours* while consuming only 156 calories per hour), the FASTER study (detailed in Chapter 4) came out, legitimizing the virtually unbelievable stories from the race course.

Bitter's fuels of choice during his record run were banana chips (which combine simple sugars and coconut oil, a medium-chain triglyceride effective at turning fat into fuel), a few handfuls of potato chips (for the salt), a bag of M&Ms, and some Gatorade and Mountain Dew. Just a little kindling—a random assortment of Bitter's personal preferences really—to stoke the impressive fat-burning inferno that Bitter patiently built with devoted training and dietary habits. "Fueling is a hassle, and the less you have to do it, the better," asserts Bitter.

**LARISA DANNIS:** Larisa, a New Hampshire hiker who found her calling as a trail runner at age twenty-one in 2009, is a good example of what can happen when you combine youth, talent, and balanced primal eating and training principles. The result: She is emerging as one of the country's best endurance runners on any surface, with her 2h:44:41 time at the 2014 Boston Marathon making her 33rd female finisher overall and the day's top non-elite female.

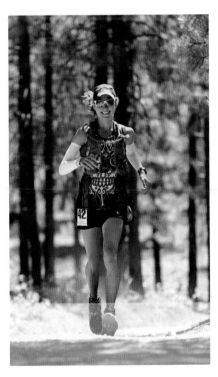

Dannis loved running the day she first laced up her running shoes in 2009 because she was good at it, and because—back to that familiar old runner's refrain—"running allowed me eat anything!" But within a year of logging miles and chowing indiscriminately, Dannis grew tired of her poor recovery, aching ankles, and significant gastrointestinal discomfort. In late 2011, upon stumbling upon MarksDailyApple.com, she learned about the havoc that inflammation can wreak on your system, and that she might have a particular sensitivity to the grain-based conventional-wisdom diet. Inspired accordingly, Dannis decided to go "cold-turkey primal."

Within a month of dumping pasta, bread, gels, and sugary sports drinks in favor of grass-fed beef, coconut oil, marrow-bone/celery/carrot broth, and other primal fare, Dannis's life-long chunkiness was gone, her stomachaches and nagging pains had resolved, and she had greater energy and quicker recovery. By the third month of primal eating, Dannis was so lean that a man stopped her on the street one day. "You look like a runner," he said. She broke into a big smile—she'd never heard that before.

But Dannis's primal dietary practices offered far more value than just physique improvements. "After I became fat-adapted, I was absolutely faster," Dannis says. She noticed better finishing times while eating just a third of the calories she needed before going primal. At the Boston Marathon, she filled her tank with a pre-race meal of three bananas, one Generation UCAN SuperStarch supplement, and one maple-bacon flavored VFuel gel. She popped two fudge brownie VFuels during the 26.2-mile event and nothing else besides water.

Dannis's training and eating strategy is designed to keep her strength and speed high and injuries low. Dannis runs sixty to seventy miles a week max (low for an ultrarunner), and does every run in a fasted state to further improve fat-adaptation (she also runs on empty for the first two hours of every race). She finds benefit in cycling in high nutrient value carbohydrates (parsnips, squash, sweet potatoes, bananas, and berries) after a hard or long run to restock muscle glycogen. She does a once-a-week interval session and three to five days a week of kettlebell strength training, focusing on compound movements that provide overall functional strength for running.

In 2013, Dannis won four fifty-milers and took second and third at two hundred-milers. In 2014, she finished fourth at the USA Ultra 100-Mile Championships and broke her previous marathon time by almost eleven minutes at Boston. And she's just getting started. A big entry on her to-do list: Qualify to run in the 2016 U.S. Olympic Marathon Trials.

**JOHNNY G:** Jonathan "Johnny G" Goldberg is widely known in the fitness world as the creator of Spinning, the original indoor group cycling workout that he started in his garage and that quickly spread to health clubs across the world, as well as Krankcycle—a cycling-inspired upper body cardio workout. In the late 1980s, years before Johnny became internationally recognized for Spinning, he was a personal trainer in Los Angeles aspiring to compete in ultradistance cycling races, such as the epic three-thousand-mile non-stop coast-to-coast bicycle Race Across America (RAAM).

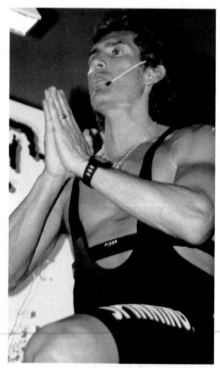

A sincere enthusiast of healthy living and natural eating, Johnny was an aggressive experimenter on innovative training methods and dietary practices throughout his competitive career. After suffering extreme digestive difficulties consuming mass quantities of carbohydrate calories around the clock during the 1987 RAAM (he had a tooth dissolve somewhere in Nebraska due to constant exposure to sugar…you might call that a "difficulty"—ouch), Johnny had to drop out in Indiana and go back to the drawing board.

After a period of intensive nutrition research and self-experimentation, Johnny became perhaps the first elite ultra-endurance athlete to implement fat fueled ultra-endurance workouts. By 1989, he had dialed in a fueling strategy for his long training rides. These included routine hundred-milers whenever he had some free time, and a *weekly* twenty-four-hour session of some 350 miles that started Friday evening and continued through Saturday evening. Brad was a frequent training partner for those weekend rides, joining Johnny on Saturday mornings to complete the last 150 or 200 miles of the route. Brad recalls that he could never complain about these journeys, knowing Johnny had been at it the previous night while he slept; and furthermore he needed to come prepared with some entertaining monologues during the afternoon hours, to prevent Johnny from nodding off while pedaling!

Johnny's performance fuel of choice was Ziploc baggies filled with smushed avocado mixed with MCT (medium chain triglyceride) oil. Today, MCT oil is a popular ingredient with paleo coffee enthusiasts and in sports supplements, lauded as an easily accessible energy source that cannot be stored as body fat. Back then, Johnny had to pay a fortune to have large drums of this strange commodity shipped in from Germany, and essentially smuggled the non-FDA approved contraband past US customs.

With his fueling challenges solved, Johnny experienced amazing performance breakthroughs. He blew the field away at the 1989 508-mile RAAM qualifying race across the California desert, and took his high fat strategy to the 1989 starting line, eager to finish what he had started in 1987. Things started well for Johnny in 1989, and he battled it out with the leaders across the American Southwest and into Texas. After a thousand miles of basically non-stop riding from the California coast, Johnny finally went down for a proper night's sleep in Texas.

It was then that Johnny realized RAAM was a contest not only of cycling prowess, but of sleep deprivation. When Johnny woke up and remounted around six hours later, he had dropped out of the top 10! The leading RAAM solo riders of the day adhered to a pattern of 22.5 hours on the bike to every 1.5 hours of rest. That meant if you ever decided to get off the bike for a nice meal, shower, and brief nap, you would wake up fifty miles behind your competition! *Note*: In 2006, RAAM changed the rules to mandate that solo riders accumulate a total of forty hours of rest along the route, a safety measure taken in response to two rider fatalities where sleep deprivation was a contributing factor (good thing Brad could tell entertaining monologues to Johnny during those training rides).

Johnny G went on to complete the 1989 RAAM in ten days and change. In 1995, with his company primed to introduce Spinning to the public at a San Francisco fitness industry trade show, Johnny called upon his endurance background, and called attention to his booth, by riding his stationary Spinning bike *all day*, for each of the four days at the trade show! For the first couple of days, passersby just thought it was a coincidence the same guy was pedaling, often by himself amidst rows of empty Spinner bikes, when they passed the booth. By the final day, a throng of a couple hundred people encircled Johnny's Spinning booth and the demo bikes were packed with a constant rotation of eager enthusiasts.

Johnny was definitely way ahead of his time, and his RAAM exploits were an inspiration in the eventual questioning of the endurance community's obsession with high carbohydrate eating and deep reliance on carbohydrate performance fuels during exercise. However, it took many more years for the endurance community to embrace the secret of fat-adapted training as a way out of the carbohydrate dependency trap, and for it to spread to a critical mass of athletes. You can't will yourself off of carbs during long training sessions; ask anyone who's bonked the folly of trying to diet and perform at the same time. No, the secret to escaping carbohydrate dependency and becoming a fat-burning beast is primarily a modification of dietary habits to ditch refined carbohydrates and moderate insulin production. As we discussed in the early chapters, you also have to cease chronic exercise patterns, but the gateway starts at the breakfast table (or the fasting window as the case may be) every day—departing from the All-American sugar bomb breakfast that sets you up to operate in sugar-burning mode all day.

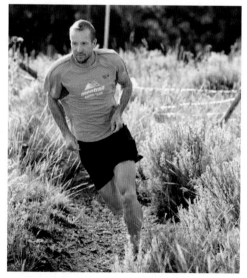

**MATT HART:** Matt, a fitness coach and ultrarunner from Boulder, knows about inflammation—it was his lifelong companion. Having grown up with drawers full of allergy pills, the constant wheeze of asthma, and an inhaler in his backpack, it would have seemed unimaginable that he'd be a champion ultrarunner someday. But in 2012, at the ripe old age of thirty-seven, Matt won his first hundred-miler, the prestigious and very challenging Tahoe Rim 100, an undulating route in the High Sierra that circles Lake Tahoe. He delivered a phenomenal time of 19h:14, besting the next runner by forty-five minutes.

Matt says that transitioning to a primal-aligned, high-fat diet was critical to his performance breakthrough. "I was always fast, but had no endurance because I only was able to use 80 percent of my lung capacity," says Hart. Hart's lung problems had plagued him since childhood, but diagnosis was a challenge. While working at Microsoft in his twenties—surrounded by free coffee, Coke, and candy bars—he was once hospitalized for waves of unattributed chest pain. He took prescription drugs to relieve the pain, but had no answers. In 2006, while competing on the winning team in a Baja adventure race, he remembers "wheezing so bad that I thought I'd die." That experience was the last straw. Resolving to do something, anything, to try and identify and eliminate the cause of his hampered lung function, Matt decided to eliminate dairy products.

As simple as that, Matt could finally breath fully. "I was 90 percent fixed, but I knew there was more," Matt remembers. "I found it on MarksDailyApple.com: cut out the gluten too." Matt's elimination of these staples of the Standard American Diet essentially eliminated lung problems, and set the stage for his ascension to the elite levels of ultrarunning and enjoying the best health of his life. Pushing forty, Matt says, "I'm stronger than I've ever been, and my primal eating patterns have made me ripped for the first time. As far as performance, a hundred-mile training week or race used to hurt—but now, it's no problem, since my inflammation is under control." Matt still carries an inhaler with him, as he has for decades, in case of emergency. "I can't remember the last time I used it!" he says.

Matt continues, "The cumulative training effect is one part of it, and the dietary modifications are the other." Matt favors avocado-turkey wraps, sweet potatoes, nut butters, and sometimes makes his own coconut-almond-raisin balls and date-raisin gels for training aids. At his fifty- and hundred-mile races, he runs right through all the regular aid stations, with their tempting Snickers bars and pierogi (boiled dough dumplings filled with meat, cheese, or potato), and runs on his own internal fuel stores or unique custom supplements. Matt will still top off his tank with carbohydrate gels when the pace gets faster in competition, but more to promote competitive success than out of the fear of bonking.

As a trainer, Matt enthusiastically recommends primal-style eating to his clients, but he is careful not to push it. He believes people must come to big lifestyle transformations at their own comfortable pace. "Primal dietary transitions have a step-by-step trickle-down effect. First cut sugar, then junk food, then do more. One elderly client lost fifty pounds. My mom, marveling that she's lighter than she was in high school, will say, 'I've been on diets my whole life, and this doesn't feel like a diet.'"

**ROB HOGAN:** This bizarre story reveals what happens when you go where few athletes have ever gone before: beyond the bonk! Rob Hogan of Galway, Ireland, has the prestigious distinction of being the world's fastest golfer. He is a world champion at the unique sport of Speedgolf, where tournament competitors not only count strokes on the course, but also add their time in minutes to generate a Speedgolf total score. For example, in the 2013 Speedgolf World Championships in Bandon, Oregon, Rob shot a 77 and completed the entire championship-length course—racing from shot to shot on foot and carrying only six clubs in a small bag—in an astonishing thirty-nine minutes. His Speedgolf score for the round was thus 77 + 39 = 116.

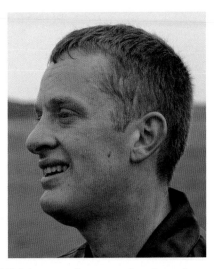

Rob is a full-time professional Speedgolfer, conducting exhibitions and competing in prize-money events across the globe against other elite runner-golfer combo athletes. As such, Rob spends hours honing his golf skills while also training with a competitive running club in his hometown. In an effort to build his endurance for tournament competition (you obviously hit better shots when you are less fatigued from running), Rob faithfully increased his weekly long run from thirteen miles, to fifteen miles, and finally up to seventeen miles. He completed a seventeen-mile run four weekends in a row, and the story starts to get juicy at the end of the fourth run...

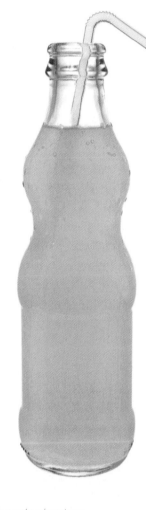

Unlike the typical distance runner adorned with a FuelBelt packed with gels, Rob completed each of these training runs on *no food or water*. When he increased his distance to seventeen miles (some three hours of running), Rob greatly enjoyed his post-run visits to a nearby convenience store to replenish with a sugary beverage of choice. Anyone who's gone long, run short on calories, and experienced the phenomenon known as *bonking* knows how that finish line treat can hit the spot like nothing else.

On his fourth consecutive weekend seventeen-mile session, Rob again ran low on fuel and hydration in the final hour, and reported that he experienced a sugar craving so intense that a vivid picture popped into his mind of a frosty cold can of Fanta orange soda. Such a vision might be benign when you're sitting in a movie theater about to go get a free refill, but during a long run it's a sign of trouble. It's your brain sending you a very powerful message that the flashing yellow "E" warning light is on, and your central nervous system is about to shut down. Being a highly driven elite competitor, Rob soldiered on through the bonking sensations—even though he was on a four-loop course and could have easily bailed before his final loop. By the time he arrived at the finish line, an extraordinary thing happened: *the vision of the Fanta can had vanished!* No trip to the convenience store necessary; just seventeen miles on no food and no water, and then on with his day (of course he quickly rehydrated with water and enjoyed an eventual delicious meal in due time). In the weeks and months that followed, Rob noticed that his general interest and appetite for sugar in his diet had completely subsided!

*Rob Hogan's phantom Fanta; the ultimate story of becoming violently—and permanently—fat-adapted*

This story has incredible implications for endurance athletes, because of the tremendous advantage offered by becoming fat- and keto-adapted for long duration efforts. As you likely know, we can only store four hundred to five hundred grams of glycogen in our bodies—enough to sustain us for around two hours at vigorous intensity before bonking occurs. In contrast, even the leanest athlete has tens of thousands of calories of stored body fat—a virtually limitless supply of energy for endurance performance. Indeed, the ability to access and burn stored body fat in the absence of dietary calories has been a central element of human survival against the harsh selection pressure that shaped evolution. For over two million years, our food supply was uncertain and sporadic. We simply would not have survived without efficient mechanisms to store energy and burn it later.

As Dr. Cate Shanahan mentions in Chapter 4, Rob's extreme effort recalibrated the function of the hormone ghrelin to the extent that he hacked the typically more arduous process of becoming fat-adapted. As Dr. Cate elaborates, "Cravings come from past learning experiences, which mediate our appetite and hormone production. When we run low on sugar, ghrelin immediately stimulates a sugar craving to feed that empty stomach and depleted brain. Athletes who come home from workouts in a depleted state perhaps have the capability to rewire their hormones to become more fat- and keto-adapted. Intense, novel, and unique experiences are very powerful signal generators. They message the body that it needs to change. Another example is a sprint workout conducted at 30 MET [metabolic equivalent task; a sprint workout revs your engine thirty times higher than you operate at rest]. Even a short workout has a profound effect on your fat metabolism, lean muscle development, hormone balance, and overall fitness progress," explains Dr. Cate.

Regarding Rob's story, I must reference the familiar admonition: *don't try this at home.* Or at least, be careful trying this at home! If you are not fat- or keto-adapted and you deplete your tank with an extreme endurance effort and insufficient calories, you'll pig out for hours afterward. You'll down a couple Fantas and the vision of a third will pop back up twenty minutes later.

We must view the entire process of Rob performing the weekend long runs again and again to appreciate the magical ending. First, Rob steadily and strategically increased his mileage each week so he was not overwhelmed by any single effort. Secondly, he carefully regulates his exercise intensity so that he remains aerobic on his long distance runs. His Irish coach Mark Davis dispenses the simple but memorable advice to "increase mileage without getting injured," which entails regulating intensity and getting plenty of rest and recovery.

Rob's steady progression on the long runs enabled his body to gradually become fat- and keto-adapted and depart from sugar dependency emphatically and for a sustained period of time afterward. Interestingly (as detailed in *The Art and Science of Low Carbohydrate Performance*), during the early phases of fat- and keto-adaptation, skeletal muscle is able to burn both ketones and fat. As you become more and more adapted, the muscles start to spare ketones for the brain and instead rely mostly on fat for fuel. Again, this story assumes that glucose levels are low from dietary restriction and/or, in Rob's case, running the tank low during extreme efforts sans sugar.

Early in the process of becoming fat- and keto-adapted, your muscles burn up ketones and fat—doing whatever they can to perform in the absence of their usual steady stream of glucose. When ketone uptake by skeletal muscle is high, blood ketone levels are low. Consequently, your brain might struggle to obtain sufficient fuel. This is why some folks report struggles with fatigue and mood disturbances in the early phases of transitioning over to a primal-style eating pattern. This is likely why Rob definitely needed to guzzle down high-sugar drinks during his earlier long runs—his muscles and brain were not yet fully adapted. Luckily, he arrived at the finish line before passing out and got his hands on a frosty soda quickly.

Over time, when you become fully fat- and keto-adapted, your muscles are fueled by mainly fat (from both fatty acids in the blood and mobilization of stored triglycerides), while ketones are reserved for use by the brain, since the brain is only capable of burning either glucose or ketones (but not fat). What you are in this case is *bonk-proof!*

Metabolically, this state of adaptation to alternative fuel sources is revealed by higher ketone levels in the blood (plenty of energy is readily available to the brain), if you are inclined to get super-techie and test such things. It's also revealed by being able to go longer on fewer calories, and with less sensation of depletion, fatigue, and sugar cravings after workouts.

We might also mention once again Dr. Peter Attia as perhaps the world's foremost expert on this stuff. He's a physician, ultra-endurance swimmer, and willing human guinea pig who has tested the concept of ketosis and endurance performance more diligently than anyone in the world. If you visit his website, peterattia.com, and check out the link "My Personal Journey," you will find further insights from a scientific perspective, tracking a storyline similar to Rob Hogan's Fanta experience.

**SAMI INKINEN:** Sami, a native of Finland, is a prominent Silicon Valley entrepreneur (co-founder of the Trulia.com real estate website) who has achieved some endurance performances that represent some of the most astonishing breakthroughs and validation of fat-adaption ever recorded.

In 2011, Sami gained notoriety for his unorthodox approach when he won the Ironman 70.3 World Triathlon Championship in the 35–39 age group, and took second in the age group at the Hawaii Ironman World Championships, despite training only twelve hours per week. This is about half of the weekly training volume of the average starter at these championship events. Numerous endurance athletes have demonstrated the ability (perhaps *folly* is a better word than ability here?) to *finish* ultra distance events on minimal training, but winning the most competitive triathlon on the planet in a professional-caliber sub-nine-hour time is another story. The endurance world started wondering just what this guy was doing to shatter conventional beliefs about what type of training and lifestyle were required to become a champion.

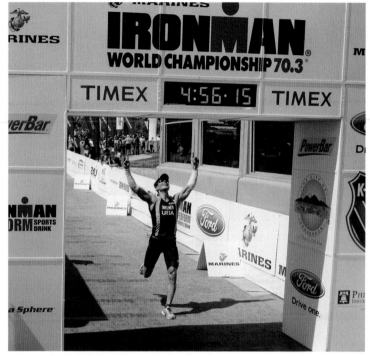

*Sami winning his age group in a low key local event. Oh, it's actually the World Championships at the 70.3 (half-Ironman) distance!*

Due to his busy work schedule, what this self-proclaimed "incurable data geek" was doing was looking at all potential angles to maximize the efficiency of his limited training time. Consequently, Sami decided to cut out the chronic type of workouts that triathletes favor (kinda long, kinda hard, kinda too frequent) in favor of shorter, high intensity sessions (both cardio and explosive power activities), combined with slower, comfortably paced aerobic workouts. He also was inspired to modify his diet after learning he was pre-diabetic despite his athletic ways and seemingly healthy (low-fat, high carb) eating habits. "I was in shock when I heard that [pre-diabetic] news," Sami explained in a *USA Today* interview. "Ever since then, I've switched to eating things from either the ground or a tree. You can't go wrong if you go that route."

Sami has engaged in extensive physiological testing in his quest to achieve peak performance. A 2009 test at the Stanford human perfor-

*Results of Sami Inkinen's initial performance test from 2009. At 300 watts, he is burning almost all carbohydrates—destined to bonk after a couple hours, maybe three if he can slam down some gels en route.*

mance lab revealed that he was a highly efficient sugar-burning machine, thanks to his ten-year devotion to that low-fat, "super high carb" (thanks to his training volume) diet and five years of diligent triathlon training by that time. Sami's test revealed that he could push an impressive 300 watts on the bike (again, around 25 mph on a flat road), while burning approximately 95 percent carbs (900–1,000 calories of carbs per hour). The performance test revealed that, like other sugar dependent endurance athletes, he would predictably bonk after two to three hours at that pace. This was not promising news for someone with ambitions to race for over eight hours at an Ironman.

In tandem with his highly focused, stress-balanced training schedule, Sami implemented a primal-style eating pattern featuring eggs, grass-fed beef, butter, nuts, fish, coconut oil, leafy vegetables, some fruits, and dark chocolate. Before and after his high intensity sessions, Sami did some targeted carbo loading with stuff like fruits, rice, and potatoes. He threw down these extra carbs only in the vicinity of these high glycolytic sessions, to ensure he was primed for peak performance and recovered quickly afterwards.

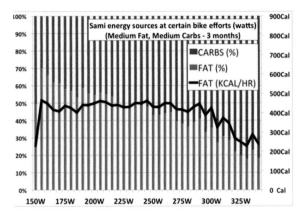

After his great 2011 Ironman win, Inkinen was quoted in a 2012 issue of *Triathlete* magazine as saying that his diet gave him an "unfair advantage." He guessed that his diet and his efficient, stress-balanced training program had increased the size and efficiency of his aerobic engine—that is, the density and ability of his muscles' mitochondria to process fat into energy.

*Sami's second performance test at Stanford, coming off three months of devoted carb restriction and fat emphasis in the diet. Here, at 300 watts, Sami has doubled his fat oxidation to over 400 calories per hour, going from burning almost all carbs to about half carbs, half fat.*

He reckons that his tiny cellular fat-burning engines became so numerous and efficient that they allowed him to "double or triple" the maximum amount of fat he could process for fuel per hour.

This insight was confirmed at Sami's second performance test at Stanford three months after the first. This time, he tested on the heels of a three-month "pretty high fat, moderate carb" eating pattern, where he replaced his sugar habits with "large quantities of nuts, oil, and avocado." Despite no differences in his training, his fat oxidation doubled to over 400 calories per hour at that 300-watt test pace. "Yes, fat adaptation happened quickly!" explains Sami.

While Sami's minimalist Hawaii Ironman victory was remarkable, even more amazing performances were in store. At the 2014 Wildflower half-Ironman distance triathlon, he won the amateur title with a stunning 4h:28 performance—again despite extremely minimal and unusual training methods for a long course triathlete. What was amazing is that Sami was barely training for triathlon (you'll learn why in a moment; no, it wasn't because he was selling Trulia to Zillow—something way more exciting than a routine acquisition windfall in Silicon Valley!). He was weighing in at 201 pounds (at 6 feet tall, this was some twenty pounds over his usual race weight), running a minute per mile slower in training than normal, and thinking he had no chance of being competitive at this classic event that annually draws the best amateurs from around the country and even internationally.

Sami needed a hack here, and so here's what he did in the final four weeks leading up to the race:

**Muscular conditioning**: Ran 10–15 minutes every day to condition the muscles to the pounding of the 13.1 mile race.

**High Intensity**: Performed a once-weekly session of ten times one-minute all-out, with one-minute recovery intervals (on a treadmill).

**Plyometrics**: Optimized running efficiency with a five-minute box jump routine, three times per week: 3 x 12 box jumps and 3 x 12 max vertical jumps.

**Endurance**: Performed once-weekly aerobic session of 50–65 minutes, including hill work at a steady but still comfortable pace.

In a total running time of less than two hours per week, Sami primed himself for the Wildflower victory, which was all the more amazing considering how 90°F+ temperatures handicap heavier athletes in particular. After the Wildflower victory, Sami performed a third cycling test in the lab, which revealed a peak fat-burning rate of 750 calories per hour (this at the low intensity rate of 150 watts) and a fat utilization rate at 300 watts of over 50 percent of total energy usage. For this test, he was holding steady for six months with a carb intake of perhaps less than 10 percent of total calories (mainly vegetables and nuts). He ditched all the sports supplements endurance athletes live and die by and instead did all workouts under three hours cowboy style—water only. As we learned in Chapters 3 and 4, this greatly enhanced his fat-adaptation and optimized his appetite hormones. If Sami went longer than three or four hours, he'd refuel with real foods like bananas or cashews.

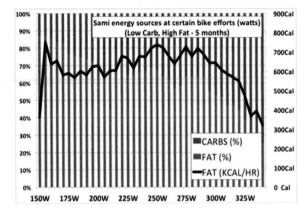

Sami energy sources at certain bike efforts (watts)
(Low Carb, High Fat - 5 months)

CARBS (%)
FAT (%)
FAT (KCAL/HR)

150W 175W 200W 225W 250W 275W 300W 325W

*Sami's third performance test, on the heels of his amazing Clydesdale-style Wildflower victory. Notice the fat utilization at low intensity of around 85 percent of total energy and 750 calories per hour—triple that of the levels he delivered on his first test!*

Buoyed by the success of his fat-adapted endurance exploits, and pondering a higher calling to spread the word about the dangers of high carbohydrate eating, Sami and his wife, Meredith Loring (a longtime primal-style grain- and starch-free eater), set their sights on one of the most extreme and challenging endurance efforts ever attempted: a 2,400-mile trans-Pacific Ocean row from San Francisco to Hawaii in the summer of 2014. Now you know what compromised Sami's triathlon training in 2014: he and Meredith were rowing like crazy to get ready for the test of a lifetime!

After months of diligent preparation and diligent primal style eating, he and Meredith paddled their specially designed two-person, twenty-foot rowboat for up to twenty hours per day (taking turns, with one rowing and the other sleeping for a couple hours at a time) and reached the shores of Hawaii forty-five days and two hours later. Their efforts raised some $300,000 for the Institute of Responsible Nutrition, an advocacy group headed by Dr. Robert Lustig, anti-sugar crusader, UC San Francisco research professor, and author of *Fat Chance: Beating the Odds Against Sugar, Processed Food, Obesity, and Disease.*

Sami and Meredith's nutritional intake during the row offers a pretty powerful testimonial to the benefits of fat-adapted endurance. Because their journey was entirely unsupported, the couple carried nearly *one million calories* on board to fuel their human engines. Despite the unimaginable daily workload, they subsisted on ultra low carb fare like dehydrated beef, salmon, and vegetables, along with fruit, nuts, and olive oil. A desalination machine met their hydration needs.

As the "bonk-proof" graph reveals, Sami extended his time-to-bonking at low intensity from a predicted 5.6 hours (extrapolated from his substrate utilization while pedaling at a comfortable 200 watts

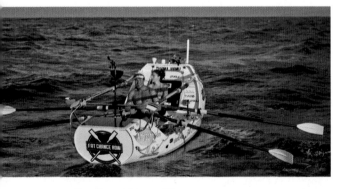

*Sami and Meredith rowing to Hawaii to raise $300,000 for the Institute of Responsible Nutrition, and testing the limits of fat-adapted endurance performance.*

during his 2009 performance test) to a phenomenal *87 hours* (predicted from his third performance test) by the time he was fully fat-adapted. Obviously, with a moderate amount of caloric intake, this enabled Sami and Meredith to become literally bonk-proof.

In fact, Sami ended up losing twenty-six pounds over the course of the journey. This indicates that his caloric intake, while prodigious by ordinary life standards, did not match up with the massive caloric expenditure of round-the-clock rowing. However, rather than bonking and drifting away to the deep blue forever (as a carb-dependent, poorly fat-adapted individual might), Sami and Meredith were able to efficiently tap into the huge reservoirs of stored energy on their bodies to be able to complete the trip. *Note*: a significant portion of Sami's total weight loss was lean mass, due to the atrophy of lower extremity muscles that were unnecessary and unused on the boat. Contrast this with the typical SAD pattern of not even being able to get through an afternoon at the office without a quick energy carbohydrate snack and a Diet Coke!

Sami and Meredith joked beforehand that their effort would test the limits of human endurance *and* marriage! When they landed in Hawaii, the couple were happy to report: "Still married! Divorce papers are untouched in a waterproof container and Divorce-o-meter at zero at the bottom of the Pacific Ocean."

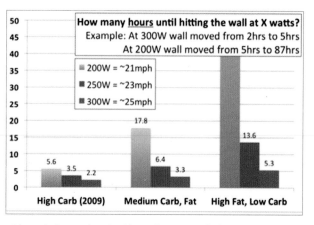

How many <u>hours</u> until hitting the wall at X watts?
Example: At 300W wall moved from 2hrs to 5hrs
At 200W wall moved from 5hrs to 87hrs

- 200W = ~21mph
- 250W = ~23mph
- 300W = ~25mph

High Carb (2009): 5.6, 3.5, 2.2
Medium Carb, Fat: 17.8, 6.4, 3.3
High Fat, Low Carb: 13.6, 5.3

*You ain't rowing to Hawaii as a carb burner!*

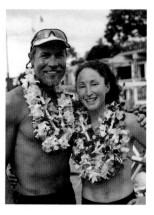

*You think you're happy when a race finish line comes into view? Imagine the feeling for Sami and Meredith when the Hawaiian islands appeared on the horizon after forty-five days on the high seas!*

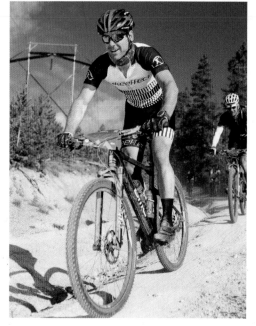

**TED MCDONALD:** Ted's initial immersion into a life of healthy, fit, clean living happened through yoga. During a time of personal and career struggles, he joined a friend, checked his ego at the door, and unfurled a mat for his first ever sun salutation. "I felt like the class was a physical, emotional, mental and spiritual cleanse all in one. Up to that day, I thought that lifting weights was the only way to get strong, and yet here I was shaking during every move in my first class. I was so confused! Afterward, I felt refreshed and revitalized, but I was sore for four days! I knew there was something there, and right away I was hooked," Ted remembers.

Ted's love affair with yoga would eventually take him from student to teacher. Today you can find him giving classes at his studio, 5 Point Yoga, in Malibu, California; leading members of the professional cycling team, BMC, through apres-ride poses during their winter and spring training camps in Spain; and even taking willing participants on yoga adventure retreats around the world a few times a year.

Before Ted found yoga, he ate typical SAD fare: Fast food, hot dogs, soda, bread, pizza, pasta, and lots of dessert. "As I began to do yoga, I became much more sensitive to what I put in my body. I cut back on the junk food, quit smoking and moderated my habit of excessive coffee intake," Ted remembers.

It wasn't long before the endurance part of Ted's journey began, with an impromptu participation in the San Diego Rock & Roll Marathon that he was suckered into by friends. The emotional experience of conquering a 26-mile run on minimal preparation awakened a latent passion for exploring his limits in a variety of endurance endeavors over the past decade—triathlons, multi-day adventure races, and ultra endurance events like the Leadville 100 mountain bike race. Ted fueled his performances with a cleaned up, but still high-carb, low-fat, borderline vegan diet. Mornings of steel cut oatmeal, nuts, bananas, and perhaps a smoothie of fruit and sweetened almond milk. Pounding gels, bars, and sweet drinks during workouts, and recovering with another sugar bomb smoothie. Chips, ice cream, and other heavily processed snacks made regular appearances. No worries from Ted's perspective; after all, he was a top-10-percent finisher in his age group!

Then one day, BMC team nutritionist Barry Murray took Ted on a long run, insisting he start the effort fasted—a common practice among the BMC pro riders to promote fat loss and fat adaptation. Despite Ted's constant anxiety, he completed the two-hour run without bonking. The experience piqued his interest in low carb, but some blood tests a few months later really got him motivated. This lean, highly competitive ultra endurance machine was showing early signs of insulin resistance. It was time for a proper 21-day transformation to primal-style eating, which Ted achieved with the help of his wife, Lauren Lobley, a professional nutrition coach, chef, and author.

At Ted's first fat-adapted trail half marathon, he beat his previous time from three years prior and finished seventh overall—becoming a true believer in the process. These days, Ted's training day diet consists of water or green tea in the morning. He doesn't take gels with him on his runs anymore, but if he trains for more than two hours, he'll pack one of the cleaner energy bars and start nibbling after two hours. His post-workout nutrition is a lower carb, higher protein shake and an omclet filled with cheese, avocado, and veggies. Still a non-meat eater, the rest of Ted's diet is made up of nuts, seeds, lots of non-starchy veggies, and, of course, fish.

Not only have Ted's performances improved since becoming a fat burner, so too has his blood work. Only three months into his new diet, Ted did another blood test, which revealed significant improvements in HDL cholesterol, triglycerides, and insulin resistance markers. "I'm literally bonk-proof now!" Ted exclaims. "Whether I'm training or racing, I'm more alert and steady, and I even get subtle bursts of energy here and there. When I was fueling on sugar and carbs, I always needed a gel to pick me up, and if I didn't get one, I would bonk. Not any more."

Ted's 2015 athletic feat was to tackle the Inca Trail in Peru, a 20-mile journey with over 9,000 feet (2,750 meters) of elevation gain that is normally done in four days. He and his friend, Rami Ghandour, had to be granted special permission from the government to do the trail in one day, and they finished in just over ten hours. Unlike his early ultra competitions where he powered down the sugar supplements throughout, Ted needed only to nibble on an energy bar (after three and a half hours of fasted exercise) now and then, and sip a third of a gel packet and discard the rest. Ted has truly found the perfect trifecta: yoga, endurance athletics, and a primal-style eating pattern, adapted to his vegetarian preferences. Tried. Tested. True. Namaste.

**TIMOTHY OLSON:** Timothy is one of the pioneers of low-carb, primal-style eating for elite endurance performance. Known as the "conscious mountain ultrarunner," Timothy has an evolved, spiritual approach to endurance running that he has leveraged to some world-beating performances. He won the prestigious Western States 100-Mile Endurance Run two years in a row (setting a phenomenal course record time of 14h:46 in 2012), and was named 2014 Male Ultra Runner of the Year.

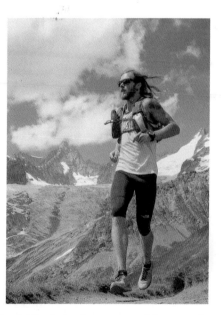

Timothy and his family's eventual transition to a primal-style eating pattern was a long time in the works. As a teenage distance runner, Timothy suffered from various digestive problems that, unbeknownst to him at the time, were largely driven by a traditional high-carbohydrate diet. His wife, Krista, had a lifelong case of juvenile rheumatoid arthritis that was serious enough to warrant long-term prescription medication. Motivated by Krista's health concerns, the couple drifted further toward low-carb, primal-aligned eating habits over time, with excellent results. Krista dramatically improved her condition to the extent that she could ditch prescription drugs. Timothy noticed that his longtime GI distress subsided when pizza went off the menu.

There was a whole 'nuther level of health and performance awaiting Timothy through dietary modification, an idea he awakened to after some big gastrointestinal trouble on the 2011 Western States race course. He delivered a respectable sixth place finish, but had to stop twenty times to empty his bowels during the second half of the race, and felt wasted for weeks afterward. In the aftermath of that ordeal, Timothy eliminated grains from his diet, started eating more green vegetables, and went to organic chicken, beef, and eggs. He cut grain-based carbs down to twice-a-month tortillas. During training runs, he went off the gel train and integrated more wholesome options like nut butters, dried fruits, or honey based gels. When racing for the big bucks, Timothy (and other elite fat-adapted ultra athletes) will still use gels or other forms of sugar, but at much lower volume and frequency. This helps reduce the inflammation and digestive distress that often accompanies high sugar consumption during grueling endurance efforts, when the digestive tract is traumatized by lack of normal bloodflow and (in the case of running) impact trauma.

Timothy reports that since that comprehensive dietary cleanup in 2011, he feels better, recovers faster, and enjoys an overall improved quality of life. His dietary centerpieces are healthy fats like nuts, avocadoes, and coconut oil. To ensure his glycogen stores are replenished, he incorporates sweet potatoes as needed with his high volume training. Timothy also embodies other primal-aligned training strategies like giving his body the proper amount of rest, not pushing the limits, and being more intuitive in what he needs for running and training, which has taken him farther than any of the previous carb loading practices that he's cast to the wayside.

With a year of momentum behind his dietary shift, Timothy went wild on the race course with some epic performances. At the 2012 Western States, Olson set a new course record of 14h:46:44—a full twenty-five minutes faster than anyone in history. He also won two other hundred-milers that year. Then in 2013, he won Western States again, in 15h:17:27. He experienced no GI or bowel problems either time.

"From 2011 to 2012, I learned how to use fat as fuel, and use carbs strategically," explained Timothy. "At the 2012 Western States, I went a couple of hours with no food at all, just water, while I was climbing thousands of feet. I moderated my pace and trusted that my body had plenty of fuel in it. It did. I hit mile sixty feeling very strong, passed people, got passed myself at mile seventy, but had enough energy left to regain the lead in the final twenty miles and hold it to the finish."

Besides the advantageous metabolic shift from carb dependency to being fat- and keto-adapted, Timothy is also quick to point out another key advantage of primal-style eating: it limits the damage caused by carb-induced inflammation. "My goal is to eliminate inflammation as much as possible, especially with the miles I put in," he said. The proof is the recovery. "After the 2011 Western States, I was destroyed for a month. In 2012, I was recovered in a week."

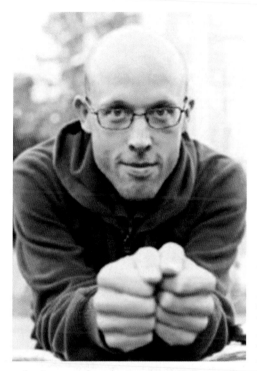

**DR. KLEMEN ROJNIK:** Klemen is a lab rat's lab rat, a data-crunching swim-bike-run cyborg who practically wrote a dissertation on his experiences, which he has shared online. A pharmaceutical researcher and triathlete since 2010, the "Slovenian Sledgehammer" obliterated his 2012 Hawaii time of 9h:26:12 (done with a high-carb diet) by nearly thirty-eight minutes in 2013 (done with a low-carb diet), when he finished in a pro-caliber time of 8h:48—good for second place in the thirty to thirty-four amateur age group.

Rojnik did it with bike and run training volumes 18 percent lower than in 2012 while eating a daily diet composed of 69 percent fat (360g), 18 percent protein (210g), and 13 percent carbs (143g). He consumed 4,700 calories per day, which by nutrient groups included 870g of vegetables, 424g of milk (about 35 gallons), 685g of other dairy products (especially plain yogurt), 273g of fruit, 284g of meat, and 130g of fish. He burned up an average of 1,680 calories per day during his workouts, leaving a basal daily metabolic rate of around 3,000 calories.

Rojnik used a diet strategy of "Train Low/Race High." That means that he follows a low-carb, primal-aligned eating pattern, but uses gels and other sugar sources in races, and carbo-loads the day before the race. "It doesn't affect my fat-burning ability to a great degree," he says.

Interestingly, Rojnik experimented with ketogenic training but did not achieve the success that other athletes report. His chronicles suggest that optimizing carb intake or adapting to an extreme dietary modification like going ketogenic is highly individualized. Trial and error should govern your decisions rather than adhering to an arbitrary template. In Rojnik's case, he spent seven weeks limiting his carb intake to 50 grams per day or less, and also being diligent to limit his protein consumption to less than 140 grams per day.

**DID YOU KNOW?** *Primal Endurance is about utilizing a giant gas tank of clean burning, internally derived fuel. Carb dependent endurance training means relying on a tiny, dirty burning gas tank requiring constant refilling.*

# BEWARE THE HIGH PROTEIN DIET

Rojnik's efforts to regulate carb intake as well as protein intake is an important take-home point, because many an athlete's efforts to eat "low carb" become compromised by high protein intake. Once your body has the protein it requires for essential function and muscle repair/preservation, it becomes averse to excessive intake. If you eschew carbs but pound the protein, your body will work hard to excrete the nitrogen waste products and/or quickly convert those excess protein calories into carbohydrates via the pro-

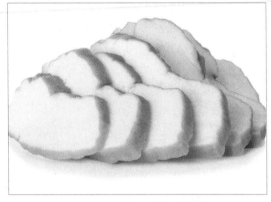

cess of gluconeogenesis (the conversion of either ingested amino acids or stored amino acids in lean tissue into glucose for quick energy—a central component of the fight-or-flight response). In short, excess protein intake (the default approach of the old-school bodybuilders and their six daily meals of turkey breasts and egg whites) will promote excess body fat (via gluconeogenesis—then you know what your body does with excess carbs), stress your kidneys, accelerate cell division and aging, and increase the risk of certain cancers.

· The ideal strategy is to emphasize healthy sources of fat as your predominant calorie source, limit carb intake by ditching sugars and grains and calibrating average daily carb intake to your personal body composition goals, recovery, and hormonal particulars, or perhaps interest in ketosis, and finally to consume the protein you need to support health and recovery. Experts are in agreement that protein requirements range from .7 to 1.0 grams per pound of lean body mass—the range depending on your activity level.

During his ketogenic experiment, Rojnik reported that he felt miserable and de-motivated on long training runs and rides, freezing in the pool, unable to produce max efforts on intervals, making excuses to miss workouts, and wracked with thirst and food cravings. "I could only explain these cravings as my body's cry for some carbs!" he concluded. His problems disappeared when he went back to his normal, but still relatively low-carb diet.

With the rise in notoriety of low carb athletes, many are speculating that ketogenic training works at lower intensities, such as-all day ultras or rowing for forty-five days from San Francisco to Hawaii.

A key takeaway of Rojnik's experience and the aforementioned stories of the ultrarunners earlier in this chapter and in various studies may be that hard and/or extra-long efforts appear to require some carbs—even "bad" carbs. Therefore, if you are going to cut workout time by ramping up the interval training, you may require judiciously targeted use of carbs.

## CHECK THE GAS TANK

As we reflect on the growing popularity of fat-adapted endurance training and racing, and perhaps gloat about being on the cutting edge of something revolutionary (and evolutionary!), we might also reflect on how sorta dumb we've been for a long time. From a metabolic perspective, endurance sports has been all about expertly managing the dispensation of fuel from a two-thousand-calorie (glycogen) storage tank. Meanwhile, we have largely ignored how to best utilize this extremely large, clean-burning fat storage tank that is fifteen to thirty times the size of the glycogen tank!

Think about Sami and Meredith's row for a moment, and athletes contemplating this feat while locked into the carbohydrate paradigm. They would set off from the California coast packing all of their own food, hoping—with life or death risks—that they wouldn't bonk or have adverse digestive reactions to consuming all those pro-inflammatory and oxidative carbohydrates. Recall Johnny G dissolving a tooth in the Midwest, and having his digestive system conk out during RAAM? At least he could get off his bike and hitch a ride home, unlike a maladapted Sami and Meredith drifting off course in a bonked state.

Clearly, operating in a fat-adapted state is a far superior choice to being stuck in a carbohydrate dependency state—at rest and during endurance exercise. As discussed in the diet chapters, it's okay to try to trend in that direction at a rate that's comfortable to you. Ditch the highly offensive processed foods from your diet and start emphasizing more primal-aligned foods. Wait a bit until you get hungry for breakfast. Try snacking on high fat foods instead of quick energy carb foods. Try waiting during your extended workouts until you really need a blood sugar boost—instead of habitually slamming the sugary gels and drinks every time your watch beeps on the fifteen minutes.

Slowly but surely, or quickly if you are inclined to really go for it, you will start to experience the amazing benefits of being fat-adapted.

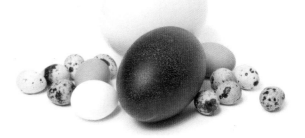

# COMPLEMENTARY MOVEMENT AND LIFESTYLE PRACTICES

*Complementary, but mandatory if you want to perform well and preserve health*

# CHAPTER 8

## IN THIS CHAPTER

Complementary movement and lifestyle practices are essential to peak performance, injury prevention, and the preservation of health. Sleep is of primary importance to athletes, and insufficiencies here can render all your other training efforts ineffective. The key to optimal sleep is to create mellow, dark evenings of minimal artificial light and digital stimulation after dark. This will enable circadian-influenced melatonin to flood your bloodstream on cue, make you sleepy soon after dark, and facilitate a good night's sleep. The top priority is to keep evenings dark and mellow—turning those screens off long before bedtime.

Efforts must be made to increase all forms of general everyday movement, because the many sedentary forces of modern life have negative health consequences—even for devoted fitness enthusiasts. Walk everywhere you can instead of always opting for motorized transport. Take frequent breaks from periods of stillness and peak cognitive function—even five minutes of movement several times per day can make great progress against the active couch potato syndrome. Resist the temptation to be lazy just because you performed an impressive workout; this mindset is unfortunately common among endurance performers.

Endurance athletes should devote significant attention to mobility and movement practices like yoga or Pilates. These efforts can help balance out the extreme and narrow focus of endurance training, improving muscular balance, strength, and flexibility. Deliberate movement practices can also improve mental focus and generate a necessary calming influence to counter the high-stress nature of endurance training.

Play is a fundamental element of healthy living that is often overlooked in hectic modern life. Getting outside for some spontaneous, unstructured physical activity provides a perfect escape from the pressures and responsibilities of daily life, and the regimented and repetitive nature of endurance workouts. Pursuing a well-managed primal thrill can deliver a good old-fashioned adrenalin rush that is sorely missing in predictable, confined modern life. The possibilities are numerous, so pursue endeavors that seem interesting and just a tiny bit outside of your comfort zone.

. . . . . . . . . . . . . .

**WE'VE SPENT ALL THIS TIME** talking about your training, which comprises only a small percentage of time in the big picture of how you live your life. Even if you train five, ten, or even twenty hours a week, you are still moving for a very small fraction of the total time in a 168-hour week! Here, briefly, are some important additional areas of focus that we will cover in more detail throughout the chapter:

**Sleep**: This is the top priority (so important it's out of alphabetical order here!) for any athlete to ensure all that hard work in training pays off, and that you preserve your health in pursuit of ambitious fitness goals. It's not as simple as the tired maxim of "get eight hours a night." Numerous training, life-stress, and circadian variables can alter your sleep requirements over the course of a year and a lifetime.

**Increase general everyday movement:** The assorted sedentary forces of modern life can create cellular dysfunction and metabolic disease risk factors, even for devoted fitness enthusiasts. Ward off the active couch potato syndrome by walking more in daily life and taking frequent breaks from prolonged periods of sitting or stillness.

**Mobility and movement practices:** The narrow and often extreme physical demands of endurance training need to be balanced out with whole-body movement practices like yoga or Pilates that synchronize muscle groups, broaden overall strength, increase flexibility, improve your ability to focus, and deliver a peaceful, yin balance to the excessive fight-or-flight yang stimulation of endurance training.

**Play**: A fundamental element of human evolution and our genetic expectations for health, adding more play into your life can help keep you motivated, inspired, and refreshed to complete the challenging workouts that support peak endurance performance—not to mention the many other challenges and obligations of hectic modern life.

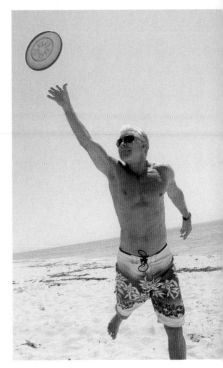

## SLEEP

You've probably seen some of the sobering stats that Americans and others in high-tech cultures are chronically sleep deprived. Harvard School of Public Health researchers found that 40 percent of Americans get fewer than five hours of sleep per night, and 75 percent suffer from some form of sleep disorder. We're violently disrupting our circadian rhythms—closely synchronized to the rising and setting of the sun for millions of years—with excess artificial light and digital stimulation after dark, assorted medications (including sleep meds, which knock you unconscious but interfere with true hormonal restoration), ill-advised food choices (especially excess carbs in the evening), the use of alcohol, caffeine, tobacco, and other health-compromising substances, shift work, jet travel, inconsistent bed and wake times, and consequent mornings of blaring alarms, foggy brains, and caffeine slams.

40 PERCENT OF AMERICANS GET FEWER THAN FIVE HOURS OF SLEEP PER NIGHT, AND 75 PERCENT SUFFER FROM SOME FORM OF SLEEP DISORDER.

It's as simple as this: sleep is the top priority for your fitness progress and preservation of health. If you are short on sleep, consider everything you have read so far in the book to be irrelevant. Insufficient sleep compromises fat burning, and disturbs appetite and satiety hormones so you overeat and store the excess calories as fat instead of burning them. It adversely affects mood, concentration, memory retention, and productivity, and can lead to hypertension, increased stress hormone levels, irregular heartbeat, a compromised immune system, obesity, sexual dysfunction, premature aging, certain cancers, and heart disease.

Optimal sleeping habits enable testosterone and other adaptive hormones to repair organs, strengthen and rebuild muscles, and rejuvenate all body systems. The immune system's white blood cells kick into high gear during restful sleep, and macrophages and leukocytes multiply rap-

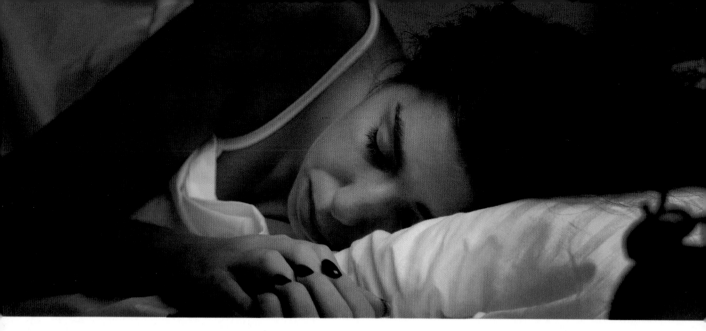

idly and induce healthy flora to prevail over harmful bacteria. Sleep also activates the release of human growth hormone, which helps your body burn fat and build or tone lean muscle. As you sleep, regions of the brain responsible for emotional and social function are rejuvenated so that you can face the day excited and refreshed. The 2008 Forum of European Neuroscience presented a study that indicated that a restorative night's sleep helps the brain solidify weak memories that might otherwise fade over time.

You're likely familiar with some of the terminology describing different sleep cycles or stages, like REM (rapid eye movement) sleep and deep sleep. The labeling can get a little alpha beta gamma hella confusing, but it's important to understand that you require not only good sleep duration, but also to cycle smoothly and completely through the various stages of sleep. REM sleep is where your brain sorts out the tremendous amount of stimuli faced each day, hones your spatial, perceptual, and visual skills, sorts out emotional experiences and stressful events, replenishes neurotransmitters like serotonin and dopamine, and refreshes the sodium-potassium pumps in your brain neurons that are easily depleted as you tackle cognitive challenges during the day.

As you drift into deeper sleep, you hardwire complex motor skills into long-term memory in a process known as *long-term potentiation* (LTP). Deep sleep is when growth hormone and other restoration processes kick into high gear. A complete sleep cycle from REM to the deepest stage and back to the start of another REM cycle lasts approximately ninety minutes and is repeated throughout the night. Earlier in the night, you spent more of that time in deep sleep and less in REM—

that's why it's so important to get to bed on time! In the morning, REM time predominates, making it easier to rise from bed and get into your morning activities.

How much sleep is enough? You've probably heard the oft-touted maxim that "eight hours a night" represents the ideal, but it's not as simple as that. Your sleep needs will vary according to your training patterns, your levels of overall life stress, and circadian influences. The harder you train and/or the more stress of all forms you have in daily life, the greater your need for sleep to try and recover, or at least hang on by a thread till things normalize.

Your sleep requirements also vary according to seasonal sunlight exposure at your latitude. In the excellent book *Lights Out: Sleep, Sugar, and Survival*, authors T.S. Wiley and Bent Formby urge us to obtain "9.5 hours of sleep for at least seven months of the year," when days are shorter. During the longer summer months, the authors acknowledge that your sleep requirements are minimized due to the longer, sunnier days. Of course, those who live in tropical regions will have less seasonal variation in sleep hours, whereas those who live in polar climates will have more variation between their summer and winter patterns. Our Canadian editor Penelope Jackson reports that in Yellowknife, Northwest Territories, Canada (latitude 62°N, almost to the 66°N Arctic Circle), "It's basically impossible to sleep on June 21!"

To ensure proper restoration, you must get back to an authentic circadian rhythm, synching your sleep habits with the rising and setting of the sun like your ancestors did. This means dealing with the foremost modern offenders of excess artificial light and digital stimulation after dark. The hormones that govern sleep and wakefulness, like melatonin (the hormone that makes you feel sleepy), serotonin (the "feel good" hormone that gets you going in the morning) and cortisol (the primary stress hormone we've discussed at length as a component of the fight-or-flight response) are incredibly sensitive to light. When you blast your retinas with TV or computer screen emissions late into the night, you immediately suppress melatonin and experience a second wind of energy and alertness thanks to the quick energy boosters of sugar and stress hormones.

Circadian disruptors also throw off ghrelin, the primary hunger hormone, and leptin, the primary satiety and fat-storage hormone. Hence, your late nights will likely feature increased hunger along with an increased propensity to store those extra calories as fat. *Lights Out* explains why in detail: unnaturally lengthening your days with excess light after dark tricks your body into thinking it's summertime year round. Our genes are programmed in summertime to consume a lot of carbohydrates (since that's when fruit ripens) and to store those carbohydrate calories as fat (to prepare for the long winters, when food is scarce). Your innocent use of a computer or TV after dark is directly contributing to you holding onto excess body fat instead of burning it off.

Beyond the metabolic consequences, routinely overriding your circadian rhythm impairs your ability to manage even moderate levels of oxidative stress, which leads to accelerated aging and measurable neurological decline. Unfortunately, this type of behavior is a given in modern life. For over two million years, our ancestors went to sleep soon after it got dark. Today, we power up when it gets dark, and create one of the most profound disconnects from our genetic expectation for health imaginable.

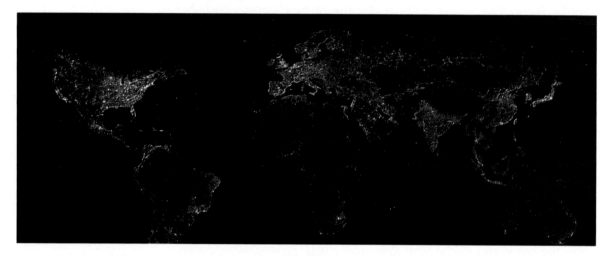

*The earth at night, courtesy of the US government's Defense Meteorological Satellite Program (DMSP) Operational Linescan System (OLS). A cool photo to be sure, but a disturbing representation of the level of light pollution in urbanized areas across the globe.*

You don't have to completely eliminate your after-dark screen engagements; screens are involved in some of the most popular leisure activities we use to balance our hectic days. However, we all deserve to make some devoted efforts to bringing things back in balance in this area. Enjoying a show or a movie after dinner is one thing, but routinely grinding away on email from 11:00 p.m. to midnight is quite another.

When you reconnect with your circadian rhythm, your hormones work as intended to make you sleepy soon after it gets dark, and help you awaken naturally refreshed and energized near sunrise. In fact, if you wonder if you are getting enough sleep, you could start by asking if you are able to awaken each day, near sunrise, naturally refreshed and energized, without an alarm clock. Not many people can give an emphatic yes to this simple and essential health scorecard entry.

Soon after it gets dark (or these days we should say, soon after you *make it dark* in your environment), circadian rhythm mechanisms cause the sleep hormone melatonin, manufactured in the pineal gland near the center of the brain, to increase in the bloodstream. This process, referred to as "dim light melatonin onset (DLMO)," relaxes brain waves and muscles, and lowers body temperature, blood pressure, heart rate, and respiration. You eventually drift off to sleep, commencing a sequence of sleep cycles that helps you achieve full restoration by morning.

When the sun rises, your circadian rhythm responds to the onset of light by decreasing melatonin and raising serotonin levels so that you wake up alert, refreshed, and ready to tackle the day. Light is registered first through the retina; the signal travels through the optic nerve to other regions of the brain, including the pineal gland that activates the release of serotonin. Levels of the stress hormone cortisol increase within the first thirty minutes of waking. This morning cortisol influx is a desirable genetic mechanism that prepares us for the energy demands of a busy day. The serotonin-cortisol effect is most effective closest to dawn, another reason to rise with the light of day.

The various stages of light to deep sleep help the brain organize short- and long-term memory and fine-tune cognitive functioning, a process called *synaptic homeostasis*. Synapses, the spaces located between nerve cells that allow the cells to communicate with each other, respond to myriad, often overwhelming stimulation during waking hours. The more enriched our days are, the more synapses grow, but our synapses can only take so much before they peter out with exhaustion. Sleep is critical to allowing the synapses to restore and recalibrate to face more stimulation the following day.

Here are some practical steps you can take to optimize your sleeping habits and environment:

**Minimize screen use:** It's hard to put it more plainly than this: the more screen time you engage in after dark, the more you compromise your health and restoration. Light bulbs and electronic gadgets, from computers to televisions to all things digital, emit *blue light*, a sustained and vivid hue on the electromagnetic spectrum. The bluer the light, the more intense it registers on the Kelvin (K) temperature scale. For instance, incandescent indoor light bulbs burn at 3,000K, ultraviolet sunlight at peak midday intensity burns at 5,500K, and the blue light emitted from most computer monitors burns at 6,500K! Exposure to excessive blue light after dark spikes cortisol and ghrelin, hampers leptin signaling, increases insulin production, and suppresses melatonin. Habitual screen use after dark makes you tired, fat, and vulnerable to oxidative damage and accelerated aging. It can also contribute to degenerative eye disease and elevated risk for certain cancers. Shut the screens off ideally two hours before bedtime and absolutely no less than one hour before bedtime.

## HABITUAL SCREEN USE AFTER DARK MAKES YOU TIRED, FAT, AND VULNERABLE TO OXIDATIVE DAMAGE AND ACCELERATED AGING.

**Mellow evenings:** Honor your circadian rhythm and start mellowing things out soon after the sun sets. Minimize indoor light use, favoring candlelight or firelight. Consider switching out some of your regular light bulbs for orange "insect" bulbs sold at home supply stores. Get yourself a pair of yellow or orange-tinted UV protection sunglasses. Low temperature light that falls in the red-orange-yellow spectrum (candlelight, fire, UV protected lenses, orange bulbs) instead of the blue spectrum does not interfere with melatonin production and can actually facilitate relaxation of the central nervous system.

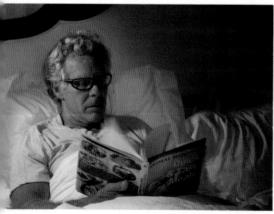

*These funky shades from a photo shoot years ago were borrowed from Brad. They take a while to get used to, but now Mark digs yellow lenses, and dim bulbs (as long as he don't have to do business with them).*

If you must work on your computer after sunset, do so earlier in the evening, and take regular screen breaks to rest your eyes and brain. Also, download a free software program called f.lux (available for all platforms at justgetflux.com) and install it onto all machines you might use after dark. f.lux adjusts the color temperature (like brightness but not quite the same) of your computer display to synchronize with the ambient light in your environment. If you are working during the time sunset occurs at your latitude, you will notice your computer screen automatically change to a more mellow, pink-tinted hue at the strike of sunset.

Make your final hours truly calming. Take an evening stroll with the dog, chat or play board games with loved ones, engage in hobbies like drawing or arts and crafts, do some leisure reading (but not work reading, disturbing news reading, or anything that requires extra cognitive power), or just enjoy some quiet reflection time, perhaps gazing at the stars outside.

**Simple, dark environment:** Strive to create a simple, clean, minimalist bedroom that is used for sleeping only. Absolutely no computers, TVs, pads, or smartphone screens allowed, and definitely no makeshift office setups in the corner either. Eliminate clutter such as excess clothing, stacks of books, magazines, or paperwork, or remnants of partially completed home improvement projects. Add a live houseplant to improve air quality and eliminate toxins. We are hardwired to sleep in colder temperatures, with experts recommending a range of 60°F to 68°F (16°C to 20°C) for evening sleep.

To prevent interference with melatonin and other hormonal processes, your sleeping quarters must be absolutely, completely dark. Eliminate nightlights and any LED screen emissions, even tiny ones like power indicators on charger plugs. Electrical tape works well for those annoying little emissions. Instead of plug-in nightlights, keep a small flashlight by your bed in case you have to get up. If you are a shift worker sleeping when it's not dark, have a partner who stays up later than you, or otherwise have light sneaking into your scene when you are trying to sleep, a quality eye mask can be helpful. However, it's important to realize that it's not just our retinas that are sensitive to light. We have light receptors in every one of our skin cells, and they will register light and send the message directly to your pineal gland, the endocrine gland in the brain where melatonin is secreted.

One University of Chicago study showed that flashing a beam of light on the back of the knee is enough to disrupt normal melatonin release. Another study delivered two-millisecond (.002—imperceptible to the naked eye) flashes of light every thirty seconds for an hour, between two and three hours after normal bedtime. These brief pulses of light penetrated the eyelids (proven by EEG data) and delayed the normal salivary melatonin rhythm.

A quiet environment is also essential for uninterrupted sleep. If you have challenges in your outside environment, get a noise-cancelling sound machine, a fan, a humidifier, or even a smartphone app of nature sounds (Sleepmaker Rain Pro for iPhone is great) to cancel out disruptive and unpredictable outside sounds.

**Consistent times:** Strive to get to bed at a similar time each evening, something that your DLMO will facilitate for you over time as you implement good habits. As you strive to sync your sleep habits with your circadian rhythm, you will actually shift your bedtime and wake times gradually to align with the lengthening or shortening of the days by season. Perhaps you will feel sleepy and achieve a bedtime of 9:00 p.m. in the dead of winter, experience a gradual extension out to 10:30 p.m. by the time of the summer solstice, and then start gradually getting to bed a bit earlier over the fall to again reach your earliest annual bedtime in the winter.

If you awaken in the middle of the night, don't be overly troubled. As we cycle though the various stages of sleep, it's not uncommon to awaken at the conclusion of an REM cycle. Just try to do some calming behaviors such as deep breathing, a quick stroll outside to gaze at the stars, fixing a cup of herbal tea, or write a journal entry, especially if something particular is troubling you. If you must read to help get back to sleep, do so with a very dim light, like a miner's headlamp. Relax, lie back down when you are ready, and hopefully you will proceed with your cycling through the sleep phases.

In tandem with your goal of creating mellow evenings and a consistent bedtime, strive to wake up near sunrise. This will allow you to take full advantage of the hormonal processes that refresh and energize you, namely the lowering of melatonin in tandem with the elevation of serotonin, as well as a healthy spike in cortisol—processes that are triggered by the rising of the sun. If you claim to not be a morning person or otherwise sleep in a manner that is highly incongruent with what is described here, make an effort to expose yourself to direct sunlight as soon as you wake up. In tandem with exerting more discipline about making your evenings dark and mellow, your hormones will soon recalibrate to these genetically optimal sleep practices—no matter who you are! Remember, anyone's night-owl tendencies are fueled not by some unique genetic particulars but rather by powerful fight-or-flight hormonal processes that are universally in conflict with what our genes expect for good health and restoration.

> Claim to be a night owl? Don't blame it all on genetics; there are light-influenced fight-or-flight hormonal processes that hinder optimal gene expression and health.

Obviously, we want disruptive alarms completely out of the picture in hopes that you will awaken naturally. When it's time to get up, move slowly and gracefully, allowing a few minutes to sit in bed, perhaps record your resting heart rate and heart rate variability (more in Chapter 9), talk quietly with your mate, or jot down some thoughts, such as doing a gratitude exercise.

Don't bother with your smartphone or other communication devices first thing in the morning. Exposure to news or personal communication—even if the content is pleasant—can throw you into a reactive, overstimulated mode, triggering an undesirable activation of the stress response that will contribute to burnout later. Instead, take control of your morning with some deliberate and pleasing rituals, such as a quick sun salute sequence outdoors, taking a warm shower, making a cup of herbal tea, taking the dog out for a quick morning outing, or simply strolling down the driveway to get the newspaper. We're all typically pressed for time in the morning, but engaging in deliberate, self-initiated, mellow morning behaviors will help you preserve a disciplined, proactive mindset when you are exposed to all kinds of distracting and stressful stimulus over the course of the day.

On the rare occasion that you need to use an alarm to wake up earlier than normal, get a special clock or smartphone app that features nature sounds and progressive tones for a gentle reminder to get up.

**Nap when you need to**: Afternoon siestas are commonplace among cultures in warm-weather countries, such as Latin America, Asia, the Mediterranean, North Africa, and the Middle East. Unfortunately, the fast pace of American and other go-go Western cultures stigmatizes afternoon naps as a sign of laziness.

A brief nap of even just twenty minutes helps you catch up on REM or non-REM sleep cycle deficiencies from the previous night, will refresh and rebalance the sodium-potassium pumps (recall our discussion of the sodium-potassium pump in muscle recovery from Chapter 6) in your brain neurons, and generate a pulse of human growth hormone and other adaptive hormones into the bloodstream. When you feel "fried" and in need of a nap, this is a literal truth, because long periods of peak cognitive function have depleted the important chemical balance in your brain cells and compromised the snappy electrical signaling needed for peak cognitive performance. When you wake up feeling refreshed and energized, this is also a literal truth, because the replenished chemicals have restored these blown circuits back to peak function.

Whenever you experience an afternoon energy lull or decline in peak cognitive function, try to take a nap and build this behavior into a habit. Don't worry about all the questionable chatter about the optimal duration and time of day for napping, nor the dire warnings that napping can interfere with evening sleep. Dr. Sara Mednick, one of the world's leading sleep experts, a Harvard-trained psychologist, and currently Assistant Professor of Psychology at University of California, Riverside, asserts that napping is unlikely to compromise your ability to fall asleep successfully, and can even help you combat conditions like nighttime insomnia. Yep, even when you take these fog-inducing deep sleep catch-up naps later in the afternoon.

Brad claims to be a professional-caliber napper. He reports benefits from taking a quick morning nap (ten to twenty minutes) when he isn't feeling sharp, a lengthy afternoon nap (thirty to forty-five minutes) when his energy is flagging, and even just lying down and closing his eyes for ten minutes after a high-intensity sprint or strength workout to facilitate relaxation and promote recovery. Tim DiFrancesco, the Director of Strength and Conditioning for the Los Angeles Lakers, keeps his players fit not only in the gym but also by looking after their diet and lifestyle habits, in association with Dr. Cate Shanahan's novel meal-planning program she dispenses to the Lakers. DiFrancesco reveals that napping is huge in the NBA. "On game day, players have a nice midday lunch and then go down for nap from 1:00 p.m. to 4:00 p.m. without fail—every one of them, before every game. It's an essential element of their lifestyle, and it helps them recover from the grueling game schedule and jet lag from crazy road trips."

Look, it's no secret that we go through life not getting enough sleep, not getting enough general rest and downtime, and not recovering optimally from stress. For the posers, paper pushers, and playahs of the planet who have minimal regard for health, and no regard for fitness or peak performance, these might not be fatal flaws. For an athlete or peak performance enthusiast of any kind at any level, even a slight deficiency in sleep is highly destructive to your goals and your overall health. It's not uncommon to hear pointed pushback on this matter from naysayers and heavy hitters who favor the quote attributed to assorted luminaries, including NBA basketball legend Charles Barkley: "I'll sleep when I'm dead." It's time to reframe any notions that sleeping and napping are for slackers. Sleep is for peak performers—in athletics, in cognitive pursuits, and in life. Do whatever it takes to get your fair share and then some.

## INCREASE GENERAL DAILY MOVEMENT

The "active couch potato syndrome" is an actual observed scientific phenomenon whereby devoted fitness enthusiasts—who conduct daily workouts but live otherwise inactivity-dominant lifestyles—are not immune to the cellular dysfunction and metabolic disease patterns driven by inactivity. Statistics referenced by James Levine, MD, PhD, a Mayo Clinic researcher, international expert on obesity, and author of *Get Up! Why Your Chair is Killing You and What You Can Do About It,* suggests that the average Westerner working in an office environment sits for some thirteen hours per day (at work and at leisure), sleeps for eight, and moves for only three. It's clear that the health risks of desk work, commuting, and digital leisure time are so extreme that they are simply not mitigated by even a devoted workout regimen of five, ten, or fifteen hours a week.

Musculoskeletally, prolonged sitting weakens your gluteal muscles by deactivating them from supporting bodyweight and essentially putting them into a prolonged static stretch. Sitting also shortens and tightens up your hamstrings and hip flexors. The glutes, hamstrings, and hip flexors comprise the foundation of all manner of daily activity, from basic leaning or crouching all the way through the movements involved in competitive sports. The typically hunched upper-body position that we use for driving and interacting with screens large and small creates an assortment of muscular and spinal imbalances in the upper body, promoting chronic neck and back pain.

Prolonged stillness also leads to metabolic and hormonal imbalances that inhibit fat metabolism, elevate triglyceride levels, elevate blood pressure, and promote excess body-fat storage. In particular, leptin signaling is compromised by inactivity. This causes you to eat more, and be more likely to store those extra calories as fat than burn them. Prolonged stillness also triggers chemical changes in the brain that impair cognitive function and promote further inactivity by diminishing motivation and energy levels at rest. These changes can be quantified by measuring *Non-Exercise Activity Thermogenesis*—caloric expenditure outside of sleeping, eating, and exercising. Lower readings indicate a more sluggish functional state, while higher readings result in more energy and motivation to move.

Again, the fact that you swam morning Masters or ran your six-mile loop does not exempt you from the dialog here. We can all attest to suffering from the afternoon blues after being stuck at a desk for many hours—no matter how active we were earlier in the day. Furthermore, if there is even a whiff of chronic patterns in your training, you might even experience more severe active couch potato symptoms because of the imbalances and burnout caused by chronic exercise.

Our genes thrive on frequent and varied movement over the course of the day. Even our workout patterns do not support this goal, because they are often rote: an hour on the treadmill, two circuits through the weight machine stations, or fifty laps in the pool. Workouts improve your fitness in those specific endeavors, and deliver a bit of a cardiovascular cross-training effect as well, but they do little to address your genetic requirements for frequent varied movement. Increasing general everyday movement will help prevent the musculoskeletal, hormonal, metabolic, and cognitive problems discussed, improving both your general health and your athletic performance as a consequence.

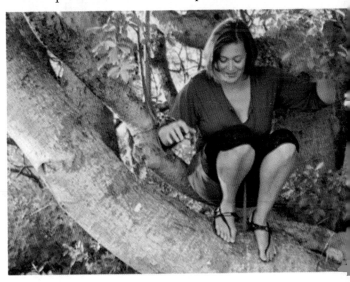

No need for a massive lifestyle overhaul here; you don't have to resign your position at the firm and get into the mail-delivery business. Even a minimal increase in your movement habits can have a big impact. One Mayo Clinic study revealed that a leisurely (1 mph) fifteen-minute walk after a meal lowered by half the two-hour-long blood sugar spike that occurs after a typical meal. Dr. Levine cites research that performing an activity as simple as standing up at your desk instead of sitting increases caloric expenditure by 10 percent, while taking frequent movement breaks during the day can add up to an additional thousand calories burned or more, as well as promoting hormonal changes that encourage fat burning instead of fat storage.

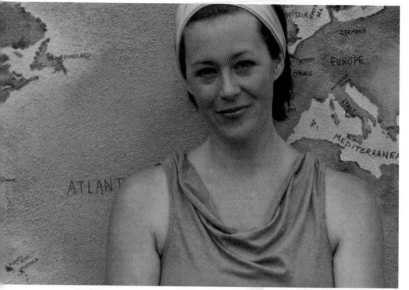

One of the world's leading experts on the importance of frequent movement and variation in your daily routine is Katy Bowman, MS, founder of Nutritious Movement, author of *Move Your DNA: Restore Your Health Through Natural Movement,* and popular blogger (Katysays.com) and podcast host (Katy Says). Katy is a *biomechanist,* someone who studies the movement of living creatures, like humans. Her focus extends beyond fitness and into the realm of overall vitality and cellular health—what she calls *movement nutrition.* Katy's goal is to help you counterbalance the assorted forces in modern life that inhibit natural movement (e.g., your propensity to sit in one spot for a long time and focus your eyes on a screen a fixed distance away). Interestingly, Katy's approach is short on hard and fast rules and precise movement techniques, and instead emphasizes being more active and varied throughout your day in any way that you please.

*Biomechanist Katy Bowman is polite about it, but she's not too impressed with your endurance superpowers. She urges you to pursue a broader sense of health by adding more movement variation to your daily routine.*

Katy's favorite form of movement nutrition is walking, and she believes you should walk anywhere and everywhere you possibly can. At our 2014 PrimalCon health and fitness retreat in Oxnard, CA, participants were amazed to learn that Katy rose before sunrise and walked *six miles* to the event venue from a friend's house to deliver her morning keynote presentation. Meanwhile, the authors actually drove the quarter-mile from the hotel to the talk venue at an adjacent beach park...Ouch!

Katy chastises endurance athletes for training so hard that they have a tendency to become lazy in everyday life: "If your hobby sucks too much energy out of you, you can fall short of your basic movement nutrition requirements. You tell yourself that because you ran ten miles or whatever, you've earned the right to slothfulness. This 'athlete's mindset,' coupled with a society that has outsourced routine movement to technology, is extremely destructive to your health at the cellular level. When you use a single position repetitively, such as curling your body into a comfortable work chair for hours every day, muscles, joints, and arteries will adapt to this repetitive positioning by changing their cellular makeup and becoming literally 'stiff,' with reduced ranges of motion and an actual hardening of the arterial walls in those areas."

Katy continues, "Granted, it's absolutely a natural human instinct to want to do as little as possible and to find the most comfortable positions. There is no doubt our ancestors were wired accordingly, but they didn't have modern luxuries to actualize their slothful tendencies. This means that today, we have to be especially vigilant to give ourselves the movement and variation we need to optimize health."

It's hard to deny that this slothful mindset is entrenched in the endurance community. When we are off the bike or off the road, we revel in reclining and indulging in assorted dietary treats that we might otherwise declare taboo. Peruse any bonafide endurance athlete's Instagram account and you'll find epic nature photography from the trails mixed in with foot-high pancake stacks, giant bowls of guacamole and chips, festive gatherings with everyone clutching an alcoholic beverage, on-location shots of the best gelato or donut shops in cities across the land, and plenty of smiling people reclining on couches, lounge chairs, and beaches.

Even as the evidence accumulates, starting with Jim Fixx and indiscriminate dietary habits and continuing to Dr. O'Keefe detailing heart damage caused by serious training, we still see lots of denial behavior in action. Not to be a party pooper again, and we've talked enough about dietary habits already, but let's consider for a moment that it's simply not enough to log your miles and then return to the habit patterns of the fattest, laziest population in the history of the human race. Instead, let's look at how some simple, painless changes to your daily routine can pay big health dividends and leverage all that hard training into further fitness improvements.

First, we need to understand that cardiovascular fitness is not the same as cardiovascular health. You might be fit enough to peg that heart rate at 165 and climb for an hour to the top of a mountain, but, as Katy Bowman explains, "cardiovascular health comes when your entire circulatory system is used in a variety of ways, to deliver oxygen to 100 percent of the cells in your body." In essence, endurance athletes are extreme specialists—good at pumping blood to the legs for cycling or the lats for swimming (if you have good stroke mechanics; otherwise it's biceps and triceps if you swim like Mark…), but severely deficient in overall arterial health due to extensive sedentary behavior and a lack of variety in workouts.

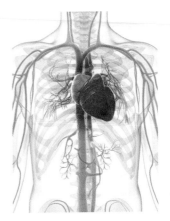

*Cardiovascular fitness is different than cardiovascular health. Banging intervals is great, but how's your overall arterial health and daily "movement nutrition"?*

> "CARDIOVASCULAR FITNESS IS NOT THE SAME AS CARDIOVASCULAR HEALTH; NARROWLY FOCUSED ENDURANCE WORKOUTS DO NOT PROTECT FROM ARTERIAL DYSFUNCTION RELATED TO EXTENSIVE SEDENTARY PATTERNS." — KATY BOWMAN

"Even a big-time endurance athlete can damage arteries in areas of the body that get stuck in a fixed position for too long, as when you are sitting for hours every day," explains Katy. "Endurance athletes need to realize that their narrow focus of performing well in a single activity during training does not correlate with nourishing all of the tissues throughout the body. When you engage in workout patterns that shunt blood into the same narrow areas in the extremities, you potentially compromise your overall health because of the lack of variation, and also the potential to overstress the heart and inflict damage [as detailed in Chapter 2 with O'Keefe's and Attia's commentary]. I don't care how ripped you look on the outside, you're a narrowly adapted creature who is adept at engorging your heart, and certain muscles, to perform occasionally. In fact, your narrow and extreme workout patterns are often a detriment to your overall cellular and cardiovascular health. From a cellular perspective, you are largely a couch potato, with an assortment of cellular structures that are hardened and misshapen from too much stillness."

Katy continues, "We should also recognize that the prevailing sedentary patterns of daily life make the repetitive loads of endurance training more high risk. You aren't used to doing anything for a long period except sitting! So going out and running for two hours or cycling for five hours is more stressful to the body than it might be if you led a more active and varied lifestyle." Increasing general daily movement—yes, even walking—will make you more resilient and adaptable to the loads you put your body under during proper endurance workouts.

Dr. Maffetone asserts something similar, explaining how different aerobic muscle fibers and enzymes are activated at each intensity level, from walking on up to aerobic maximum heart rate, and that activating the lowest-intensity aerobic energy production systems can improve your ability to burn fat and circulate blood at all intensity levels. Unfortunately, most endurance athletes routinely skip right over lowest-intensity aerobic energy production when they perform their workouts. These low-end aerobic muscle fibers and enzymes could and would make a significant contribution to your performance at higher intensities, but they are poorly trained because of insufficient walking in daily life, insufficient warmup and cooldown periods at a typical workout, and insufficient workouts performed at recovery heart rates (i.e., below 65 percent of max heart rate). If you find a way to add more walking into your lifestyle, you will improve your ability to perform at all paces beyond that. Remember, as we learned earlier, even an all-out one-hour race is 98 percent aerobic.

You could also jump in here with a plug for strength training. Recall Dr. Kelly Starrett's comments in Chapter 5, where he identified strength training as a way to "connect the dots and identify weaknesses that can cause your form to break down during an endurance workout." Because we have insufficient general movement, we need to make a concerted effort to put our muscles under extreme load to be able to benefit fully from endurance workouts. To optimize endurance performance and aerobic function, we can add more movement and variation to our daily routine, conduct strength training sessions per Primal Endurance guidelines, and finally spend more time walking or exercising at extremely low intensity levels. It all counts toward peak performance!

If you are inclined to go Type-A crazy here and discount the importance of this peripheral stuff, a narrow-minded, hard-trainer-but-otherwise-active-couch-potato lifestyle pattern will absolutely compromise your endurance performance. Starrett says strength training is like "free money" for endurance athletes, and now we can add walking and increased daily movement to the list of low-hanging fruit to feast upon! Here are a few tips to increase general everyday movement and variation:

**Dynamic workplace:** You likely are familiar with the burgeoning standup desk movement, where you elevate your screen and keyboard so you can operate while standing up. Standup workstations are great fun, they increase muscular load and calorie burning, but they are not the end-all for workplace health. As Katy Bowman explains, "Standing all day is no better than sitting. The only difference is you'll be more tired, stiff, and sore at the end of the day!" Instead, Katy recommends pursuing the broader goal of having more variation in your workday positioning.

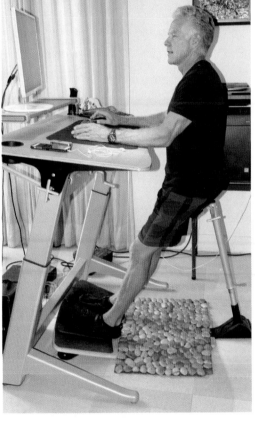

Go ahead and create a standup setting for your keyboard and monitor, but make it so you can easily switch from standup back to sitting. The fancy height-adjustable workstations from Focal Upright Furniture and VariDesk are great, but you can also create a similarly versatile low-tech setup using a footstool from a home supply store and some stacked cardboard boxes. After an appropriate standup period, you just lift the monitor and keyboard off their perches and back onto the desktop, and pull up your chair once again. Try to add as many position options as

*Mark loves his Focal Desk setup, where he can stand on a pebbled mat or ease back into a bicycle-seat-style peg chair for variation.*

possible, such as a floor option where you use a low coffee table for a desk and sit on a cushion or Bosu ball. More detailed instruction on creating a dynamic workplace is offered with a digital multimedia program called *Don't Just Sit There*, a joint effort between Mark and Katy Bowman, available at PrimalBlueprint.com.

Any time you can get away from a static position and go mobile, seize the opportunity—such as taking phone calls or personal meetings in the courtyard or while making some trips up and down stairs. Sure, there are conventions and constraints in many workplace environments, but the time for change is now. Any reasonable manager or human resources department will be supportive if you inquire about improving the ergonomics and variability of your work environment.

**Movement breaks:** Examine your current lifestyle patterns and identify prolonged periods of stillness and lack of variation. The instant and simple cure is to break these periods up by getting up and moving. You can take a walk, or do any other form of movement—take a few swings of the golf club, rattle off a set of pushups, pullups, or air squats, do some sun salute yoga movements, or descend and ascend four flights of stairs in your building.

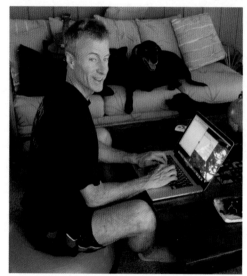

*Brad at a low desk with a Bosu ball. Can you spot the two stealth animals who crashed the shot?*

In the workplace, we are talking about taking a short break for every twenty minutes of peak cognitive focus to move your body and give your neurons a breather. Brain science confirms that we are simply incapable of sustaining intense focus for longer than twenty minutes. If you don't take frequent breaks, you will take them unwittingly, as when you absentmindedly click on a YouTube video link or jump on live chat instead of finishing your proposal. Ideally, your breaks will expose you to fresh air, open space, and direct sunlight to energize your body with electrically charged air particles called *negative ions*. This will balance out excessive exposure to indoor air, which is literally stale and de-energized—dominant in energy-zapping positive ions.

For every two to three hours of diligent cognitive effort, you should take a longer break of fifteen to twenty minutes where you change your environment, do some significant physical movement, and perhaps perform some specialized exercises to counterbalance the time your body has spent in fixed positions. Get outside and stroll a few laps of the courtyard, focusing your eyes on assorted distant objects to counter the fatigue of screen-gazing. Do some arm circles and mini-lunges to reactivate muscles that have been locked in fixed, unnatural positions at your desk.

If you want to argue that you're deserving of sedentary screen entertainment at the end of a busy, stressful day, at least alter your positions frequently while you enjoy your shows: Spend some time sitting on the floor, doing some standing stretches, sitting upright on the couch, and then returning to your reclining position.

**Walking**: In the name of your health and your devotion to total fitness, it's time to increase your mileage—and we're not talking about what's in your training log! Start parking at the outer edges of every parking lot, instead of always trolling for a primo spot. Swear off elevators, escalators, and people movers and use the stairs every time it's practical. Run errands to the post office, bank, or farmers' market on foot, or perhaps by bicycle (strap on a huge basket—you'll be surprised how many groceries can fit!), instead of always defaulting to a motor option.

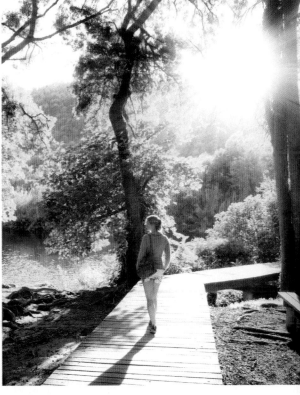

If you have a dog, honor your commitment as an owner by giving the animal a good, healthy outing every single day—ideally twice a day—no matter what the weather or how busy you are. If you find it difficult to make tiny little habit changes like increased walking, take a stroll as the very first thing you do every morning upon waking up—before the coffee pot, the shower, or the smartphone. Taking a five-minute walk to begin the day will build momentum for you to progress with all manner of personal goals that require focus and motivation.

You might have an environment of such convenience that you have to manufacture walking opportunities, so start getting creative. Virtually any phone or live conversation can probably be handled while you are walking, so when you jump up to get the phone, head right out the door in the same motion. Little things add up to big changes. If you find a way to add three minutes of walking each day (as in your new parking lot strategy), that's eighteen hours over a year's time!

# "LIFE IS LIKE RIDING A BICYCLE. TO KEEP YOUR BALANCE YOU MUST KEEP MOVING." —ALBERT EINSTEIN

## MOBILITY AND MOVEMENT PRACTICES

Stretching, foam rolling, preventative or rehabilitative exercises, yoga, Pilates, and other cool stuff that most endurance athletes "don't have time for" can mean the difference between peak performance and health, and injury, burnout, or technique dysfunction.

While you will indeed be devoting some additional precious time to complementary movement and mobility practices as needed, you can make a straight swap for reduced training hours and become a faster athlete. As Dr. Starrett discussed at length in Chapter 5, you must always be mindful of exhibiting correct technique and fatiguing into safe mechanical positions. If you develop chronic tightness and/or muscle imbalances from hard training and don't do anything to help rebalance your body, you will compromise technique efficiency and power generation to the extent that you will work just as hard but go slower.

Yoga, Pilates and other programs focused on flexibility, balance, and stretching help balance the extremely repetitive and narrow movement planes of traditional endurance workouts. We all know how the impact trauma of running can be assuaged by mobility and flexibility work, but even low- or no-impact endurance sports like swimming, cycling, or paddling sports bring a high risk of muscle imbalance and injury.

Going through the sequences of a good yoga or Pilates session requires not only the major muscle groups, but the smaller stabilizer muscle groups that are underused when you perform gross motor work like pedaling a bike, swimming, or running. Improving your balance, flexibility, and broad overall strength will not only make you fitter and more resilient for the physical challenges of daily life, it will help you preserve good technique as your large muscle groups fatigue during challenging workouts. Because of your improved proprioception honed through deliberate movement practices, you will be able to better notice and correct when your technique does falter on the road. Furthermore, your nuanced movements in the studio will help you identify a strength imbalance in a certain leg, or expose your weak feet that quiver under the stress of simply balancing for a bit on one leg. Also, the breathing awareness, counting, and precise movements demanded during a yoga or Pilates session can help improve your ability to focus during challenging endurance efforts, and also to stay relaxed and maintain control over your emotions when you fatigue.

Experts familiar with both yoga and endurance sports assert that your yoga or Pilates efforts will counterbalance the constant compression and contractions of endurance training. Improving your range of motion and muscle suppleness while at the same time building your endurance through training will enable you to preserve optimal technique and that all important maximum power output during workouts. This is particularly true for the core musculature, which is essential to good technique in every sport but doesn't get much of a training effect in endurance sessions. Building awesome core strength through yoga or Pilates will generate a noticeable improvement in your technique in a very short time, and will help prevent common injuries to the lower back and hamstrings that are triggered by a weak core.

Beyond the physical benefits, yoga and the like offer a calming, yin balance to the extreme, full-gas-pedal, yang nature of endurance training. Recall Dr. Starrett talking in Chapter 5 about athletes grinding their teeth at night, unable to recalibrate their autonomic nervous system due to the overstimulation of the sympathetic from hard training. Even a physically challenging class proceeds to a conclusion where your body and mind are feeling calm, relaxed, and peaceful. Frankly, it's hard for many athletes to get to this state without participating in a very focused and guided movement class. It's not the same as plopping yourself down on the couch after a hard training day and proclaiming yourself "relaxed."

If you are skeptical, take a single yoga class and take note of how you feel by the time of the restorative poses and breathing sequences at the end. You have just oxygenated the organs and tissues throughout your entire body, improved your respiratory capacity, put your joints and connective tissue through full-range-of-motion exercises, and smoothly synchronized the contracting of certain muscles and length-

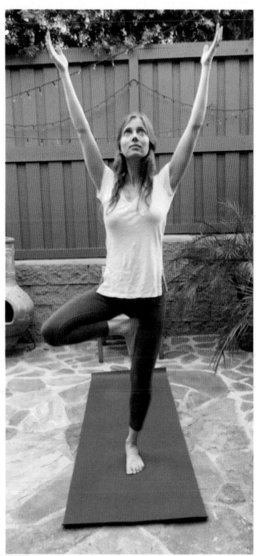

*Malibu, CA, health coach, primal chef, and author Lauren Lobley demonstrating excellent yoga technique and exuding calmness in general*

ening of others to perform assorted complex movements, promoting muscle equilibrium and movement efficiency throughout the body.

In contrast, consider what you do during an endurance workout. As Katy Bowman said, "…you engorged your heart and certain muscles to deliver an extreme and narrow performance, possibly to the detriment of your overall cellular and cardiovascular health." No need for a knee-jerk defense of endurance workouts here; we can all admit to the pleasure and satisfaction that comes from pursuing our passions. We're simply advocating for a little balance in the form of activities that will make you not only a better athlete, but a healthier, more stress-balanced person.

## PLAY

While it's clear your endurance workouts provide an effective balance to sedentary patterns, give you some valuable exposure to nature, and provide a sense of satisfaction from pushing your performance limits, it's hard to categorize them as truly playful. In fact, due to their structured nature and physical effort required, they can easily become drudgery to some extent—yet another addition to your never-ending, constantly challenging "to do list" of daily life.

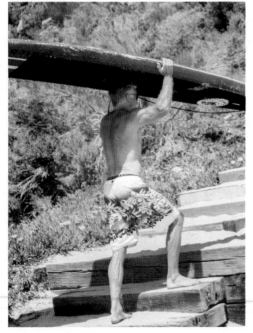

*Um, is this why everyone says standup paddling is a great upper body workout?*

Rediscovering your childlike inclinations and aptitudes to just get outside and enjoy spontaneous, unstructured outdoor physical activity—true play—will help you balance the many constraints, conventions, and sedentary forces that define our hectic modern lives. Introducing more play into your life will make you a happier, more creative, more productive, more sensitive, more balanced, and more playful human being.

This assertion is not just playful banter; we have a hardwired genetic need for play that stems from our evolution under constant and withering life-or-death selection pressure. It's clear from anthropological and archaeological evidence that play was a vital component of our primal ancestors' lives. While it obviously provided a needed escape from the hazards and harshness of primal life, play has offered humans numerous other benefits. Play contributed to communal living and social cohesion, nurtured creative energies, and strengthened problem-solving skills—as it still does today!

Play necessitates mental modeling, critical thinking, and creative innovation, through which we develop behavioral, intellectual, and emotional creativity and flexibility. Play has been scientifically proven to increase work productivity, improve stress management, and enhance self-esteem, social competency, and creativity.

Play can be loosely defined as activity that is fun, perhaps has an element of spontaneity, deemphasizes formal structure and tangible measurements of accomplishment, and gets you out of the focused, rational mindset that you exist in for most of the day. Play has you completely absorbed in the moment and the pure joy of the experience. Sitting on a weight machine in the gym and counting reps is a workout, while playing chase games with your dog or children in a park is play.

Unfortunately, humans have been so heavily socialized into regimented, technological, industrialized life that time for play is widely neglected. As the challenges and responsibilities of making a living or managing a family accumulate, we collectively adopt the belief that play is for youth. The truth is that play is for everyone, particularly those absorbed in the incredible complexity and breakneck pace of work, family, and home responsibilities, and, oh, the obligations of your training schedule.

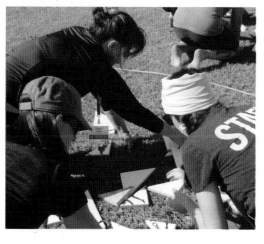

*The final task at the PrimalCon Survivor team challenge—complete the Grok puzzle!*

Psychiatrist Stuart Brown has spent his career studying the role of lifelong play. In his book *Play: How it Shapes the Brain, Opens the Imagination, and Invigorates the Soul*, Brown presents evidence that play, across the span of a lifetime, literally shapes our brains—forming new connections, creating new circuits, and organizing existing connections. The free-flowing, risk-free nature of play allows us to test out skills and scenarios that prepare us for real-life challenges. The exploration and spontaneity that characterize play help us form new neural circuits and mold new and improved connections and behavior patterns.

When humans are deprived of play they can suffer from multiple dysfunctional symptoms, including lack of curiosity, diminished social competency, and uncontrollable emotions. The net result is a narrowing of social, emotional, and cognitive intelligence. We've discussed some of the physical markers of accelerated aging, and this "narrowing" of perspective is also a profound marker of accelerated aging as well.

Today, play promotes the development and maintenance of a "cognitively fluid mind," a wonderful attribute with which to navigate the extremely complex and high-tech nature of modern life. This same attribute—a cognitively fluid mind—is believed by anthropologists to

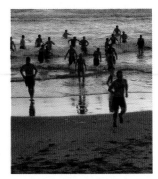

*Primal enthusiasts came from all over the globe to experience the PrimalCon evening ocean plunge/Jacuzzi sprint in Oxnard, CA. Water temp: low 60s. Resort Jacuzzi: sixty-second sprint up the beach (capacity 45, except for PrimalCon: capacity 90)*

represent one of the most profound breakthroughs in human evolution that occurred around sixty thousand years ago. Around this time, human cognitive function took a quantum leap and we were consequently able to increase the sophistication of our hunter-gatherer existence, invent culture, and successfully populate the globe with continually advancing societies.

The attachment to the outcome we assign to our core daily responsibilities, such as gaining a promotion at work, getting on the podium at a race, or receiving external approval for tangible achievements of any kind, can easily compromise our happiness, increase our risk for mortality, and may quite possibly even compromise our ability to perform in competitive settings with a calm, relaxed, focused mindset. Researchers have discovered that centenarians the world over possess a common ability to roll with the punches and release attachments to outcomes. Whether it's getting over the disappointment of a bad race, or moving forward after the death of a loved one, the ability to go with the flow is an important strategy for living a long, happy, productive life—and play can help you get to this exalted mindset and disposition.

Play is a loosely defined term that can encompass many endeavors. Because of our confined, predictable, indoor-dominant modern life, it's best to try to emphasize endeavors that balance these forces—namely spontaneous, unstructured, outdoor physical activity, as well as primal thrills that deliver jolts of adrenalin that we are sorely deficient in these days. Following are an assortment of ideas for play that will hopefully get you motivated and inspired to get out there and have some fun.

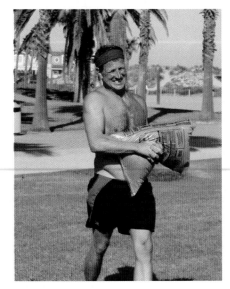

**Primal thrills:** Let's face it, modern life is incredibly safe, predictable, and often mundane. As we talk at length about the health hazards of excess fight-or-flight stimulation, it's easy to forget that our genes crave brief, intense stressful events that trigger a healthy, hormetic fight-or-flight stimulation. Inspector Clouseau knew this when he commanded his assistant to launch recurrent surprise attacks upon him in order to keep him sharp and alert at all times.

What about you? When's the last time you got a real rush from an intense challenge? We cannot disregard the reality that we evolved facing threat for millions of years, nor the possibility that our predictable, anesthetized modern life might be making us bored at the very deepest level. It's time to honor the legacy of your bold and adventurous ancestors and introduce some more thrills into your life! Don't worry, you don't have to take foolish, dangerous risks, like zig-zagging your motorcycle down the freeway at 100 mph, but rather engaging in calculated, well-managed challenges that will nevertheless deliver a similar charge to what the foolish motorcyclist or extreme sport athlete enjoys.

To access the exalted and oft-discussed flow state or "zone," your ideal challenge is just slightly outside your comfort zone—not too freaky or stupid to paralyze you with fear, and not so routine that it fails to stimulate an adrenalin buzz. For example, Mark loves snowboarding, and gets a thrill out of challenging the limits of his abilities—trying to keep pace with his speed-demon son, Kyle, or tackling an unfamiliar double black diamond slope. He accepts the calculated risks of sliding down a mountain slope, and does his very best to mitigate these inherent risks by staying totally focused and cognizant of where the limits of his abilities lie.

It's highly probable that the vast majority of "accidents," not only in extreme sports but in all areas of routine daily life, result from stupid mistakes rather than a natural consequence of the inherent risk—think texting and driving, or cleaning out your rain gutters on a flimsy ladder during a storm. Often, the stupid mistake involved is the initial decision to attempt an endeavor with excessive risk. While respecting and marveling at big-wave surfers, extreme skiers, and mountaineers, you can reject exceeding the limits of skill and common sense in the name of generating a viral YouTube video or bagging a peak for your resumé.

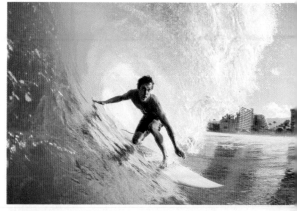

*Surfing offers a direct connection with nature, the yin/yang blend of calmness on the water against aggressive wave riding, time outdoors in fresh air and open space, and a killer total body workout—not a bad option for play!*

That said, we must also admit that no matter how sensible and prudent you are, pursuing primal thrills still involves a certain level of physical risk and danger. That's just the realities of gravity, random bad luck, and of course pilot error. However, physical risk and danger will also arise any time you zone out in daily life due to a bored, restless, under-utilized mind—right? Any fender benders involving a smartphone come to mind?

When you access the flow state and test your boundaries, you invariably improve your ability to focus, heighten your awareness of risk and danger, and access an elevated mental and physical state where your attention becomes focused instead of scattered. What sounds interesting, a little scary, but definitely do-able for you? Is it skydiving, scuba diving, or bungee jumping? How about taking your first rock-climbing or surfing lesson, going on a river-rafting excursion, or just taking a boogie board out into the ocean for the first time in years? Go for it!

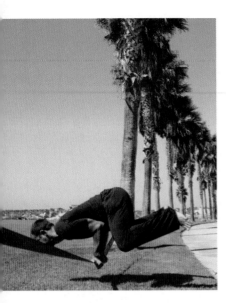

**Amusement parks:** Your genes don't know the difference between a real life-or-death adrenaline rush and a simulated one at the amusement park. Granted, the long lines and cotton-candy stands might not be as badass as racing your mountain bike down an expert level trail, or a solo yachtsman racing in the epic round-the-world Vendeé Globe race. However, the waterslides, the roller coasters, ziplines, and the ever-more-sophisticated and gasp-inducing contraptions rising from your nearest amusement park are a legitimate way to break up your routine with some gravity-defying, scream-inducing craziness.

**Comfort zone expansion:** Forget about the grand excursions for a moment; consider the opportunities you pass by every day in spectator mode. How about getting up off your folding chair and actually participating at your kid's soccer practice, or jumping into your club's lunchtime pickup basketball game instead of doing another hour in the lap pool? How about going off the front of your group ride for as long as you possibly can, knowing you're gonna blow up and disappear off the back at some point, but living for the moment for once?

Similarly, while competitive events might depart a bit from the core definition of play as spontaneous and unstructured, venturing beyond your primary competitive outlets to try some new stuff can definitely feel playful and comfort-zone-expanding. If you're a runner, why not try a mini-triathlon? If you're a triathlete, how about entering a mud run? You'll toe the start line feeling buoyant and excited in a different way from the pressurized feeling you get on the start line of your core competitive events.

*Paleo Primer author Keris Marsden (L) and Kitchen Intuition author Devyn Sisson race their cardboard boat to the finish line at PrimalCon New York in 2014. They won a free case of dark chocolate for dusting the competition with their innovative square hull craft.*

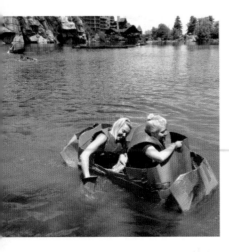

**Group activities:** When we play with friends and family members, we infuse these intimate relationships with humor, lightheartedness, vulnerability, and a stronger sense of connection. At our PrimalCon health and fitness retreats, we've always balanced the formal expert presentations with unusual challenge activities designed to bring out the playful spirit in everyone. These fun interludes often turn out to be the event highlight for many participants—the ocean plunge/Jacuzzi sprint at sunset; jumping off a fifteen-foot granite perch into a mountain lake; playing the PrimalCon Survivor Team Challenge game—a mix of scavenger hunt, brainteaser challenges, and team-building exercises; and enjoying Mark's personal favorite play endeavor of Ultimate Frisbee. Plan a play outing and rally your favorite group!

**Jump off something:** There is just something about jumping from an elevated perch into water—it's hard to think of anything more primal. Find a river, lake, or ocean with rocky shorelines and a suitable perch from which to launch. Failing these options, go for the high diving board at a local swimming pool. Caution and good sense are advised here. First, if you haven't seen anyone else jump from the spot, don't be the first! Second, always go feet-first when jumping into any body of water besides a swimming pool. If the water is not crystal clear, first dive down and thoroughly examine the underwater landing area to ensure it's of a safe depth and there is no debris or any slightly submerged hidden objects.

While it's hard to do damage jumping from ten feet or less, anything over that height requires correct form to prevent injury. For example, even something as innocuous as hitting the surface with your arms outstretched can tear a rotator cuff when you are a couple stories high and beyond. Also, it's a great idea to wear Vibrams or sneakers to protect your bare feet from impact trauma.

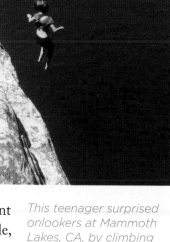

*This teenager surprised onlookers at Mammoth Lakes, CA, by climbing to the high rock jump and letting it fly without hesitation.*

**Mini adventure race:** Choose three or more modes of transportation and establish a challenge to go from point A to point B using various forms of human-powered locomotion. For example, bike ride to a lake, swim to the opposite shore, hike the perimeter to return to your bike, and then ride back home. Throw in a skateboard, scooter, or—if you have winter conditions—snowshoes, cross-country skis, or ice skates. City-dwellers can try this: hike a few blocks to a tall building, climb and descend the staircase, then hike to the next skyscraper and repeat.

**Nature challenges:** Mountain climbing, rock climbing, water sports (swimming, surfing, standup paddling, waterskiing, wakeboarding, wakesurfing), and winter sports (downhill and cross-country skiing, ice skating, snowshoeing) all entail synchronizing your physical efforts with natural forces—going with the flow. You haven't lived until you have tried standup paddling or wake surfing (yep, sans rope behind a ski boat). Moving within a naturally varied environment like water virtually demands that you transition out of an analytical state into a flow-like state.

**Night workout:** You have your local trail system so wired that those runs, bike rides, or cross-country ski sessions can be performed unconsciously, or at least while fully distracted by music or an audiobook. How about shaking things up a bit and doing your workout at night? Today's high-powered portable headlamps are quite impressive, and allow for safe passage over even a technical mountain bike route. Even with high-tech modern lighting, venturing out in the dark will awaken your senses like never before. You can expect sweaty palms, a more elevated heart rate, and jittery nerves as you enter into the unfamiliar world of darkness. This is a good outing to do with a group, or at least another training buddy.

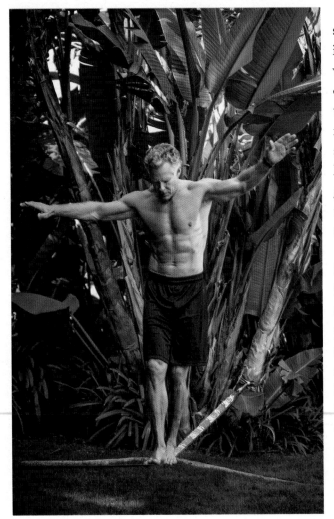

As you proceed with your adventure, a sense of focus and peace will edge out your initial fears. In a short while, your hard-wired instinct and sensory acuity will take over and you'll realize you're somehow able to balance your body deftly along a dark, rocky trail. You'll hear every small sound and identify the exact source. As other long-buried, primal abilities awaken, you'll gain courage and confidence that is hard to acquire via the quarterly sales contest or adult softball league playoffs.

**Slacklining**: Another one of Mark's favorite play endeavors, and something he does several times every single day in his backyard to clear his head from work matters, such as his high maintenance writing partner. Slacklining is such a simple endeavor, but one of powerful symbolism. A slackline is a flat nylon tightrope a couple inches wide that you suspend from two anchor points, such as trees, or strong posts or poles. As the name suggests, the line is not taut under the user's weight; rather it will stretch and recoil under load. It looks easy, but it's a tremendous challenge to simply mount the line and keep your footing. The dynamic tension in the line can send you flying off with the slightest disturbance to your center of gravity.

Slacklining is an activity that engrosses you immediately. An approach that's too casual will spit you off the line before both feet even leave the ground. Try too hard and you'll tense up and experience the dreaded sewing machine legs (uncontrollable twitching). But when you can get into the sweet spot of balance and start taking steps up and down the line, it's a blissful, connected feeling. Search YouTube for "Slackline World Cup" and you'll see the amazing exploits of "trickliners" who use the line like a trampoline, launching to perform aerial tricks and then landing gracefully back on the skinny line.

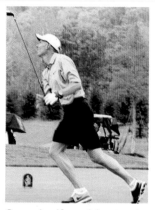

*Speedgolf world record holder Christopher Smith tees off (search YouTube for "Speedgolf Christopher Smith" and see one of the greatest golf rounds ever on high-speed camera).*

**Speedgolf:** Brad plugging for his favorite sport! Speedgolf can take the deliberate and often frustrating game of golf and make it playful in an instant. When you try to play as fast as you can *and* score the best you can, you enter an intuitive, reactive state that is the essence of flow. If you deliberate like usual, you'll play too slowly; if you get rushed and frenzied, you'll score poorly. You have to empty your mind, run to your ball, visualize your shot, and take a swing—simple as that! What's absolutely shocking is that virtually all participants in Speedgolf tournaments—despite playing with only five or six clubs (since you have to lug them around; any more and you'll run too slowly) play *as good or better* during these frenzied one-hour rounds than they do during the typical four-to-five-hour rounds with a full set of fourteen clubs. This is a good insight to apply to many other areas of life where our over-analytical, paralysis-by-analysis approach gets in the way of our natural, intuitive abilities.

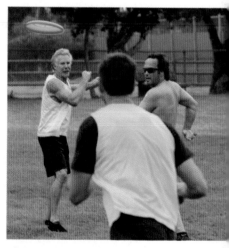

*If you wanna join Mark at a weekend Ultimate Frisbee match in Malibu, come right out—but bring your A-game. These guys are good!*

**Ultimate Frisbee**: If you haven't tried it, you are missing out on one of the most enjoyable games around. All ages and ability levels can play safely together, with minimal equipment or logistics, in groups of varied numbers. The game (the proper term is simply "Ultimate," since Frisbee is actually a brand name) is somewhat like soccer with a flying disc. Teams try to score a goal by covering the length of the field passing the disc and crossing the end line. It's free flowing, creative, and unencumbered by the abundance of complex rules, play stoppages, potential competitive imbalances, and physical dangers that inhibit the ability to engage in casual pickup games in other sports.

# CHAPTER SUMMARY

- **Sleep is king—turn off screens after dark!**
- **Yoga, Pilates, etc. counter narrow physical pursuits**
- **Movement builds fitness, burns fat, speeds recovery**
- **Bust loose and enjoy some play time!**

Complementary movement and lifestyle practices can help you achieve peak performance in endurance competition and preserve your health while you follow a challenging training regimen. The practices discussed in this chapter are sleep, increasing general everyday movement, mobility and movement practices, play, and optimizing recovery.

**Sleep**: Modern society suffers from epidemic sleep deprivation, so endurance athletes have to be especially vigilant about getting optimal sleep. Insufficient sleep can compromise immune function, cognitive function, and mood and energy levels during waking hours, and also significantly hamper fat metabolism and efforts to achieve ideal body composition. The best tip for optimizing sleep is to do whatever you can to **live in closer alignment with your natural circadian rhythm**, which is guided by the rising and setting of the sun each day. Depending on what latitude you live at, this allows for longer wake times during the summer months when days are longer, and for more sleep in the winter months. Winters of more sleep and less activity also promote optimal gene expression, as it gives us ample recovery from the temperate periods of the year where activity is increased.

**Minimize artificial light and digital stimulation after dark**, instead creating mellow evenings of reading, socializing, or neighborhood strolls. **Create an optimal sleeping environment (dark, cold, clutter-free), and observe consistent bed and wake time habits.** Be sure that your room is completely dark, because even a small amount of light (as in an LED clock screen or plug-in nightlight) can suppress melatonin release.

Take advantage of napping when the inevitable sleep deficiencies arise. Solid efforts in these areas will hopefully enable you to awaken naturally near sunrise, feeling refreshed and energized. **If you struggle to awaken easily and full of energy in the morning, expose yourself to direct sunlight as soon as you wake up**. This will stimulate the mood-elevating hormone serotonin as well as the stress hormone cortisol.

**Increase general everyday movement:** The active couch potato syndrome suggests than **even devoted fitness enthusiasts are not immune to the assorted serious health consequences of inactivity-dominant lifestyles (commuting, desk work, digital leisure time).** Prolonged sitting and stillness create muscle weakness and imbalances, disrupt healthy metabolic and hormone function, impair cognitive function, and make you more likely to overeat and store the excess calories as fat. **Taking numerous brief breaks for movement throughout your day can greatly reduce the negative effects of prolonged stillness.** Take a five-minute movement break for every twenty minutes of peak cognitive function, and take longer breaks of fifteen to twenty minutes after a few hours of focused cognitive effort to get outside into fresh air, open space, and sunlight.

Choose movement over motor whenever possible, such as parking far away in lots, taking stairs instead of elevators, and taking phone calls or personal meetings on the move. Movement expert Katy Bowman warns against the "athlete mindset" where slothfulness is justified by your impressive workout accomplishments. Also be aware that cardiovascular fitness (ability to deliver extreme and narrowly focused peak performances) differs from cardiovascular health (efficient delivery of blood and oxygen to cells throughout the body).

Creating a dynamic workplace is a wonderful way to increase daily movement. Focus on variation in your positions rather than just swapping a chair for a standup setup.

**Movement and mobility practices:** Stretching, foam rolling, preventative/rehabilitative exercises, yoga, and Pilates are perfect complements to the narrowly focused training patterns of endurance athletes. **Yoga, Pilates, and the like help address the imbalances and weaknesses that can arise from extreme repetitive training.** You'll build stabilizer muscles and improve balance and proprioception so you can preserve good technique and power output even as your large muscle groups fatigue during tough workouts. **The breathing awareness, counting, and precise movements of a yoga or Pilates class will improve your ability to focus**, and also help you enter a relaxed, parasympathetic-dominant state—an effective counter to the excessive fight-or-flight stimulation of endurance workouts.

**Play:** Play is an essential element of human health, stress management, and peak cognitive performance. Unfortunately, it has been widely disregarded by the hectic, confined, and structured nature of modern life. **Play supports the development of a "cognitively fluid mind,"** priming our brains for peak performance in core endeavors and helping to delay the aging process by keeping us enthusiastic and curious.

Due to the many sedentary and confining forces of daily life, the best forms of play might be spontaneous, unstructured outdoor physical activity. In particular, **pursuing primal thrills that give you a brief, healthy fight-or-flight charge will help add some spark to your often mundane daily routines.** Make sure your challenges are sensible and calculated, so you can experience your thrills without the negativity and anxiety of real fear. Break out of your comfort zone by trying stuff you've hesitated on—new competitive events, learning new skills, and especially tackling challenges that require you to synch with nature, such as water and winter sports.

# TIPS TO OPTIMIZE RECOVERY

*Strategies ranging from simple, common sense lifestyle behaviors to ultra high-tech contraptions*

9

## IN THIS CHAPTER

Some effective strategies to speed recovery include cold therapy (largely psychological—to reset the central nervous system back to a calm and cool state), compression gear (to assist the lymphatic and circulatory systems in pumping out waste products and improving blood and oxygen delivery), hydration (to ensure that recovery processes are not disrupted by immediate hydration issues), increased movement (an often overlooked but critical element of muscle repair and rejuvenation), refueling (with good nutrition, not empty calories), the new RTX cooling glove (to quickly cool core temperature and extend workout duration or speed recovery), self-myofascial release (working trigger points can alleviate referred pain elsewhere, and reduce injury risks), getting adequate sleep, and finally releasing your attachment to the outcome to relieve psychological stress.

An innovative way to monitor the success of your recovery efforts, protect against overstress and burnout, and track fitness progress is measuring Heart Rate Variability (HRV). HRV measures the variation in beat-to-beat intervals of your heart. While resting heart rate has long been the gold standard to measure an athlete's general state of stress and recovery, HRV takes biofeedback to the next level by providing a direct window into the functional state of your autonomic nervous system, delivering nuanced readings that accurately reveal conditions like hyper-arousal or burnout.

• • • • • • • • • • • • •

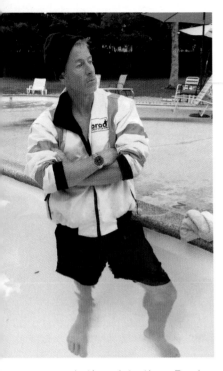

In the wintertime, Brad uses a cold swimming pool (temp 50-55F, 10-13C) after high intensity workouts. He dives in, swims one lap, towels off, bundles up, and moves his legs gently for ~5 minutes. Even after a few minutes of hot tub to rewarm, he'll experience a minor chill/shiver for a few hours—possibly helping enhance fat metabolism and speeding recovery.

*Hair:* Laurén of Beverly Hills ($77). **Embroidered beanie:** PrimalBlueprint.com ($15). **Parka:** Auburn City Public Works Dept ($100). **Trunks:** Emporio Armani ($125). **Towel:** Matouk Milagro ($45). **1991 National Champion watch:** USA Triathlon (Priceless).

**RECOVERING OPTIMALLY FROM WORKOUTS** is a complex challenge requiring an assortment of good decisions and lifestyle behaviors. It starts with a sensible, stress-balanced, periodized, aerobic-emphasis training schedule. If you are immersed in a chronic pattern, you should first address your ill-advised workout decisions before worrying about getting compression socks or a twelve-thousand-dollar hyperbaric chamber. If you are training sensibly and looking to cover all your bases to optimize recovery, here are some tips and aids you can use to recover from training stress as fast as possible: Cold therapy, compression, hydration, movement, refueling, the new RTX cooling glove, self-myofascial release, and last but perhaps most important, sleep!

**Cold therapy:** There is some difference of opinion on the use of ice, cold water, and cold air cryotherapy to promote recovery and injury healing. Everyone agrees that icing an acute injury right away, and continuing with ice applications for the first twenty-four to forty-eight hours, can help reduce the severity of the injury. Outside of the initial acute treatment, the application of ice is known to reduce inflammation and injury pain. However, these "benefits" are now being second-guessed as potentially problematic.

The new thinking suggests that the acute inflammatory responses to injury, and the general inflammatory chemical responses to exercise, are necessary for healing, and to stimulating fitness adaptations. When you apply ice to an inflamed area, you inhibit the function of the lymphatic system in clearing toxins out of the injured area, potentially delaying your recovery and even interfering with your ultimate ability to adapt and become stronger from training stress. Dr. Starrett and other thought leaders are swapping out the familiar RICE (Rest, Ice, Compression, Elevation) acronym with a new one called ECM—Elevate, Compress, and Move—as the best way to heal injured or overworked tissues. The ECM protocol helps increase bloodflow to the injured area, supporting the hardworking vascular and lymphatic systems in clearing out toxins and accelerating the healing process.

Ice, cold water, and cold air cryotherapy still have an interesting place in the recovery formula, but in a way that's different from conventional understanding. Cold therapy is not about reducing inflammation after workouts to speed recovery, because inflammation is a necessary component of recovery. Instead, it is believed that exposure to cold after workouts might provide more of a psychological benefit than a cellular benefit.

After a strenuous workout, exposure to cold air or water will lower your core temperature (which was elevated by the workout), increase oxygenation to tissues exposed to cold, help reduce hemoglobin volume and muscle metabolic activity back to resting levels, elicit an "enhanced antioxidative defense," boost immune function through enhanced T cell activity, and give you a hormetic boost of norepinephrine to provide a bit of sustained pain relief.

When you plunge your overheated muscle enzymes and overheated, hyped-up central nervous system into an icy river at the conclusion of a tough workout, you are going to get a reset effect to the extent that you emerge feeling like you are suddenly in a calm-central-nervous-system, mellow-muscle-metabolic-activity, moderate-body-temperature state. You feel refreshed and invigorated instead of overheated and fried as you might when puttering around in the hours after a tough workout.

The refreshing sensation of cold exposure has a profound psychological impact that cannot be discounted when you are looking to speed recovery, an impact that has been confirmed in an assortment of studies. Basketball players report feeling less fatigued and can jump higher twenty-four hours after post-exercise cold exposure. Cyclists recorded higher HRV readings right after cold-water immersion, and better maintenance of sprint power after consecutive days of training. Rugby players reported less muscle soreness and improved muscle contractions with cold-water immersion.

Don't worry about following strict rules and guidelines when it comes to post-workout cold exposure. Just a few minutes of immersion in a cold river, ice bath, winter swimming pool, one of the new high-tech cryotherapy chambers (commercial facilities are popping up all over the place), or using the RTX cooling glove that we will discuss shortly will generate that refreshing psychological impact, and avoid the delayed recovery risks of excessive or chronic cold exposure—like an all-day icing regimen for an injury. Don't worry about it being super cold; you don't want to injure sensitive tissues—or dread going in, for that matter. Some experts mention an ideal water temperature range of 50° to 60°F (10° to 15°C), and an ideal exposure period of five to ten minutes—never exceeding ten minutes at 50°F or below.

Some evidence suggests that whole-body exposure is most effective, but you can just immerse your legs if you are dealing with really cold water, perhaps with a quick full-body submersion right at the end. In the winter months, an outdoor swimming pool works well (uh, at least in California. Hopefully you can find some water that's not frozen in the winter!) for quick full-body plunges. A pool, river, or lake that's well above freezing allows you to move around for a few minutes instead of just sitting there shivering miserably. If your outdoor game is hindered by ice and snow, a cold shower works fine too. If you want to get serious and make an ice bath or ice barrel, take care to not stay in too long, especially with your face, hands, and feet. You want to exit long before you start to go numb.

**Compression**: Compression gear such as tight socks or wraps enhances the ability of the lymphatic and circulatory systems in clearing out the extracellular waste products and excess fluid that accumulate in tired muscles after strenuous workouts. Compression garments or wraps act like pumps to squeeze blood vessels open with force, allowing more blood and oxygen into the area to remove waste and excess fluid. This pumping effect is greatly enhanced when combined with elevation of the traumatized area above the heart, and also with movement while wearing the garment. Hence, a post-workout recovery strategy might be to plunge into a cold river for a few minutes, throw on some compression socks, and hang your feet on the edge of the couch while you watch a show. Over the ensuing hours, frequent brief walks would ideally break up extended lounging periods. Many elite athletes will keep their compression socks on overnight, and especially when traveling on an airplane to counter high risks of edema (fluid pooling in extremities) on long flights.

There is some good science on the effectiveness of compression garments, with reports of improved performance and diminished fatigue when sprinting, reduced DOMS (delayed onset muscle soreness), reduced muscle damage as measured by CK (creatine kinase) levels, and improved absolute power output and anaerobic threshold power output for cyclists wearing compression while pedaling. Wearing compression socks while running is believed to minimize the muscle vibrations that occur upon impact and contribute to post-exercise soreness.

As with cold therapy, many of the compression benefits might be categorized as psychological, but no less relevant to the user who feels better when using socks. Yes, socks are the best because they originate at the point farthest away from the heart, thereby starting the pumping process from the bottom. Whether you get socks or tights, find a quality pair that has graduated tightness (tighter at the bottom, easing up as you rise toward the heart) and is rated at a pressure of 22-32 mmHg.

**Hydration**: Rehydrate immediately after workouts, so you can ensure the body's recovery mechanisms kick into gear right away. If you are in a slightly dehydrated state after your workout—which is easy to get to—this will inhibit the recovery process until you deal with the urgency of rehydrating. You've probably heard about the dangers of overhydrating and throwing off your delicate sodium balance (hyponatremia), so be reasonable with your consumption. Add a pinch or two of sea salt if you are drinking plain water, or consider a naturally electrolyte-rich beverage like coconut water. Don't bother with the colorful sports drinks loaded with chemicals and added sugars.

**Movement**: Coming on the heels of our discussion about adding more movement and variation to daily life, this concept is especially important to respect in the hours after workouts. If you open up the throttle with a good session, do a perfunctory cooldown of five or ten minutes, and then plunge right into cubicle life for hours on end, you are going to significantly hamper your recovery. You'll realize this when you feel stiff and congested when you do get up and move for the first time, or even the following morning. If you make an effort to move more frequently—even for a few minutes at a time and especially in the hours after your workout, you will soon notice that you are a more fluid, flexible, and energetic human at all times. This will be especially apparent if you monitor your condition first thing in the morning, a time when you can really notice the effects of insufficient movement patterns, overtraining, and inflammatory dietary habits.

The goal is to wake up in the morning and feel pretty decent—like you don't need a ten-minute hot shower or two cups of coffee to get your creaky joints moving. If you move more in daily life per the guidelines discussed in Chapter 8, you will progress steadily toward eventually hopping out of bed with fluid and limber joints.

When you are dealing with an actual injury instead of just trying to accelerate recovery, you need to make sure that your movement efforts are appropriate and don't contribute to any backsliding. For example, rehabbing a sprained ankle might involve some circular range of motion work, then progressing to working through range of motion with resistance bands, followed by actual weight-bearing activities. If your ankle feels worse the following day, it's possible that you were too aggressive with your exercises and you need to back down to the previous step. Ditto for your progression from injury to returning to training. If you do a workout that makes your injury feel worse the next day, you need to slow the pace of your progression.

**Refueling**: Eat something real and nutritious within an hour after your workout. My favorite post-workout recovery meal is a salad. If you're pressed for time you can make a recovery smoothie, using whey protein powder and natural ingredients like fruits and vegetables. Forget the manufactured foods like bars, gels, and sweets—exactly what you don't need to feed an athlete after a workout. Even the healthiest-sounding bars deliver a major sugar bomb (does that sound harsher than "organic brown rice syrup," "organic evaporated cane juice," "barley malt syrup," "organic agave nectar," etc.?), and kick you back into the carbohydrate dependency we worked so hard to escape back in Chapter 3.

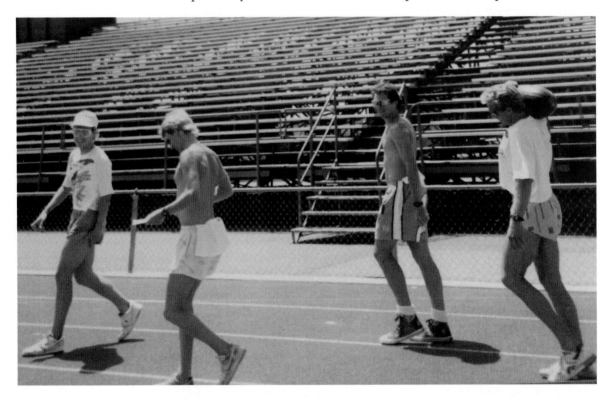

*Provo, UT, circa 1988. Four athletes pull off a heist of a watermelon from the post-race buffet, in the interest of optimal rehydration and refueling after an oppressively hot competition. Can you identify any legendary old timers in the photo?*

**RTX cooling glove:** A new product called the RTX (Rapid Thermal Exchange) cooling glove has the potential to make a tremendous impact on recovery from exercise by quickly and easily lowering an elevated core temperature. Overheating is one of the most, if not *the* most, significant limiters of physical performance. When you become overheated during exercise (which happens easily even in a temperate environment during a moderate workout, and happens dramatically when you perform in a warm environment and/or at high intensity or prolonged duration), a key enzyme involved in energy production called *pyruvate kinase* becomes misshapen and malfunctioning. This inhibits the production of ATP in the muscles, causing you to become fatigued, slow down, cramp up, and eventually just stop. Breaking a sweat is the first indication that you are becoming overheated. Sweating is functional, and a critical survival mechanism, but it's obviously a metabolically expensive, last resort mechanism. If you're exercising in hot ambient temperatures, sweating isn't even that effective, causing further performance limitations.

More than a decade ago, biology researchers at Stanford University made a stunning discovery in the exercise laboratory: by merely sticking your hand into a specially designed glove, enclosed in a chamber that circulates cold water while applying gentle vacuum pressure, you can quickly cool your core temperature. This cooling glove works by acting on the *arteriovenous anastomoses*—AVAs—an extremely temperature sensitive network of veins concentrated in the palms of your hands that regulate body temperature with a highly variable bloodflow based on environmental temps (AVAs are also concentrated on the soles of your feet and non-hairy facial areas.)

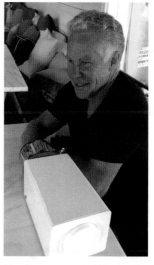

*Feeling pretty chill testing out a prototype of the RTX cooling glove, a scaled down model of the original invention that is suitable for individual use*

AVAs are your body's radiators—they attract heated blood from your inner body and exchange it with cooler blood from the atmosphere to recirculate (think how an overheated dog extends her tongue to generate an evaporative cooling effect). Your brain will always cool first, followed by internal organs and then muscles. If you become overheated during a workout (the glove also has industrial applications for soldiers, laborers, etc.), you can use the glove for a few minutes and dramatically accelerate the natural, homeostatic cooling process. You will likely notice that you stop sweating—a sign that your internal temperature has returned to normal. This allows you to continue your workout and perform well beyond your natural limitations caused by overheating. When you use the glove while overheated at the conclusion of your workout, it can likely accelerate recovery in the same manner as discussed in the cold therapy section.

Studies with mice show that cooling down immediately after a workout can suppress the accumulation of the inflammatory cytokine Interleukin-6, which is one of the agents that drives muscle soreness. As discussed in the cold therapy section, the benefits of cooling down quickly after a workout might be more anecdotal than scientific, but it's reasonable to project that you can minimize muscle damage and experience an important psychological refresher by accelerating and enhancing what your body is trying to do anyway. If you've ever lain around after a long workout feeling fried—like you're too tired to relax or fall asleep come bedtime—you can acknowledge the potential benefits of teleporting right into a cool, restful physiological and psychological state.

One of the researchers at Stanford performed 180 pullups in a single workout as a baseline before working with the glove. After training with the glove for six weeks (taking three-minute breaks between sets of 50 pullups—yes, this dude was fit!) he was able to perform a mind blowing *620 pullups* at a single session!

So, why not just jam your hands into a bucket of ice mid-workout to cool down? This would have the opposite of the intended effect, because the excessively cold ice water would shock the AVAs and cause them to constrict, again as a safety mechanism from an environmental threat perceived as too cold. This was validated by Stanford researchers who had athletes exercise indoors until they were sweating heavily, then ushered them into a room air conditioned to 62°F (17°F). The room was too cold to facilitate a lowering of core temperature, instead causing their AVAs to constrict instead of radiate. Ditto for splashing your face with cold water during a hot workout; you'll get a temporary psychological refresher, but do nothing to promote a cooling of your core temperature.

Interestingly, you can't get too cold using the glove. After all, the water temp is only around 60°F (15°C), and it's not even directly touching the skin—it's circulating around outside the glove. Once your internal body temperature has stabilized, the glove will just be cooling your hand a bit. It follows that the glove is useless unless you have an elevated core temperature (one professional team testing the glove proclaimed that it didn't work—athletes were trying it some twenty minutes after their workout concluded, when natural cooling had already been achieved). If you live in an exceptionally hot climate, conduct frequent indoor workouts where you really sweat, or otherwise feel like overheating is hampering your workout enjoyment and fitness progress, consider trying this item out. The RTX glove retails for $399. More information at avacore.com.

**Self-myofascial release:** The tremendous popularity of foam rollers and therapy balls and other torture contraptions used for self-myofascial release is a testament to their ability to speed the healing of tight or stressed muscles through deep, dynamic compression. Self-myofascial release can go beyond stretching by applying deep pressure to areas known as trigger points that represent the origination of stiffness and

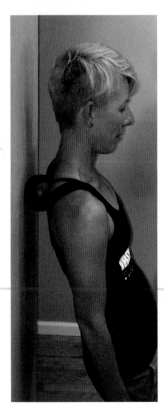

*Coach Kimmie Smith of Kinesis Movement Studio in Culver City, CA, demonstrates one of her innovative therapy ball movements*

mobility problems that might be symptomatic elsewhere. For example, you may have Achilles tendon pain or the dreaded iliotibial (IT) band syndrome, where sharp pain is often localized on the outside of the knee when running. The cause of IT band syndrome might be extreme tightness all the way up at the top of the quadriceps muscles near your hip and pelvis—the upper insertion point of the IT band (which extends all the way down to the pain point outside the knee.) A tight, inflamed Achilles might be strongly influenced by tightness higher up the leg in the gastrocnemius calf muscle.

By rolling hard along the side of your upper leg or smashing away at your gastroc muscle with a lacrosse ball or rolling device, you can break up adhesions and scar tissue formed between layers of muscle and connective tissue in these areas, increase bloodflow and lymphatic function, and promote a speedy return to healthy tissue function. With the trigger point areas released and revitalized, often the referred pain (Achilles, etc.) resolves.

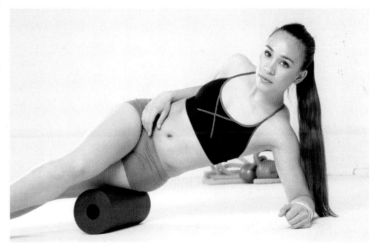

*Foam roller in action. This debonair model is obviously not going deep enough for maximum benefit. You have to go deep and break down those adhesions— hurts so good!*

Self-myofascial release delivers an added benefit of stimulating the parasympathetic nervous system to help relax and unwind both brain and muscles from the stress of workouts or a busy day in general. As you apply the pressure and breathe through the discomfort, calming, relaxing neurotransmitters are released into your bloodstream to leave you feeling blissful when your session is over. Spend some time each evening working with balls and rollers as you relax in front of the TV or visit with family and you'll discover the true meaning of the word *relaxed*. And by the way, if you see that foam roller stacked in the corner and are too tired to commence a session, you are most likely overtrained!

Keep in mind that a finely tuned, mobile, flexible physical specimen should not experience pain anywhere on the body, even when pushing or rolling tissues with significant force. That's right, you should be able to lower your hamstrings right down onto a hard ball or roller, with most of your bodyweight applying force, and not wince in pain. Ditto for grinding a ball into those commonly touch-sensitive calf muscles, or lowering down onto a roller at the location of your thoracic spine. If you do experience pain in certain areas—and it's highly likely that you will—this is an indication that the area needs myofascial release. Work diligently on your most sensitive areas every day and soon you will go from the immediate "ouch" upon a light application of pressure to a catlike state where you can press all the way down to the bone without pain.

Effective self-myofascial release will definitely be uncomfortable, even painful, but in a good way. Breathe and work through the application of pressure on those trigger points and you will often experience immediate relief from muscle tightness when you finish the effort. Focus on finding the tight trigger points instead of applying pressure directly to the referred pain area (e.g., the Achilles or the outside of the knee in our examples), as this could exacerbate the acute inflammation in those areas. Experts recommend rolling around at a deliberate pace, probing for those particularly sensitive trigger points, and holding the pressure in place for fifteen to thirty seconds.

Know the difference between the desirable pain of working hard to release trigger points and excessive pain, pain from working directly on injured areas, or pain caused by hitting nerves, bones, or joints. Avoid rolling on your lower back because there is insufficient muscular protection for the spine in that area. If you have low back tightness, work around the area by grinding on the mid-back, quads, glutes, and even the abdominal area.

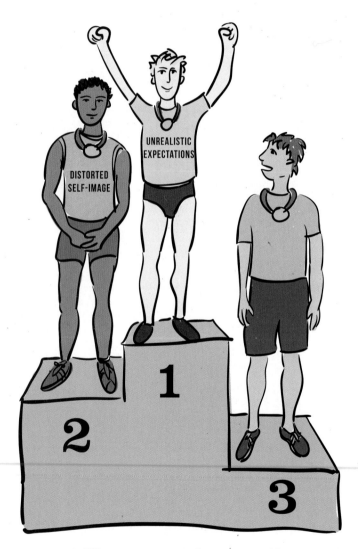

*"You guys are tough opponents!"*

**Release attachment to outcome**: Time to add a recovery tip for your mindset to all this practical stuff! The worst-kept secret in the endurance scene is the inner anguish caused by missing workouts, performing below standard in races, or losing precious weeks or months of training to injury. Psychological stress can definitely impact your rate of recovery, and inhibit you from delivering peak performance.

Yep, endurance athletes can choke due to an unhealthy mindset. It's not the same choke as a pro golfer whose nerves get the better of him as he sweats over a putt to make the rent payment. A results-obsessed triathlete will make poor decisions in training and competition that lead to overtraining or blowing up on the racecourse. Behaving in conflict with their stated goals and values ("peak for important race," "explore my potential as an athlete," "be a role model to my kids," etc.) to sabotage competitive performance, fitness progress, and general health is the way that endurance athletes choke.

IT'S ALWAYS POSSIBLE TO GO TO THE WELL AND FORCE THINGS TO HAPPEN UNNATURALLY, BUT YOU WILL PAY A LONG-TERM PRICE FOR AN UNNATURAL, IMBALANCED APPROACH.

It's essential to govern your competitive instincts on a day-to-day basis and be patient with the process of fitness. Relax, trust in your approach, and let competitive excellence happen naturally. Take what your body gives you every day and nothing more. Remember, it's always possible to go to the well and force things to happen unnaturally—we'll discuss this in detail in Chapter 10—but you will always pay a long-term price for an unnatural, imbalanced approach. Focus on enjoyment of the process of becoming fit—even if things don't work out exactly as planned—and resist the temptation to drift into an obsessive/compulsive, outcome-oriented mindset.

**Sleep**: You can't emphasize sleep enough, and it's highly likely that your sleep requirements will increase in concert with the total energy expended in your training. Be sure to utilize napping, particularly in conjunction with high-intensity workouts, to accelerate recovery. Review the Chapter 8 sleep section and own it!

## USING HEART RATE VARIABILITY TO MONITOR RECOVERY AND PREVENT OVERTRAINING

So, how to track whether all your recovery efforts and gadgets are really working? How to tell if you really are recovered and ready for another breakthrough workout? Heart Rate Variability (HRV) is some incredibly exciting technology that has only recently been made available outside a clinical cardiology setting or sophisticated Olympic training center. HRV measures the variation in the intervals between your heartbeats as a stress indicator. When the parasympathetic and sympathetic factions of the autonomic nervous system are working in harmonious balance, you have a greater variation in beat-to-beat intervals, delivering a high HRV score. When you are under stress and thus sympathetic dominant, your heart beats in a more metronomic fashion, leading to a lower HRV score.

You may think that a heart rate of 60 beats per minute means your heart is beating once every second, but in fact there is a certain amount of variation in the time interval between heartbeats. So inside that heart rate of 60 bpm, you might see an interval of 1.15 seconds here, 0.98 there, 1.10 next, 0.92 next, and so forth, to total sixty. Surprisingly and perhaps counter-intuitively, variation in beat-to-beat intervals (technically known as "r-r" intervals, revealed as the spikes on a familiar EKG readout) is actually a good thing and indicative of a harmonious interaction between the sympathetic (fight-or-flight) and parasympathetic (rest-and-digest) components that comprise your autonomic nervous system. This delicate synchronicity that is reflected in beat-to-beat interval variation happens, imperceptibly, in response to all sorts of environmental stimulation, such as standing up from a seated position, or upon each inhalation and exhalation. The sympathetic nervous system stimulates a very slight increase in heart rate upon each energizing inhalation, while the parasympathetic stimulates a tiny decrease upon each relaxing exhale.

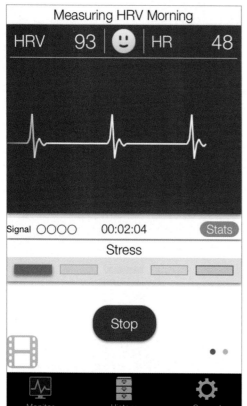

*Screenshot of the PrimalBeat HRV application in action. The main screen shows both HRV reading (93) on a 1-100 scale, and resting heart rate (48). Brad tracked HRV patiently for six months to deliver this new PR of 93 for the book!*

The more variation in beat-to-beat intervals, the higher your HRV score and generally the more fit and healthy your cardiovascular system. This seems at odds with the image of a powerful heart pumping out blood with metronomic efficiency. HRV is a measurement that has the most relevance when measured in a rested state at the same time of day, such as before getting out of bed in the morning—similar to the strategy for tracking resting heart rate. When you start exercising and place an extreme demand on the heart to go to 10, 20, or 30 MET, your HRV nosedives as your heartbeat indeed becomes more metronomic to keep up with the exercise demand, which is what's supposed to happen.

To get started with HRV monitoring, obtain an HRV reading each morning before getting out of bed, taking care to assume a completely

SURPRISINGLY AND PERHAPS COUNTER-INTUITIVELY, A GREATER VARIATION IN BEAT-TO-BEAT INTERVALS IS INDICATIVE OF A HEALTHY, STRONG CARDIOVASCULAR SYSTEM.

relaxed body position and mindset. Spend a few minutes to allow your values to stabilize and then archive the data with the push of a button. Over a period of months, you will see your HRV values land into a normal "baseline" range that's indicative of you feeling rested and recovered. With a reliable baseline established, you can be alert for trends of lower-than-baseline values, which are associated with overstress or insufficient recovery. You'll also have occasional days where you generate numbers higher than your baseline, suggesting you are exceptionally relaxed and recovered!

For example, over a few months' time, you might see your HRV scores commonly ranging from 65 to 75. When you have a day or sequence of days where HRV is in the 55 to 60 range, this is a strong sign of overstress or insufficient recovery. In this example, you will want to scale back workouts and other forms of life stress until values return to normal. Keep in mind that a suppressed HRV is indicative of a stressed cardiovascular system, so it's expected that you will see temporary dips in HRV the day after performing a difficult workout or when you are stressed by jet travel or insufficient sleep. This is a good indicator to take it easy until you generate baseline HRV numbers.

Going a little deeper, a sustained pattern of low resting heart rates could suggest you are a badass with a world-class aerobic engine, or it could mean big trouble. As Dr. Phil Maffetone explains, a suppressed resting heart rate can be a sign of the third and most severe stage of overtraining, parasympathetic overtraining. Here, your chronically excessive production of fight-or-flight hormones finally exhausts your endocrine system and you start producing insufficient levels of important energy-regulating hormones like cortisol, DHEA, and testosterone.

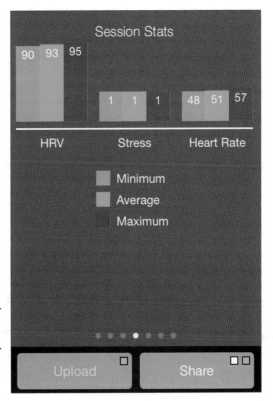

*After each HRV session, PrimalBeat HRV delivers summary screens that show averages and ranges for the various values. You can archive each session with a push of a button and view graphic presentations of long-term HRV trends.*

You feel exhausted in daily life and in no condition to train, despite your impressive resting heart rate value. On the flip side, an elevated resting heart rate is commonly associated with overtraining, and can indeed be a sign of overstimulation of the sympathetic fight-or-flight response. It can also be a sign that you are just temporarily excited (stressed) by thoughts of the workout or the hectic day ahead, or simply have to use the bathroom.

HRV takes biofeedback tracking to the next level of sophistication by revealing the nuances of the sympathetic and parasympathetic interaction, something that can easily be thrown out of harmonious balance through high-stress training. For example, a chronic overstimulation of the sympathetic nervous system can fool you into an overtraining spiral, because your bloodstream is bathed in stress hormones that help you awaken each day feeling energized and psyched for another big training session. Here, a lower-than-baseline HRV score will provide a graphic indicator that you are in a state of overstress, indicative of a metronomic, sympathetic-dominant heartbeat. A reduction in training load and other forms of stress, along with increased rest and recovery, is imperative to allowing HRV values to return to normal levels.

## WHY HRV IS BETTER THAN RESTING HEART RATE TO MONITOR STRESS AND RECOVERY

As you probably know, resting heart rate has long been used by endurance athletes to track recovery. A low number suggests the cardiovascular system is rested and pumping at a strong stroke volume, while a high number suggests that the heart is tired and needing more beats per minute to keep up with energy demands at rest. These characterizations are generally accurate, but there are an assortment of variables and unique circumstances that can result in resting heart rate being an incomplete and potentially inaccurate indicator of your stress and recovery.

For one thing, HRV is a much more sensitive and sophisticated indicator of cardiovascular stress than resting heart rate, so it will reveal more variation in response to workout and life stress variation. For a great example of the informative power of HRV beyond resting heart rate, take a look at a few days of Brad's data relating to how resting heart rate and HRV were affected by a challenging sprint workout.

**Tues a.m.** (twelve hours before workout, feeling rested): Resting HR 48, HRV 74. HF 1,700 and .2 HF/LF ratio. **p.m.** Did ten minutes of challenging high jump and running technique drills, followed by 4 x 100 meters (all-out, from a track start), in 97-degree heat.

**Wed a.m.** (twelve hours after workout): Resting HR 47, HRV 75. HF 1,700 and .3 HF/LF. Felt okay considering the previous evening's session.

**Thurs a.m.** (thirty-six hours after the workout): Resting HR 47, HRV 54. HF 300 and 1.0 HF/LF. Felt tired and sore, much more so than Wednesday.

Interestingly, Brad reported feeling surprisingly fresh right after the sprint session and even the morning after the session, as he was probably still bathed in the feel-good chemicals of an endorphin high. Essentially, it took thirty-six hours for the fatigue to set in and register with a nosedive HRV score, vastly lower power spectrum readings for HF and LF, a vastly elevated HF/LF ratio, and a subjective report of more fatigue and muscle soreness. Meanwhile, the fatigue from the session didn't register at all in resting heart rate. Accordingly, an athlete training by resting heart rate might only conclude they were "recovered," but in reality their body has been severely stressed and recovery is recommended until HRV and power readings return to normal range.

Brad's subjective report of feeling fine and delivering a normal resting heart rate and HRV score the morning after the sprint session illustrates a common situation that trips up endurance athletes—the initial window of *resistance response* to exercise stress. Your body loves rising to the occasion when you tackle a challenge, and will stay in a heightened state of arousal for a certain period of time after it's over—as evidenced by Brad's high-functioning cardiovascular system twelve hours after the sprint session. In this example, fatigue set in by the thirty-six-hour reading, with the tanked HRV numbers and increased stiffness and subjective fatigue.

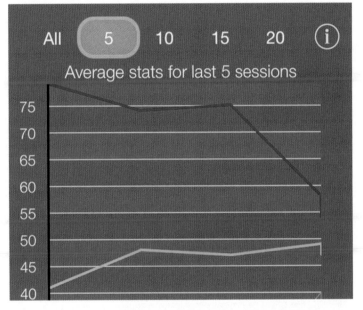

Brad's HRV report from PrimalBeat HRV iPhone app. A nosedive in HRV score occurred thirty-six hours after an intense sprint workout, but with no corresponding change in resting heart rate.

This simple example might play out on a bigger scale, where you deliver three months, or even three years, of excellent training, leveraging a brain and bloodstream drugged by stress hormones to feel strong, fresh, enthusiastic, and energized. Unfortunately, you are headed for a burnout when your sympathetic nervous system and fight-or-flight hormones become exhausted from chronic stimulation. A 2015 article in *Outside* magazine titled "Running on Empty" details an alarming frequency of extreme and sudden burnout experienced by elite ultradistance runners. One year a guy is shattering records at assorted hundred-kilometer and hundred-mile events all over the globe, and the next year has disappeared from competition to run an organic farm in New Mexico—literally. Dr. David Nieman, professor of health and exercise science at Appalachian State University (NC) and former vice president of the American College of Sports Medicine, says, "Overtraining syndrome is one of the scariest things I've ever seen in my thirty-plus years of working with athletes. To watch someone go from that degree of proficiency to a shell of their former self is unbelievably painful and frustrating."

Fortunately, HRV is a relatively rapid early indicator (more responsive than resting heart rate, as evidenced with Brad's example) of you being in resistance response, rather than being truly recovered and stress balanced. Monitoring HRV and the HF and LF power spectrums can give you an objective view of something you might not have the ability to be very objective about. After all, if you feel fine, who's to say you shouldn't go out there and rack up some more miles? HRV—that's who!

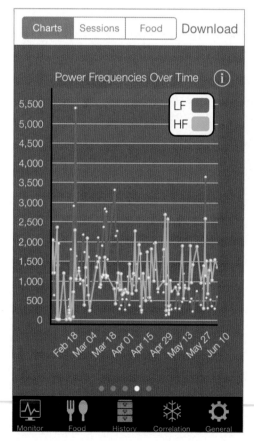

While "high HRV = good" and "low HRV = burnout" are simple and generally accurate maxims, overtraining and burnout are complex issues that can manifest in different forms. Further insights can be obtained by learning that there are two bands of the HRV power spectrum, known as LF (low frequency) and HF (high frequency). The LF power spectrum is representative mainly of sympathetic activity. The HF power spectrum represents the parasympathetic nervous system's influence on HRV. A well-functioning nervous system and cardiovascular system will reveal high power levels for both LF and HF, as the intensity of the electrical signal emitted by the heart is strong.

When you are stress balanced, you will have a favorable LF-to-HF ratio, ideally with HF higher than LF. For example, an athlete delivering an LF score of 2,000 and an HF score of 4,000 will have a LF:HF ratio of 0.5. When you are in a state of fight-or-flight/sympathetic dominance, you might see a flip-flop of these values, delivering an LF (4,000):HF (2,000) ratio of 2.0, along with a lower-than-baseline HRV score. When you

*A PrimalBeat HRV chart of Brad's LF and HF power frequency values over several month's time. Notice in the early months how LF predominated (including a freaky outlier fight-or-flight morning reading up at 5,500), corresponding with a period of Brad's overly stressful training patterns and sympathetic overstimulation. Come April and May, HF values started to predominate over LF as Brad's stress levels moderated and he returned to a healthy autonomic nervous system balance.*

are in a burnout state, you might deliver a low HRV score along with low absolute power spectrum scores and LF dominance, such as an LF of 400 and HF of 200. Here, the fight-or-flight response has been exhausted, the adrenal glands are producing less than normal levels of cortisol in the bloodstream, and the parasympathetic and sympathetic nervous systems are in dysfunction. Ideally, you would like to see a high HRV score (parasympathetic and sympathetic nervous systems working in balance), a high HF value, and favorable LF:HF ratio (stress response and stress hormones moderated/optimized), and of course a low resting heart rate.

While the maxim that "higher is better" with HRV, LF, and HF values is valid, HRV is highly individualized, and there is no sense comparing your values to those produced by other athletes. Yes, it's likely that an elite athlete might deliver an HRV of 90, and LF and HF values in the 6,000 to 8,000 range; an ordinary fitness enthusiast might deliver an HRV of 65, and LF and HF values in the 1,000 range; and a sedentary subject might have an HRV of 50 and low LF and HF values. But your main concern should be tracking your own baseline over time, and making sound training and lifestyle decisions based on daily values that depart from baseline. Regardless of the absolute values, an athlete or ordinary person who is stressed will deliver a lower HRV score than normal, and likely a higher than usual LF:HF ratio.

IDEALLY, YOU WOULD LIKE TO SEE A HIGH HRV SCORE (PARASYMPATHETIC AND SYMPATHETIC BALANCE), A HIGH HF ABSOLUTE VALUE, A FAVORABLE LF:HF RATIO (STRESS RESPONSE AND STRESS HORMONES MODERATED/OPTIMIZED), AND OF COURSE A LOW RESTING HEART RATE.

It's also interesting to note that when one is functioning in a heightened state or peak performance zone due to positive and enjoyable stressors, such as workplace or athletic challenges, this might be reflected in increased levels of both LF and HF power, and deliver (consequent to the complex HRV score calculations) a high HRV score. This is true even when the sympathetic nervous system is dominating because of the high stimulatory environment. Conversely, when burnout occurs due to the overtaxing of the fight-or-flight response and sympathetic nervous system due to prolonged heightened stimulation with insufficient rest and relaxation to balance, this is reflected in lower-than-normal power levels for both LF and HF, and the aforementioned high LF value in relation to HF value. This condition is reflected in a lower HRV score.

As you gain more appreciation for and experience with biofeedback, you will notice that calming behaviors can generate an immediate impact on HRV, and thus help you balance stress and speed recovery. Breathing exercises (studies show inhaling to a three count and exhaling to a six count will raise HRV), meditation, yoga, assorted other mindfulness practices, or simply relaxing in the backyard, gazing at the clouds or the stars, can stimulate the parasympathetic nervous system and immediately make you feel more calm and relaxed, especially if you are coming off a stressful experience like an intense workout, gnarly commute, or argument with a loved one.

As an endurance athlete, it's critical for you to respect the importance of stress and rest balance, and add calming thoughts and behaviors to your repertoire. Even the most sensibly trained athlete who gets plenty of sleep and eats a nutritious diet still can't help but suffer from a chronic overstimulation of the sympathetic nervous system. Even when you stay aerobic, an endurance workout of 45 minutes is still a significant stressor to the body—more than a restorative yoga class, if you get the drift. Even when you fly first class with fully reclined seats and a silk blindfold, jet travel through time zones is still monumentally stressful to your hormonal and immune function, since your genes are totally unaccustomed to such an extreme circadian disruptor. Even if you faithfully wrap up your emails or Netflix queue and turn out the lights by 10 p.m. every night, you are still blasting several hundred hours' worth of highly stressful artificial light and digital stimulation after dark into your central nervous system over the course of a calendar year.

Even if you are super aware of your stress levels and enthusiastic about doing calming behaviors and generally staying in balance, including objective HRV data into your game is critically important, because it's difficult to tell when you are immersed in chronic stress patterns. Ronda Collier, co-founder and CEO of Sweetwater Health, explains further. "The brain acts as a pattern matcher and a filter," says Collier, a longtime Silicon Valley chip engineer who embarked on a career change and obtained a degree in holistic psychology, then blended her

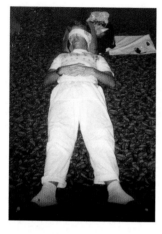

*Brad doing the fourth event on the pro triathlon circuit: sleeping—undaunted by the dirty carpet at the Honolulu airport—midway through a grueling transcontinental flight home from Australia*

passions and talents to start Sweetwater Health (with CTO Jo Beth Dow) and deliver HRV technology to the masses.

*The brain can become comfortable in a chronic fight-or-flight state because it's familiar.*

Collier continues, "The brain recognizes what's familiar and filters out other things so you can remain focused on the task at hand. If you're in a chronic fight-or-flight state, your brain recognizes this familiar operating mode (amped, emotional, reactive, harried, etc.) and you feel comfortable. The brain accepts even a dysfunctional situation or dysfunctional behavior because it's familiar. You might even feel relaxed and think everything is fine, since your familiarity filters out any negative perceptions of chronic stress. Instead, your chronically stressed state shows up in the form of absentmindedness—like the classic story of the cyclist driving into his garage with a bike on the roof rack!"

Getting started with HRV is easy thanks to mobile technology. All you need is a Bluetooth low energy (BLE 4.0)-enabled wireless chest transmitter and a smartphone app, such as the PrimalBeat HRV Tracker App for iPhone. Hopefully you already have a chest strap and heart rate monitor for training, because monitoring your training heart rate is so critical to aerobic development and aligning with the primal principles. You can purchase a chest strap monitor separately like the Polar H7 or the Wahoo ($50–$60), but as a serious endurance athlete, you should be monitoring training heart rates at all aerobic workouts by watch (and perhaps indulging in other watch features like GPS or lap-split timing), as well as monitoring HRV

daily with a smartphone app. A heart monitor watch with a Bluetooth low energy (BLE 4.0)-enabled strap can be used for both HRV and for workout heart rate monitoring. For the iOS (Apple) platform, the PrimalBeat HRV app (made by Sweetwater Health, available for ten dollars) is our favorite, obviously! For other platforms, try ithlete or Bioforce.

After a few weeks, you'll notice some baseline patterns emerging, but give it a good several months of daily monitoring to be sure you gather enough data to optimally guide your training decisions. As with making progress on your Maximum Aerobic Function test results, you should aspire to gradually elevate your

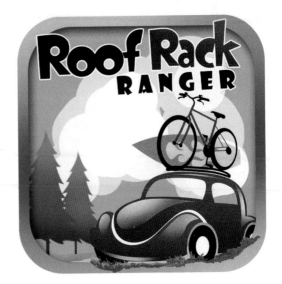

*They actually have an app (RoofRackRanger.com) to prevent overstressed athletes from one of the misfortunes of absentmindedness.*

HRV baseline over time, as well as improve your average LF:HF ratios. On the flip side, be vigilant about sustained patterns of low HRV (as opposed to the acceptable transient suppression of HRV caused by hard workouts or brief, stressful life circumstances) scores and poor LF:HF ratios, which suggest an overtraining or overstress pattern.

# CHAPTER SUMMARY

- **Cold therapy for psychological benefits**
- **Cool down, compress, rollout, move!**
- **HRV = direct window to stress/recovery**
- **No te olvides—sleep is king!**

The best way to recover quickly is to follow a **stress-balanced training program that avoids chronic patterns**. Beyond that, there are numerous cutting-edge strategies that can help you optimize recovery and minimize breakdown, including:

*Cold therapy*: Not to reduce inflammation (since inflammation is critical to the recovery and adaptation process), but more for **resetting the central nervous system and muscle metabolic activity back to a calm and cool state**, which delivers a significant psychological effect. Five to ten minutes of full immersion into 50°F to 60°F water will deliver optimum results.

*Compression gear:* Compression socks and tights help the lymphatic and circulatory systems remove extracellular waste products and excess fluid from traumatized tissues, and improve the delivery of blood and oxygen. **Compression gear acts like a pump to squeeze blood vessels open with force,** an effect that is enhanced by elevation of the traumatized area above the heart. There is some scientific support for compression helping relieve muscle soreness, but the psychological effect is also prominent.

*Hydration*: Rehydrating immediately after workouts will **ensure that the assorted recovery functions are not interrupted by the immediate urgency of dehydration**. Water with a bit of sea salt is fine—no need for sugary sports drinks.

*Movement*: Advanced recovery theory emphasizes movement as absolutely critical to muscle repair and rejuvenation. **Stillness is the enemy of muscle recovery**, while more walking and daily movement can help you become a more fluid, flexible, and energetic human at all times. Move more and track your progress by measuring improvements in your level of morning stiffness.

*Refueling*: Focus on high-nutrient-value whole foods, and **reject the heavily processed beverages, bars, and snack foods** that offer minimal nutrition and a big sugar bomb that promotes carbohydrate dependency.

*RTX cooling glove:* This novel contraption allows an exerciser to **quickly lower core body temperature** and keep going! While heat is not a performance limiting factor when exercising at super low heart rates, in water or in cold weather, overheating muscles and core temperature is a severe performance limiter in many activities, including indoor gym exercise, prolonged endurance workouts, or exercising in hot outdoor conditions.

*Self-myofascial release:* Foam rollers, therapy balls, and other self-care tools apply deep pressure to trigger points that represent the proximate cause of assorted aches, pains, stiffness, and injuries. **Self-myofascial release breaks up adhesions, improves blood and lymphatic flow, greatly reduces injury risk, and also helps stimulate the parasympathetic nervous system**—critical to helping you unwind fully after workouts.

*Sleep:* As discussed at length in Chapter 8, sleep is king for recovery and health. Athletes might benefit from more napping efforts, particularly in conjunction with stressful workouts.

*Release attachment to outcome:* Reduce the psychological stress of training by focusing on the enjoyment of the process of getting fit, and minimizing the importance of measured results. **Take what your body gives you every day and nothing more**, and be satisfied, and patient, with the natural progression of fitness.

**Heart Rate Variability (HRV)** is an outstanding way to monitor overtraining, recovery, cardiovascular health, and fitness progress, as it tracks the harmonious interaction between the sympathetic and parasympathetic nervous systems. HRV measures the variation in beat-to-beat intervals of your heart. **A high HRV value suggests a healthy, fit, stress-balanced subject.** A sustained pattern of low HRV readings suggests a state of overstress or exhaustion. The LF (sympathetic) and HF (parasympathetic) power spectrums provide further insights into your stress levels and recovery status. High absolute values (relative to one's individual historical baseline) represent a strong, well-functioning cardiovascular system, while a high HF value in relation to LF suggests a harmonious balance between fight-or-flight and rest-and-digest. Tracking HRV along with resting heart rate each morning and establishing baseline values can help inform correct training decisions and prevent chronic stress hormone stimulation.

# CHAPTER 10

# HITTING THE SHOWERS

*The delicate balance between pursuing peak performance and promoting longevity*

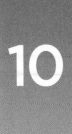
**10**

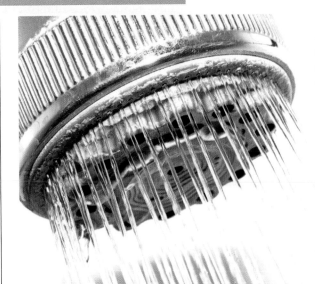

*The cortisol showerhead has an assortment of settings to support your peak performance and longevity goals.*

As you pursue endurance goals in hectic modern life, it might be helpful for you to envision a reservoir residing in your body that stores the precious fight-or-flight hormone cortisol. You were born with this tank, and your genetics have a big influence on the size of your tank, how easily it is depleted, and how efficiently it is refilled. However, like other genetic attributes influenced by environmental signals, you have tremendous control on how you spend, save, or squander this precious resource that gives you heightened physical and cognitive performance on demand.

Imagine the cortisol is dispensed though one of those super-deluxe showerheads with numerous adjustment options. You have everything from the full-blast power setting down to a fine mist. Just like with a real shower dispensing energized negative ion air particles and invigorating the nervous system, you get a pleasant boost of energy every time you turn on the nozzle. This cortisol showerhead analogy summarizes everything Mark and Brad have bantered about for the past twenty-seven years related to balancing training with recovery, balancing health while you pursue ambitious fitness goals, and, perhaps most profoundly, balancing peak performance ambitions with longevity.

• • • • • • • • • • • •

**A FAVORITE PRIMAL BLUEPRINT TAG LINE** for weight-loss enthusiasts is that when you go primal, losing weight is as simple as having your hand on a dial. Dial back your total dietary insulin production, and you reduce body fat quickly. In this discussion, instead of a dial, your hand is on the showerhead, ready to adjust your spray option any time. How are you going to handle the tremendous power and responsibility that comes from controlling your showerhead? There are no right or wrong answers here. The NFL and NBA guys who play hard by day, club hard by night, and earn a lifetime fortune in a seven-year career probably wouldn't have it any other way. Even many of the aged, crippled, cognitively declined football warhorses assert that their journey was worth it.

The desire to seize the day and pursue the limit of your human potential can be all-consuming, and it's a gift to have a goal so compelling that you give your heart and soul to the effort every day for years and years. The elite Ironman triathletes training for six hours a day and jetting around the globe to drop the hammer for eight hours in competition might have a vague notion that they're compromising their long-term health and longevity, but that doesn't stop them from fulfilling their destiny. Ditto for the roadie going on an eleven-year run with Pearl Jam, or the associate at an elite law firm grinding for seventy-five hours a week to ascend to partner one day. Strike when the iron is hot, leverage years of methodical preparation, and unleash the highest expression of your talents during your peak years of productivity. This is the essence of the continued progress of humanity in every peak performance arena.

Most of us are presented with less extreme life path options than the all-consuming and health-challenging careers mentioned, but the question of how to best dispense the cortisol coming out of our showerhead is no less relevant. There are many well-meaning folks who enter the world of endurance sports, become intoxicated by the low-hanging fruit (the endorphin buzz after vigorous workouts, the satisfaction of the finisher medal), and proceed with all manner of wickedly imbalanced, ill-advised approaches. What happens at first, due to the dynamics of how the spray nozzle affects your body, is they succeed. They might have a two-year ride, or a five-year ride, but eventually the repercussions of an imbalanced, overly stressful approach start to accumulate. It seems that the endurance scene today is booming like crazy, *and* is manifesting a very high attrition rate; one that will continue to climb unless the masses radically change their approach to get the spray nozzle moderated. Perhaps not many people care about attrition risks. The people who traffic in event production, energy gels, running shoes, or triathlon wetsuits are happy to lure fresh blood into the game each year, and it's certainly not their obligation to advocate for the long-term best interests of their customers.

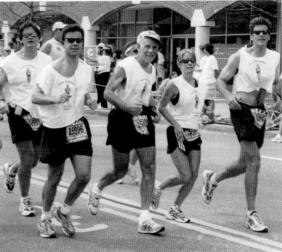

*After discovering running later in life, "Runlike" Ron Kobrine completed thirty consecutive Boston marathons, spanning from 1980 to 2010. His best time in the string was 2h:54. He's pictured here in 2004, surrounded by family members each adorned with a commemorative Ron Kobrine 25th Boston Marathon T-shirt.*

If you care about your longevity in endurance sports, and longevity on the planet, you'll want to do the best possible job managing your spray nozzle. This will enable both the actualization of your potential with challenging, appealing, and appropriate life goals, as well as the preservation of your health and longevity through the judicious balancing of stress and rest. Along those lines, it's important to recognize that there are significant differences among individuals in work capacity, stress tolerance, athletic potential, and preferences for just how much stimulus and excitement one wants to take on over the course of life. It's critical to spend a little time figuring out where you stand on the spectrum, and honor your particulars with your lifestyle decisions.

What athletic challenges are most appealing to you, and fit most conveniently with your other lifestyle circumstances? Set yourself up for success before you even think about workout particulars or race strategy. Get your attitude straight so you don't get unnecessarily stressed about your results, peer pressure, or adhering to a consistent regimented workload.

Take inspiration from athletes who manage their spray settings expertly, enjoying not only peak performance but comprehensive, long-lasting health and happiness. For example, let's meet Brad's high school running mentor, **"Runlike" Ron Kobrine**, a father of his star teammate Steven, who set the tone with a tremendous work ethic on the road, while leading a balanced life as a finance executive and father of five. Among many distinctions, Ron completed the Boston marathon *thirty years in a row*, a longevity record that seems unfathomable in today's age of epidemic running injuries and burnout.

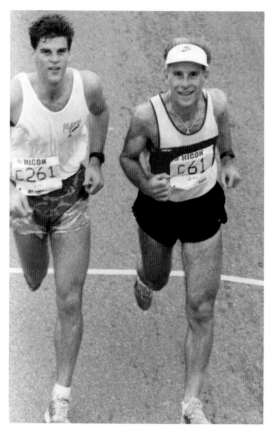

*Ron finishing the Los Angeles marathon with his son "Doctor" Dave, a former UCLA basketball player and Hawaii Iron-man finisher who inspired Brad to pursue triathlon, instead of basketball.*

Unlike many who pursue longevity streaks for the sake of the streak, Ron's approach was from the opposite angle. "The Boston streak was something that just happened; I didn't plan it. I enjoy running and the social connections of running, and things just became habit after a while. The Boston Marathon is a beautiful race in a beautiful city, so of course I signed up every year," explains Ron.

Indeed, the social aspects were central to Ron's motivation and enjoyment. His son Eric accompanied to him to Boston each year (Eric has a twenty-year Boston finishing streak going himself!), and his other children frequently joined him to watch or run Boston over the years. He was surprised by a knock on his hotel room door the night before his twenty-fifth Boston Marathon, in 2004—it was his daughter and three other sons. Ostensibly, they where there to cheer him on, but he learned otherwise while watching a television interview where Steven informed Boston viewers that each Kobrine had secretly trained and qualified over the previous year to gain official entry into the race.

Social and unstructured as he was, Ron did not fool around on the racecourse. He was good for a ballpark three-hour performance for the first fifteen or twenty years (with a best of 2h:54), before finally allowing himself to gradually get slower in the latter years. After all, he didn't discover running until his early forties, so his Boston performances came between the ages of forty-three and seventy-three.

Ron is nonchalant about his running accomplishments; everything is framed as ordinary and routine. He doesn't keep any records and didn't much care about the details at the time, either. Remember, his career predated the modern hyped era of endurance. There are no Boston marathon tattoos on his body, no "BSTN 30" vanity plates on his ride, and no Facebook posts to his fan base during the streak. His motivating force was personal satisfaction, and the camaraderie of a small, close-knit group of training partners and family members.

He even explains away his high-caliber performances with a shrug: "Running fast was just part of the culture in that day. The qualifying standards at Boston were so rigorous [3h:10 as a forty-plus runner from 1980 to 1990; then they adjusted up five minutes for every five-year age bracket] that you were compelled to run fast if you wanted a place on the start line. If ten of my training buddies and I [Ron was part of a large and notorious pack of 5:30 a.m. runners in the San Fernando Valley of Los Angeles] went to a 10K, we would all break forty minutes. But I didn't train with any methodical plan or strategy. If I felt great, I'd go long and hard. If I felt tired or sore, I'd take it easy. It wasn't a complex approach. I remember I was interviewed once by Boston television and they asked, 'How long does it take you to get ready for a marathon?' I didn't even understand the question!"

Make no mistake, Ron relished the competitive aspect of his journey, but his tangible performance goals were never put before the purity of the experience. This is likely why he never missed the Boston starting line due to injury or illness. Ron simply followed his passion where it led, rather than forcing the issue. If it's possible to convey this to you with a straight face, Ron took a "low stress" approach to running thirty consecutive Boston marathons, and set himself up gracefully for future decades of robust health, gentler exercise habits, and more modest fitness goals. The distinction is critical because we get so wrapped up in the importance of our goals, or in comparisons to others (he's called Runlike Ron because no one else can…) that we apply an overly stressful approach and bomb out.

Today, at seventy-eight, Ron has gracefully transitioned to walking as his main exercise, and he enjoys lengthy daily walks along the beach near his home in Northern California. No drama here: after battling a couple of health problems a few years back, he emerged from convalescence walking instead of running, and just never felt the inclination to return to running. Ron explains, "Upon reflection, I realize that my life in retirement is much simpler and calmer, so I don't *need* the running like I did when life was busier. Running was a form of meditation for me; it helped me clear my head and balance the assorted stresses of building a business, raising a family, and managing the faster-paced life in my younger years."

Ron's approach and perspective seem healthy and balanced, but the fact remains that running over a hundred marathons—the vast majority of them *fast* marathons!—requires a tremendous commitment to decades of extremely hard training—a significant amount of spray coming out of the tank. However, Ron's healthy perspective and process-oriented approach clearly helped ease the stress impact of his thirty years of phenomenal dedication to fitness. It's reasonable to speculate that he likely didn't need as much spray as an amped-up, results-obsessed competitor trying to achieve the same feats.

While thirty years of Boston is a fine example of managing one's spray settings deftly, how does an eighty-year athletic career sound? Let's meet Brad's father, ninety-three-year-old **Dr. Walter Kearns.** Dr. Kearns has played amateur golf at the elite level for over eighty years and continues to go strong as the premier golfer in the world over the age of ninety.

Since he's still active at ninety-three, Walter has obviously had a life of exceptional health, enjoying many other sports and fitness activities in addition to golf. While he was never tempted to try anything extreme like a marathon, he dropped a handful of 10Ks back in the run-

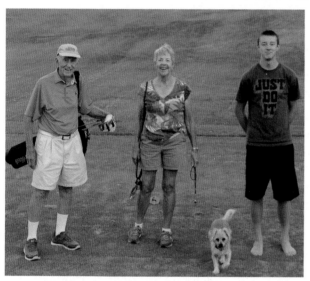

*Walter out for a quick few holes in the evening, with Gail, Quincy the ballfinder, and grandson Jack*

ning boom days, coached his kids' sports teams, and has kept himself tournament-sharp for decades. He was captain of the Princeton golf team as a youth, and qualified for the 1941 U.S. Amateur at age nineteen, *and* the U.S. Senior Amateur (ages fifty and up) at the age of sixty-seven in 1989. This forty-eight-year gap is believed to be unmatched in the history of national championship qualification.

Starting in 1989, when he shot a four-under 66 at age sixty-seven, he's shot his age over eleven hundred times and counting (basically every time out in case disaster strikes; don't smirk as you envision a ninety-three-year-old lamenting a miserable 94 on the scorecard). While no official rankings are kept in the ninety-plus category, it is very unlikely there are similar aged golfers in his stratosphere anywhere on the planet. Any challengers would be well advised to bring cash to the course. Walter can be counted on for a low 80s score any day, and will frequently post rounds in the 70s. On three occasions he has shot a stunning sixteen strokes under his age: a 71 at the age of eighty-seven, a 75 at age ninety-one, and a 76 at ninety-two (Guinness Book of World Records lists two folks shooting seventeen below as the record.) Oh, and he's had eleven holes-in-one, including a barrage of *seven in five years* once he turned eighty.

At a recent round, Walter was complaining to his playing partners about his declining vision making it hard to follow his shots. One of them fired back, "Walter, the reason you can't see your shots is because you hit the ball too damn far! Most ninety-three-year-olds see their shots just fine—ten feet off the ground." Walter is referred to by everyone he encounters out on the course and elsewhere in life as a physical marvel or genetic freak. Obviously these sentiments are delivered as compliments, but the truth is not so simple. He's made the most of his genetics for sure, having a lifelong devotion to healthy eating and exercise habits inspired by his career as a physician. But there are some additional critical insights in this story of longevity, pacing, and peak performance.

Walter is a very chill guy, period. He does not get emotional, harried, overstressed, negative, angry, or overexcited. He's level and calm in the face of everything that's come down his path in ninety-three years. Mark even tried to rattle his cage a bit by challenging his lifelong beliefs relating to conventional wisdom's lipid hypothesis of heart disease. Walter played an important role in helping get the presentation about cholesterol in the *Primal Blueprint* book completely tight and medically verifiable. He was open to hearing an opposing view, and methodically did the reading and evaluations necessary to rethink his position and approve the message in the book.

Walter is all about pacing and balance. These characterizations are preferable to "moderation," which can easily be misconstrued as, or used as license for, mediocrity. Shooting in the 70s at the championship-caliber Braemar Country Club is not a moderate golf round. Walter faithfully gets adequate sleep and downtime each day, however much he

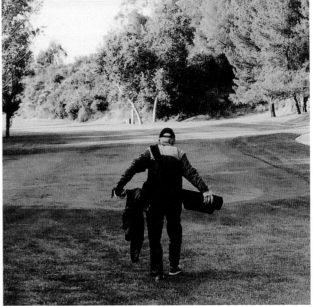

*Walter takes the long, long walk to another bombed tee shot. Yep, lugging his own sticks in a junior bag. "Carts are for old guys," says Walter.*

needs, no matter what. That's a consistent nine to ten hours a night and a leisurely afternoon period of napping/reading quietly in a darkened room that ranges from at least ninety minutes up to three hours after a busy morning or a hot day on the golf course.

Walter loves his golf outings, as you can imagine, but he's careful not to overdo it. He'll stay home if the temperature is below 50°F, or above 95°F. He's perfectly content to play nine holes instead of eighteen these days, especially if the weather is less than ideal. He often makes this snap decision at the turn (the halfway point of the golf course) if he's tired, hot, cold, or hungry… even if he's standing at one over par—really!

Walter takes a Pilates class once a week with his super-high-energy wife, Gail, seventy-eight, a part-timer at Primal Blueprint who prepares the written summaries of our podcast shows, does book editing and metric conversions, and was enlisted at PrimalCon to push her Prius through the parking lot as part of a Primal Play workshop (search YouTube for "76-year-old lady pushes car"). Sometimes Gail is concerned that the Pilates teacher is pushing Walter too hard for his age, but extending yourself a bit once a week and allowing for full recovery seems like a savvy anti-aging strategy. Jack LaLanne's fitness legacy was validated when he lived to the ripe old age of ninety-eight, and it's possible that he could have gone much longer had he not pushed himself so hard his whole life with excessive exercise—seriously!

Again, there is no right or wrong way to use your showerhead. What we are talking about here is a trade-off between peak performance and seizing the day (the turbo-pulsating-massage setting) on one side, and longevity (the fine-mist setting) on the other side. If you do things the right way—pursue your endurance goals with a primal-aligned, stress-balanced approach—these two goals don't have to be diametrically opposed. Energy is a renewable resource in the body, so an active, exciting, adventurous lifestyle can beget more energy and vibrant health. However, when your approach is flawed—either logistically or psychologically—peak performance and longevity can indeed be diametrically opposed. You are indiscriminately blasting the showerhead, enjoying the short-term peak performance boost from the all-powerful fight-or-flight response, but draining the tank—one you'll be needing for a lifetime—irresponsibly.

Sometimes severely abusing the spray nozzle causes it to jam up and shut off without warning, as discussed with the "Running on Empty" ultrarunners in Chapter 9. Article author Meaghen Brown reports that a pattern appears among the athletes studied: a steady progression to the top lasting around two years, followed by a sudden crash, with an assortment of disturbing symptoms that thoroughly confuse even the most informed physicians.

# DONATING AN APPENDIX TO CHAPTER 10

A little, okay a lot, closer to home, we must reveal how frighteningly literal the title "Appendix" is for this sidebar. You see, Brad was laid up in a hospital bed recovering from an emergency appendectomy when we started working on this final chapter. When a teenager, or even a healthy fifty-year-old male in this case, ruptures his appendix, most every physician will tell you this is a random event, apropos of nothing. Brad is not so sure, and had some post-surgical spare time in the summer of 2015 to reflect on this—with his ambitious daily fitness regimen suddenly reduced to a fifteen-minute walk, followed by a nap. We pondered whether maybe, just maybe, Brad's unintended binge of black hole cardio training in early 2015 in pursuit of Speedgolf excellence (detailed in the Chapter 1 sidebar) might have contributed to his burning up an organ one night in June. After all, Brad presented in ER just a few hours after an "awesome" sprint and basketball workout (in 106°F heat, ahem) where he was elated to Tweet out to his peeps that he grabbed the rim several times, a rare occasion for a 5'11" former pro trigeek.

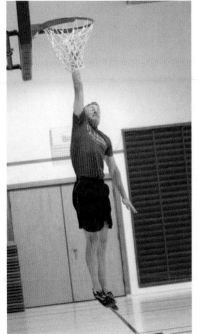

*With this kinda elevation, who needs a caption?*

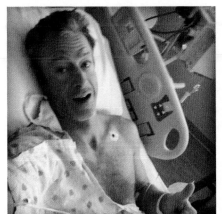

*"Nothing's random. Even if it looks that way, it's just because you don't know the causes."*
*—Johnny Rich, author of*
The Human Script

The sobering question loomed: could it be that old jocks like us were tempting fate by forcing too much spray out of a weathered showerhead? Ordinarily, our knee-jerk reply would be "no," especially when you measure Mark's game up against the sorry-ass, sad sack of bones that is the average sixty-two-year-old American male. However, at the time of Brad's inquiry (he emailed Mark a Siri-crafted, morphine-drip-influenced stream of consciousness from the hospital bed one night that was hilariously incoherent, misspelled, and malapropped by Siri, but definitely got the central question posed as a starting point), Mark was dealing with a recurring barrage of premature ventricular contractions (PVCs). These are extra, abnormal heartbeats that disrupt regular rhythm. They are quite common, usually benign, but very noticeable and annoying when emanating from one's chest.

Perhaps Mark's issue was also apropos of nothing, except a fear in the back of his mind that he had induced this condition by being overexuberant with a new rope climb simulator machine at his gym in recent months. Yeah, this Marpo unit (Marpo Kinetics) is the bomb—you go all out for, say, a one-minute effort, and it records the vertical feet accumulated. As the former world record holder in the vertical ascent on a VersaClimber (5,280'—one mile—in twenty-two minutes and change, heart rate pegged at 186 bpm), Mark was compelled to establish a fresh gym record for the young guns to gun for. After all, we occasionally advocate brief, "all-out" sprints as a fundamental element of the Primal Blueprint (law number five) and of the Primal Endurance approach, and it's important to walk one's talk. Mark's competitive intensity and dedication to healthy living has served him well for this long, so why cede to the younger generation in the name of chronology alone when he can still bring the heat?

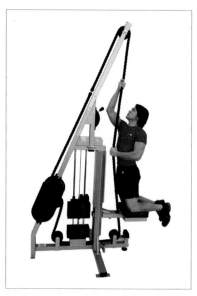

A discernible boom-boom-(space) rhythm coming out of your chest will get you second-guessing anything, though. Fortunately, extensive testing reveals Mark's condition to be benign, and—in expert medical opinion—probably not influenced by the particulars of his exercise regimen or past history as an elite endurance performer. Of course, that's what the docs said about Brad's appendix too....Nevertheless, Mark is keen to still deliver occasional brief, intense max efforts, but pay a little more attention to Maffetone's edict that you need not exceed 90 percent of max heart rate if you are going for longer than thirty seconds.

*Behold the Marpo Kinetics VLT rope trainer, and their youthful brochure model; homey don't want no part of Sisson on a one-minute vert challenge!*

Regardless of whether or not you identify with certainty a cause for your health challenges and seemingly random misfortunes, managing risk prudently, aging gracefully, and pursuing goals that are appropriate to your current age, time available for training, and overall lifestyle circumstances seem like good ideas. And hey, how about starting in high school, where our football-playing youth nonchalantly barter a few years of glory and distorted cultural significance for perhaps a lifetime of extra aches and pains, accelerated connective tissue deterioration, not to mention repetitive brain trauma—the dire consequences of which science is only scratching the surface of today. *Note:* Brad recently endured some difficult conversations with his son about the sensibleness of Jack's high school football aspirations. A showdown was temporarily averted by Brad allowing him to participate in non-contact summer conditioning drills, with a promise to reconvene later for further debate. A peaceful, natural resolution to the standoff was

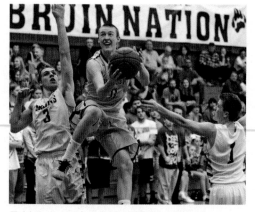

*Taking it to the rack: beats getting clotheslined after a catch over the middle...*

achieved one night in summer basketball league when Jack buried five three-pointers, reaffirming his greater love for basketball than for the sweltering conditioning drills with the football team he did the following morning for the last time.

We are still strongly in favor of brief, maximum effort strength and sprint workouts, with the emphasis on brief, and the assertion that you absolutely should not attempt any intense workouts unless you are 100 percent rested and motivated for peak performance (and also perhaps not when it's over 100°F outside...). After some reflection on Maffetone's directive to limit your prolonged anaerobic cardiovascular training sessions (intervals, hill repeats, time trials, etc.) to 90 percent of max heart rate, we have had a bit of an awakening that all those old-time, all-out slugfest endurance rides and runs—conducted under the guise of preparing for max effort racing—might have been more about feeding the group's collective ego demands and less about sensible race preparation. Says Mark:

> I can still recall my best-ever workout on the track during my marathon days, and the detrimental effect it had on my physiology and my psyche. I'm not kidding when I say this single workout permanently scarred my central governor, if not the actual muscle fibers and neurotransmitters involved. It was a set of 16 x 800 meters on the track in 2m:24 to 2m:28 each, with a lap of walk/jog recovery between. Eight miles of suffering in circles, definitely not adhering to the "consistent quality of efforts" maxim described in Chapter 6. No, this was a steady march to the gallows. After the first six or eight efforts, for which my fitness afforded a smooth on-time arrival, I donated an ever-growing amount of brain cells, free radicals, and sodium-potassium pumps in my cell membranes to the cause of keeping that watch stopping in the 2m:24 to
>
>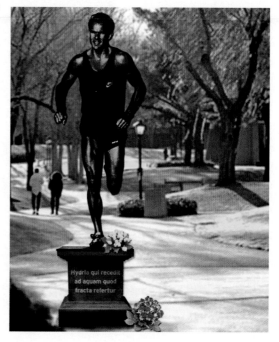
>
> 2m:28 window at the finish line. After the final effort, a strange and ominous chill ran up and down the length of my spine, signaling to me that something really was wrong. Of course I was sick in bed the following morning. But even after the minor illness cleared in two weeks, a faint sense lingered that I would never be the same as a runner. As the old proverb reads, "The pitcher who goes too often to the well is broken at last." Today, at the Foothill College track where I made my offering to the running gods with that early 1980s workout, there stands a statue of me with the proverb engraved (in Latin) in its stone base—a poignant warning to others to learn from my foibles and chart a more sensible course.

Hopefully you can keep the image of the spray nozzle in the back of your mind as you plot your future course as an athlete, and as a healthy person in general. As with the ultrarunners and many other extreme performers, you can crank up the intensity of the spray whenever you want and demand great achievements from your body, imbalanced as your approach may be. But be mindful that you are under the influence of this magic spray that has the capability to mask fatigue and distort your decision-making abilities in the process.

In conclusion, Primal Endurance gives you the go-ahead to go sign up for those ambitious goals of yours, whether it's a 70.3, a fifty-kilometer trail run, or a bike tour down the west coast of the USA. But try to adopt a chill approach, like Ron or Walter, and don't get too worked up when things go wrong, or when they go well. When you ask the maximum from your mind and body for athletic excellence, understand the consequences of your performance demands. Notice the times when you are cranking up the spray nozzle to the turbo settings, and resolve to include the necessary downtime to balance extreme peak performance demands. This might mean implementing a pattern of skipping a year of competition after two or three consecutive years.

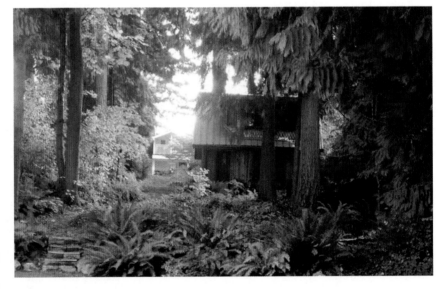

*Brad's friend "Mellow C" likes to unplug and retreat to this tiny lakeside cabin for a spell when life gets a little hectic. Departing from one's training routine, even briefly, is a novel concept for many endurance athletes—what with the ever-present fears of getting out of shape or losing the feel for the water.*

*If an endurance enthusiast landed at such a cabin by chance, their initial thoughts might be, "Open water swim!" or "Any trails around?" Have the courage and the confidence to trust the natural process of fitness, and the tremendous contribution that rest and balance offer to the equation.*

Perish the thought of missing out on something, but a year away from the race course, or at least a year pursuing an alternate, perhaps less encompassing, goal, will surely recharge your batteries; provide relief from competitive pressures; give you a chance to emphasize complementary movement, mobility, and lifestyle practices that often get pushed aside in favor of bread-and-butter mileage obligations; rekindle your enthusiasm and appreciation for core competitions when you return to the race course; and finally, give your cortisol tank a chance to refill a bit.

In the academic world, they call this a *sabbatical*, a tradition that exists for a very important reason. Sabbaticals give educators a chance to broaden their horizons and bring more energy and excitement back to their students and their research. Ditto for those in other fields requiring creativity, innovation, enthusiasm, and clear thinking—which covers just about everyone. In Mosaic law, a sabbatical, or Sabbath, was mandated every seventh year, where normal activity was ceased and "the land was to remain untilled and all debtors and slaves were to be released." This edict is thousands of years old, but any farmer today knows that leaving land untilled for a year allows it to rest and rejuvenate, and any endurance athlete knows that being a slave to the training log is no fun. So try leaving your land untilled and give the spray nozzle a break now and then. A sabbatical year is a great idea for a serious, long-term competitor, but you can take sabbaticals of a week or month any time you want with great benefit.

# APPENDIX

*Sample Annual Periodization Schedule*

Following are sample annual periodization schedules for Big George, a triathlete competing from sprint distance up to half-iron distance, and Runner Ray, a distance runner competing at 5K through marathon. Both these hypothetical folks are accomplished endurance athletes with some significant years invested in the traditional approach and will now start a new season adopting the primal approach. These workout patterns are merely examples, as I strongly recommend against adhering to any kind of predetermined workout schedule.

## TRIATHLETE BIG GEORGE

**January, February, March: Aerobic base building, 12 weeks.** All workouts at heart rate of 180 – age or below for twelve weeks. Following is a six-week sequence that represents a sensible approach to follow for the twelve-week base building period. What you will find upon close examination is a complete lack of predictability or consistency. George's primary goal is to build fitness in three events. He does this not by robotically meeting arbitrary volume goals, but by escalating the difficulty of key workouts and expertly balancing stress at all times through significant variation in his weekly patterns.

Weekly training volume spikes up and down in accordance with other lifestyle variables, the main one being the daily subjective scores of energy, motivation, and health, and general desire to train. You will notice occasional clusters of more focus on a particular sport, which may be a consequence of weather inhibiting cycling, logistics inhibiting swimming, or simply by an intuitive sense to pay more attention to running during a certain time period.

Remember, all aerobic base building period workouts are conducted at a comfortable pace, so the weekly training hours will be far greater than during intensity phases. George performs regular MAF tests in both running and cycling to monitor his aerobic development and be aware of any regression, which is likely to be caused by overtraining or overly stressful life circumstances.

### Week 1 - Aerobic
1. **Bike** 1h:30, **Run** :45m (MAF test)
2. **Swim** :45m. **Bike** 1h:30
3. **Swim** :20m
4. **Bike** :30m  (MAF test), **Run** 1h:20
5. **Swim** :20m, **Run** :20m
6. **Rest**
7. **Bike** 4h:00

Hours: 11h:20

### Week 2 - Aerobic
1. **Swim** :20m
2. **Swim** :20m, **Run** :20m
3. **Run** 1h:45
4. **Swim** :45m, **Bike** 1h:30
5. **Rest**
6. **Rest**
7. **Rest**

Hours: 5h:00

### Week 3 - Aerobic
1. **Swim** :45m, **Bike** 1h:30
2. **Bike** 4h:00
3. **Swim** :20m, **Run** 1h:20
4. **Run** 1h:45
5. **Swim** :45m, **Bike** 1h:30 (MAF test)
6. **Swim** :20m
7. **Rest**

Hours: 11h:15

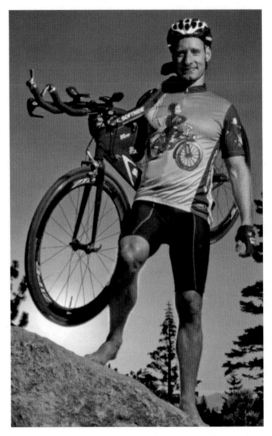

*Some say Big George is just a hypothetical athlete, others swear to have seen this creature training deep in the Tahoe National Forest, decked out in custom George attire....*

## Week 4 - Aerobic
1. **Rest**
2. **Rest**
3. **Swim** :20m, **Run** :30m (MAF test)
4. **Rest**
5. **Bike** 2h:00, **Run** :20m
6. **Swim** :20m
7. **Swim** :20m

Hours: 3h:40

## Week 5 - Aerobic
1. **Swim** :20m, **Run** 2h:00
2. **Swim** :20m, **Run** :30m
3. **Bike** 2h:00, **Run** 1h:00
4. **Swim** 1h:00, **Run** :20m
5. **Swim** :20m, **Bike** 2h:00
6. **Rest**
7. **Bike** 2h:00

Hours: 11h:50

## Week 6 - Aerobic
1. **Rest**
2. **Swim** 1h:30
3. **Swim** :45m, **Run** :45m
4. **Swim** :20m, **Run** 2h:00
5. **Swim** :20m, **Run** :45m
6. **Bike** 1h:00, **Run** :20m (MAF test)
7. **Run** 1h:30

Hours: 9h:15

**Weeks 7–12:** Continue strict aerobic period, escalating duration of key workouts in each sport with varied, intuitive workout pattern.

**April, May, June: Intensity/Competition period with mini-cycles, 12 weeks.** As the competitive season approaches, George introduces the first high-intensity workouts of the year. George realizes that a little goes a long way here, so his intensity phase lasts for only three and a half weeks before he initiates mini-cycles of rest and aerobic base building. Besides the specific workouts labeled "Intensity," the other workouts are all conducted at aerobic heart rates. The following six-week sequence represents a sensible approach to follow for the twelve-week intensity/competition period with attached rest and aerobic mini-cycles.

## Week 1 - Intensity/Competition
1. **Intensity – Run** :45m, including 4 x 3m @ AT with :30s rest intervals
2. **Swim** :45m, Bike :45m
3. **Bike** 1h:00
4. **Intensity – Swim** :20m @ 2K race pace, followed by **Bike** :45m including 5 x :04m @ AT with :40s rest intervals
5. **Rest**
6. **Rest**
7. **Swim** :20m, **Bike** 2h:00

Hours: 6h:40

## Week 2 - Intensity/Competition
1. **Swim** :30m, **Run** :45m
2. **Swim** :30m, **Run** :30m (MAF test)
3. **Intensity – Bike** 1h:00 including 2 x 10m @ AT with :05m rest interval. **Run** :25m immediately after including 10m @ 5K race pace
4. **Swim** :20m
5. **Bike** 1h:00
6. **Rest**
7. **Rest**

Hours: 5h:00

## Week 3 - Intensity/Competition
1. **Intensity – Run** :30m including :15m of :40s @ 5K race pace, :20s recovery jog, continuous
2. **Intensity – Bike** 1h:00 including :30m of :02m @ 40K race pace, :02m rest interval
3. **Swim** :20m, **Run** :20m
4. **Bike** 1h:00
5. **Rest**
6. **Rest**
7. **Competition** (5K run)

Hours: 3h:10

### Week 4 – Intensity & Rest
1. **Rest**
2. **Swim** :45m, **Bike** :45m (MAF test)
3. **Bike** 1h:00
4. **Intensity – Bike** 1h:00 including 5 x :04m @ AT with :40s rest intervals
5. **Swim** :20m, **Run** :20m
6. **Bike** 1h:00
7. **Rest**

Hours: 5h:10

### Week 5 – Rest/Aerobic
1. **Rest**
2. **Swim** :20m, **Run** :20m
3. **Bike** 1h:00
4. **Rest**
5. **Swim** :20m, **Run** :20m
6. **Rest**
7. **Bike** 1h:00

Hours: 3h:20

### Week 6 – Rest/Aerobic
1. **Swim** :30m, **Bike** 3h:00
2. **Swim** :45m
3. **Run** :30m (MAF test)
4. **Bike** 2h:00
5. **Swim** :20m, **Run** :20m
6. **Rest**
7. **Rest**

Hours: 7h:25

**Weeks 7, 8, 9:** Repeat three-week intensity/competition period
**Weeks 10, 11, 12:** Repeat three-week rest/aerobic period

**July, August: Midseason break, aerobic rebuild, six weeks.** After a successful aerobic base period of higher volume training, and a couple of intensity/competition periods, it's time for a midseason break and casual return to four weeks of aerobic base building. The midseason break entails a complete vacation from training and thinking about training for two weeks. Ideally this would occur in tandem with a real vacation, where you depart from your home environment and routine and enjoy a getaway. Mark Allen was known for taking off in the middle of the summer to participate in a spiritual retreat with the Huichol Indians. Upon return, he started his focused building for the October Hawaii Ironman, which he won six times in succession from 1989 to 2005.

You certainly don't have to sit on the couch for two weeks; the most restorative strategy is to walk frequently and engage in other forms of active leisure, like water sports. Returning from your break, you will ease into a four-week aerobic base building period. You will then be positioned for a couple more intensity/ competition periods in the latter part of the season.

## Weeks 1 & 2 – Midseason break
No formal training sessions, just walking and active leisure activities

## Week 3 – Aerobic
1. **Swim** :30m, **Bike** :30m
2. **Swim** :30m, **Run** :30m
3. **Bike** 1h:30
4. **Rest**
5. **Rest**
6. **Bike** 1h:30, **Run** :30m
7. **Run** 1h:00

Hours: 6h:30

## Week 4 – Aerobic
1. **Swim** :45m, **Bike** 2h:00
2. **Swim** :20m, **Run** 1h:15
3. **Swim** :20m, **Bike** 1h:00
4. **Rest**
5. **Bike** 2h:30
6. **Run** 1h:30
7. **Swim** :20m, **Bike** 2h:00

Hours: 12h:10

## Week 5 – Aerobic
1. **Rest**
2. **Rest**
3. **Swim** :30m, **Bike** 2h:00
4. **Rest**
5. **Swim** :30m, **Run** :30m
6. **Swim** :20m, **Run** :40m
7. **Rest**

Hours: 4h:30

### Week 6 – Aerobic
1. **Swim** :30m, **Bike** 1h:30
2. **Bike** 4h:00
3. **Rest**
4. **Rest**
5. **Swim** :30m, **Run** 1h:30
6. **Rest**
7. **Swim** :30m, **Bike** 1h:30, **Run** :30m

Hours: 10h:30

**August, September, October: Mini cycles of intensity/competition paired with equal duration rest/aerobic mini cycles, 12 weeks**

Notice that the day before a competition, it is recommended to get out and get the blood flowing with some short aerobic workouts and some brief accelerations up to anaerobic intensity. This will prime the muscles and central nervous system to perform at high intensity the next day and also keep your blood volume high (a key component to peak performance), especially in contrast to lying around for the final twenty-four to thirty-six hours before competition.

### Week 1 – Intensity/Competition
1. **Intensity – Run** :45m, including 6 x :03m @ AT with :30s rest intervals
2. **Swim** :30m, **Bike** :45m
3. **Bike** 1h:00
4. **Intensity – Swim** :20m at 2K race pace, **Run** :20m with 10 minutes of :40s @ 5K pace/:20s recovery jog
5. **Rest**
6. **Swim** :20m, **Bike** :40m, **Run** :20m at recovery heart rates
7. **Competition – Olympic distance triathlon**

Hours: 6h:40

### Week 2 – Recovery/Intensity
1. **Swim** :20m
2. **Swim** : 20m
3. **Rest**
4. **Bike** :45m
5. **Swim** :20m, **Run** :20m
6. **Intensity – Bike** 1h:00 time trial
7. **Competition – 5K road race**

Hours: 3h:35

## Week 3 – Recovery/Intensity

1. **Rest**
2. **Rest**
3. **Swim** :20m
4. **Rest**
5. **Bike** :45m
6. **Bike** 1h:00 including :30m of :02m at 40K race pace, :02m of recovery
7. **Run** :30m

Hours: 2h:35

## Week 4 – Rest

1. **Rest**
2. **Run** :30m
3. **Run** :30m, **Bike** 1h:00
4. **Swim** :30m
5. **Rest**
6. **Rest**
7. **Bike** 1h:00

Hours: 3h:30

## Week 5 – Intensity/Competition

1. **Intensity – Run** :30m, including 3 x :03m @ AT with :30s rest intervals
2. **Swim** :30m, **Bike** :45m
3. **Bike** 1h:00
4. **Intensity – Swim** :20m @ 2K race pace, **Run** :20m with 10 minutes of :40s @ 5K pace/:20s recovery jog
5. **Rest**
6. **Swim** :20m, **Bike** :40m, **Run** :20m at recovery heart rates, and a couple accelerations of :20s in each discipline
7. **Competition – 70.3-mile half-iron triathlon**

Hours: 6h:45

## Weeks 6–12 – Repeat Rest/Aerobic

**December: Season-ending rest period, 4–6 weeks**

## RUNNER RAY

Please keep in mind that this hypothetical schedule is recording formal training sessions in running or other cross training cardiovascular sessions (i.e., Bike/Swim). Since running delivers a high degree of difficulty in less time than other activities, it's especially important to spend significant additional time on cross training cardio workouts, complementary movement and mobility practices (yoga, Pilates, self-myofascial release, technique drill sessions, dynamic stretching) as well as varied forms of general everyday movement, including hiking, walking the dog around the block, and taking frequent breaks to avoid long periods of stillness.

**January/February/March: Aerobic base building, 12 weeks**

### Week 1 - Aerobic
1. **Run** :45m (MAF test)
2. **Bike/Swim** :45m
3. **Run** 1h:15
4. **Run** :20m
5. **Run** :45m
6. **Rest**
7. **Rest**

Hours: 3h:50

### Week 2 - Aerobic
1. **Run** :30m, **Bike/Swim** :30m
2. **Run** 1h:30
3. **Run** :30m
4. **Rest**
5. **Run** :30m, **Bike/Swim** :30m
6. **Rest**
7. **Run** 1h:30

Hours: 5h:30

### Week 3 - Aerobic
1. **Run** :30m, **Bike/Swim** :30m
2. **Bike/Swim** 1h:00
3. **Rest**
4. **Run** 1h:00
5. **Rest**
6. **Run** 2h:20
7. **Bike/Swim** :20m

Hours: 5h:40

### Week 4 - Aerobic
1. **Rest**
2. **Rest**
3. **Rest**
4. **Run** 1h:00 (MAF test)
5. **Bike/Swim** :30m
6. **Bike/Swim** :30m
7. **Run** 1h:00

Hours: 3h:00

### Week 5 - Aerobic
1. **Rest**
2. **Rest**
3. **Run** 1h:00
4. **Run** :30m
5. **Rest**
6. **Run** 2h:45
7. **Run** :20m

Hours: 4h:35

### Week 6 - Aerobic
1. **Bike/Swim** 1h:00
2. **Rest**
3. **Run** 1h:00 (MAF test)
4. **Run** :30m
5. **Rest**
6. **Run** 2h:15
7. **Run** :20 m

Hours: 5h:05

**Weeks 7–12:** Continue strict aerobic period, escalating duration of key workouts in each sport with varied, intuitive workout pattern.

**April, May, June: Intensity/Competition period with mini-cycles, 12 weeks.** As the competitive season approaches, Ray introduces the first high intensity workouts of the year. Ray realizes that a little goes a long way here, so his intensity phase lasts for only three and a half weeks before he initiates mini-cycles of rest and aerobic base building. Besides the specific workouts labeled "Intensity," the other workouts are all conducted at aerobic heart rates. The following six-week sequence represents a sensible approach to follow for the twelve-week intensity/competition period with attached rest and aerobic mini cycles.

## Week 1 – Intensity/Competition
1. **Intensity – Run** :45m, including 4 x :03m @ AT with :30s rest intervals
2. **Bike/Swim** :45m
3. **Rest**
4. **Intensity – Run** :30m with :10m of :40s @ 5K race pace, :20s rest, continuous
5. **Rest**
6. **Rest**
7. **Bike/Swim** :45m

Hours: 2h:45

## Week 2 - Intensity/Competition
1. **Run** 1h:00
2. **Bike/Swim** :30m
3. **Intensity – Run** :30m with :10m @ 5K race pace
4. **Bike/Swim** :30m
5. **Run** :30m
6. **Rest**
7. **Rest**

Hours: 3h:00

## Week 3 - Intensity/Competition
1. **Intensity – Run** :30m including :15m of :40s @ 5K race pace, :20s recovery jog, continuous
2. **Intensity – Bike** :30m including :10m of :02m hard, :02m recovery
3. **Run** :30m
4. **Run** :30m
5. **Rest**
6. **Rest**
7. **Intensity – Run** 1h:00 with 6 x :03m @ AT with :30s rest intervals

Hours: 3h:00

## Week 4 – Intensity/Rest
1. **Rest**
2. **Rest**
3. **Bike/Swim** :30m
4. **Run** :30m
5. **Intensity – Run** :30m with :15m of :40s @ 5K race pace, :20s recovery jog, continuous
6. **Bike/Swim** :30m
7. **Rest**

Hours: 2h:00

### Week 5 – Rest/Aerobic
1. **Rest**
2. **Run** :20m
3. **Run** 1h:00
4. **Rest**
5. **Run** :20m
6. **Rest**
7. **Bike/Swim** :30m

Hours: 2h:10

### Week 6 – Rest/Aerobic
1. **Run** 1h:00 (MAF test)
2. **Run** 1h:00
3. **Bike/Swim** 1h:00
4. **Rest**
5. **Run** :30m, **Bike/Swim** :30m
6. **Rest**
7. **Run** 1h:00

Hours: 5h:00

**Weeks 7, 8, 9:** Repeat three-week intensity/competition period
**Weeks 10, 11, 12:** Repeat three-week rest/aerobic period

**July, August: Midseason break, aerobic rebuild, six weeks.** As with George's schedule, after a successful aerobic base period of higher volume training, and a couple of intensity/competition periods, it's time for a midseason break and casual return to four weeks of aerobic base building. The midseason break entails a complete vacation from training and thinking about training for two weeks. Ideally this would occur in tandem with a real vacation, where you depart from your home environment and routine and enjoy a getaway. You certainly don't have to sit on the couch for two weeks; the most restorative strategy is to walk frequently and engage in other forms of active leisure, like water sports. Returning from your break, you will ease into a four-week aerobic base building period. You will then be positioned for a couple more intensity/competition periods in the latter part of the season.

## Weeks 1 & 2 – Midseason break
No formal training sessions, just walking, hiking, and active leisure activities

## Week 3 – Aerobic
1. **Run** :30m, **Bike/Swim** :30m
2. **Run** :30m, **Bike/Swim** :30m
3. **Run** 1h:00
4. **Rest**
5. **Run** :30m, **Bike/Swim** :30m
6. **Run** 1h:45
7. **Rest**

Hours: 5h:45

## Week 4 – Aerobic
1. **Bike/Swim** 1h:00
2. **Run** :30m, **Bike/Swim** 1h:00
3. **Run** :30m
4. **Run** :30m
5. **Run** :30m
6. **Run** 1h:00
7. **Run** :30m

Hours: 5h:30

## Week 5 – Aerobic
1. **Rest**
2. **Rest**
3. **Run** :30m, **Bike/Swim** :30m
4. **Run** 3h:00
5. **Bike/Swim** :30m
6. **Rest**
7. **Rest**

Hours: 4h:30

### Week 6 - Aerobic
1. **Run** 1h:00
2. **Run** 1h:00
3. **Bike/Swim** 1h:00
4. **Rest**
5. **Rest**
6. **Run** 2h:00
7. **Run** :30m

Hours: 5h:30

**August–November: Mini-cycles of intensity/competition paired with equal duration rest/aerobic mini-cycles, 12 weeks**

Notice that the day before a competition, it is recommended to get out and get the blood flowing with some short aerobic workouts and some brief accelerations up to anaerobic intensity. This will prime the muscles and central nervous system to perform at high intensity the next day and also keep your blood volume high (a key component to peak performance), especially in contrast to lying around for the final twenty-four to thirty-six hours before competition.

Due to the hypothetical race schedule dates, you see a bit of departure from the template here, where the intensity/competition period goes for four weeks, a week of rest is thrown in, and then another intensity/competition week, followed by another mix of rest and aerobic base training.

### Week 1 - Intensity/Competition
1. **Intensity – Run** :45m, including 6 x :03m @ AT with :30s rest intervals
2. **Bike/Swim** :20m
3. **Run** :20m
4. **Rest**
5. **Run** :45m
6. **Run** :20 with :04m of :40s @ 5K race pace, :20 recovery
7. **Competition** (5K, 10K, or 13.1mi)

Hours: 3h:30

## Week 2 – Intensity/Competition

1. **Rest**
2. **Bike/Swim** :30m
3. **Rest**
4. **Run** 1h:00
5. **Run** :30m with :10m of :40s @ 5K race pace, :20s recovery
6. **Rest**
7. **Rest**

Hours: 2h:00

## Week 3 – Intensity/Competition

1. **Run** :30m, **Bike/Swim** :30m
2. **Run** :45m with 4 x :03m @ AT with :30s rest intervals
3. **Rest**
4. **Run** :30m, **Bike/Swim** :30m
5. **Rest**
6. **Run** :20m with :04m of :40s @ 5K race pace, :20s recovery
7. **Competition** (5K, 10K, or 13.1)

Hours: 4h:00

## Week 4 – Rest

1. **Rest**
2. **Run** :30m
3. **Run** :30m, **Bike/Swim** :30m
4. **Swim** :30m
5. **Rest**
6. **Rest**
7. **Bike/Swim** :30m

Hours: 2h:30

## Week 5 – Intensity/Competition

1. **Intensity – Run** :45m, including 4 x :03m @ AT with :30s rest intervals
2. **Bike/Swim** :30m
3. **Run** :30m, **Bike/Swim** :30m
4. **Rest**
5. **Rest**
6. **Run** :20m with :04m of :40s @ 5K race pace, :20s recovery
7. **Competition** (5k, 10k or 13.1)

Hours: 3h:35

### Week 6 – Rest
1. Rest
2. Run :30, Bike/Swim :30
3. Bike/Swim :30
4. Rest
5. Rest
6. Bike/Swim :30
7. Run :30

Hours: 2h:30

### Week 7 – Rest & Peak Event

Instead of a dramatic and prolonged building and tapering to the major competitive event like a marathon (an approach that can push you in the direction of overstress and an obsessive mentality about adhering to the arbitrary schedule), the Primal Endurance philosophy keeps you always in stress/rest balance, and capable of delivering a peak performance at any time.

The "ideal" pre-race preparation pattern is highly individual and highly debatable at that, so here, for your reading pleasure, we gracefully drop in a little bomb at the end of the passage (to see if you are still reading, for one!)—time to go 26.2, baby!

1. Run :30m, Bike/Swim :30m
2. Run :30m with :10m of :40s @ 5K pace, :20s recovery
3. Rest
4. Rest
5. Bike/Swim :30m
6. Run :20m with :04m of :40s @ 5K race pace, :20s recovery
7. Competition – 26.2 marathon

Hours: 5h:30

### Weeks 8–14

The next few weeks might be a little boring to read, but I cannot emphasize strongly enough the importance of complete and total rest after a marathon. Remember the morbid description by Dr. O'Keefe in Chapter 1 about the micro-tears in your arteries and heart after running a marathon, the elevated blood inflammation markers, and how desperately your body wants to rest and repair after such a traumatic event? Often, the elation of achieving a major goal and the lingering effects of the endorphin high after a marathon mask the symptoms of fatigue and breakdown that are present inside your body.

What happens repeatedly during this post-marathon euphoric period is that runners head out for "easy" training sessions only days after the race, and start excitedly making plans for the next twenty-six-mile event to conquer. Floating along on an endorphin high, they might last for one, two, or four weeks before they totally fall apart and contract bronchitis, pneumonia, IT band syndrome, or a stress fracture. I can't count the number of times I've heard such a story play out, always accompanied by the qualifier, "it came out of nowhere."

Following is a detailed suggested post-marathon workout pattern for six weeks. Don't forget that in the absence of formal training sessions, general everyday movement is essential to speeding recovery and optimizing health. Just back off on the formal training sessions until your body is completely healed and stress balanced. After a late season marathon is obviously a great time to commence your season-ending rest period, so the following weeks might be more useful to apply to when you want to continue your competitive season after running a marathon earlier in the year.

## Week 1 - Rest

1. Rest
2. Rest
3. Rest
4. Rest
5. Rest
6. Rest
7. Rest

Hours: 0

## Week 2 - Rest

1. Rest
2. Rest
3. Rest
4. Rest
5. Rest
6. Rest
7. Rest

Hours: 0

### Week 3 – Rest

1. Rest
2. Rest
3. Rest
4. Rest
5. Rest
6. Rest
7. Rest

Hours: 0

### Week 4 – Rest/Aerobic

1. Rest
2. Rest
3. Bike/Swim :30m
4. Bike/Swim :30m
5. Run :20m
6. Rest
7. Run :30m

Hours: 1h:50

### Week 5 – Aerobic

1. Rest
2. Run :45m
3. Bike/Swim :30m
4. Bike/Swim :30m
5. Run :45m
6. Rest
7. Run :20m

Hours: 2h:50

### Week 6 – Aerobic

1. Run 1:15m
2. Run :30m
3. Bike/Swim :30m
4. Bike/Swim :30m
5. Run :20m
6. Rest
7. Run :20m

Hours: 3h:25

After you recover completely from a marathon, you can commence an aerobic base building period or even return to some intensity/competition blocks, depending on the time of year. As Ray's annual calendar is presented here, he will finish up the season with a couple of final competitions and then head into the annual rest period. Again, we are departing from the template a bit here, but the general philosophy of balancing stress and rest is looking good.

## Week 7 – Intensity/Competition

1. **Run** :45m with 4 x :03m @ AT, :30s recovery
2. **Rest**
3. **Bike/Swim** :30m
4. **Bike/Swim** :30m
5. **Rest**
6. **Run** :20m with :04m of :40s @ 5K race pace, :20s recovery
7. **Competition** (5K or 10K)

Hours: 3h:00

## Week 8 – Intensity/Competition

1. **Rest**
2. **Bike/Swim** :30m
3. **Bike/Swim** :30m
4. **Run** :30m with :10m of :40s @ 5K race pace, :20s recovery
5. **Rest**
6. **Run** :20m
7. **Competition** (5K or 10K)

Hours: 2h:45

**December: Season-ending rest period, 4–6 weeks**

# ONLINE RESOURCES AND SUGGESTED READING

## BOOKS

- *The Art and Science of Low Carbohydrate Performance* – Dr. Steven Phinney and Dr. Jeff Volek
- *Beyond Training* – Ben Greenfield
- *The Big Book of Endurance Training and Racing* – Dr. Phil Maffetone
- *Body, Mind, and Sport* – Dr. John Douillard
- *Breakthrough Triathlon Training* – Brad Kearns
- *Good Calories, Bad Calories* – Gary Taubes
- *Lights Out – Sleep, Sugar, and Survival* – Bent Formby and T.S. Wiley
- *Lore of Running* – Dr. Timothy Noakes
- *Play* – Dr. Stuart Brown
- *The Primal Blueprint* – Mark Sisson
- *The Primal Blueprint 21-Day Total Body Transformation* – Mark Sisson
- *The Primal Blueprint 90-Day Journal* – Mark Sisson
- *Wheat Belly* – Dr. William Davis
- *Why We Get Fat* – Gary Taubes

## ARTICLES/REFERENCES

Links to interesting articles and research used in the book are published at primalblueprintpublishing.com/books/primal-endurance/

# INDEX

Rojnik, Dr. Klemen, 208, 227–228
sample annual periodization schedule, 299–306
triglycerides, 101, 102, 243
type 2 diabetes, 19, 111, 131

## U

UCAN SuperStarch, 109, 125, 212
Ultimate Frisbee, 233, 256, 259
*Ultrametabolism: The Simple Plan for Automatic Weight Loss*, 190
University of Chicago melatonin study, 239

## V

vegetable oils, 103–104
vegetarian, Ted McDonald, 225
ventilatory efficiency, 159
ventilatory threshold (VT), 34
VersaClimber, 14, 294
Volek, Dr. Jeff, xvii, 18, 91, 110, 132, 135–137, 140, 144, 318

## W

walking
   after meals (Mayo Clinic study), 243
   general daily movement, 249
warmup
   importance of, 194–195
   sprinting workouts
      drills, 197, 203
      importance of, 194–195
water, 267
weather, 73–75
Weaver, Don "Dewey", xii
weekly schedules, 77–78
weight loss, 118–119
   conventional wisdom vs. Primal Endurance, 21
   sprinting, 190–191
wheat, 100, 119
   gliadin, 119
   withdrawal, 120
*Wheat Belly*, 119, 318
whole grain, 98–100
*Why We Get Fat*, 102, 318
wild rice, 107
Wiley, T.S., 235, 318
Willis, Nick, 78–79
workouts
   aligning difficulty with daily energy, motivation, and health, 58–59
   applying intuition, 15–16, 51, 57–58
   chronic cardio. *See* chronic cardio
   conventional wisdom vs. Primal Endurance, 20, 22

glycogen reloading, 92, 107
journaling, 58–59
Maximum Sustained Power (MSP), 166–168, 176–177, 180–181
   vs. blended workouts., 170–171
   blending MSP with sprints, 200
   increasing baseline weight, 181
   rest breaks, 177, 180–181
night workouts, 258
post-ketogenic training workouts, 141–142
sprinting. *See* sprinting
strength training. *See* strength training
workplace environment, 247–248

## Y

yoga
   complementary movement and mobility practices, xxiii, 51, 155, 231–232
   intensity/competition periods, 68
   McDonald, Ted, 223–235
   movement breaks, 248, 250–251

## Z

Zabriskie, Dave, 173–175